Theranostics

Editors

HOJJAT AHMADZADEHFAR
ALI GHOLAMREZANEZHAD

PET CLINICS

www.pet.theclinics.com

Consulting Editor
ABASS ALAVI

July 2021 • Volume 16 • Number 3

ELSEVIER

1600 John F. Kennedy Boulevard • Suite 1800 • Philadelphia, Pennsylvania, 19103-2899

http://www.pet.theclinics.com

PET CLINICS Volume 16, Number 3
July 2021 ISSN 1556-8598, ISBN-13: 978-0-323-81307-5

Editor: John Vassallo (j.vassallo@elsevier.com)
Developmental Editor: Karen Solomon

PET Clinics (ISSN 1556-8598) is published quarterly by Elsevier Inc., 360 Park Avenue South, New York, NY 10010-1710. Months of issue are January, April, July, and October. Periodicals postage paid at New York, NY, and additional mailing offices. Subscription prices per year are $254.00 (US individuals), $501.00 (US institutions), $100.00 (US students), $282.00 (Canadian individuals), $514.00 (Canadian institutions), $100.00 (Canadian students), $275.00 (foreign individuals), $514.00 (foreign institutions), and $140.00 (foreign students). To receive student and resident rate, orders must be accompanied by name of affiliated institution, date of term, and the signature of program/residency coordinator on institution letterhead. Orders will be billed at individual rate until proof of status is received. Foreign air speed delivery is included in all Clinics subscription prices. All prices are subject to change without notice. POSTMASTER: Send address changes to PET Clinics, Elsevier Health Sciences Division, Subscription Customer Service, 3251 Riverport Lane, Maryland Heights, MO 63043. **Customer Service: 1-800-654-2452 (U.S. and Canada); 314-447-8871 (outside U.S. and Canada). Fax: 314-447-8029. E-mail: journalscustomerservice-usa@elsevier.com (for print support); journalsonlinesupport-usa@elsevier.com (for online support).**

Reprints. For copies of 100 or more of articles in this publication, please contact the Commercial Reprints Department, Elsevier Inc., 360 Park Avenue South, New York, NY 10010-1710. Tel.: 212-633-3874; Fax: 212-633-3820; E-mail: reprints@elsevier.com.

PET Clinics is covered in MEDLINE/PubMed (Index Medicus).

Contributors

CONSULTING EDITOR

ABASS ALAVI, MD, MD (Hon), PhD (Hon), DSc (Hon)
Professor of Radiology and Neurology, Director of Research Education, Department of Radiology, Perelman School of Medicine, University of Pennsylvania, Philadelphia, Pennsylvania, USA

EDITORS

HOJJAT AHMADZADEHFAR, MD, MSc
Department of Nuclear Medicine, University Hospital Bonn, Bonn, Germany; Department of Nuclear Medicine, Klinikum Westfalen, Dortmund, Germany

ALI GHOLAMREZANEZHAD, MD, FEBNM, DABR
Assistant Professor of Clinical Radiology, Department of Diagnostic Radiology, Keck School of Medicine of USC, University of Southern California, Los Angles, California, USA

AUTHORS

FARHAD ABBASI, MD
Department of Infectious Diseases, Bushehr Medical University Hospital, School of Medicine, Bushehr University of Medical Sciences, Bushehr, Iran

MARIAM ABOIAN, MD, PhD
Department of Radiology, Yale School of Medicine, New Haven, Connecticut, USA

ALI AFSHAR-OROMIEH, MD
Professor, Department of Nuclear Medicine, Inselspital, Bern University Hospital, University of Bern, Bern, Switzerland

HOJJAT AHMADZADEHFAR, MD, MSc
Department of Nuclear Medicine, University Hospital Bonn, Bonn, Germany; Department of Nuclear Medicine, Klinikum Westfalen, Dortmund, Germany

IAN L. ALBERTS, MD, MA
Department of Nuclear Medicine, Inselspital, Bern University Hospital, University of Bern, Bern, Switzerland

ANETTE ALTMANN, MD
Department of Nuclear Medicine, University Hospital Heidelberg, Clinical Cooperation Unit Nuclear Medicine, German Cancer Research Center (DKFZ), Translational Lung Research Center Heidelberg, German Center for Lung Research (DZL), Heidelberg, Germany

ABDULLATIF AMINI, MD
Bushehr Heart Medical Center, School of Medicine, Bushehr University of Medical Sciences, Bushehr, Iran

AZAM AMINI, MD
Department of Internal Medicine, Division of Rheumatology, Bushehr Medical University Hospital, School of Medicine, Bushehr University of Medical Sciences, Bushehr, Iran

MAJID ASSADI, MD, FASNC
Department of Molecular Imaging and Radionuclide Therapy (MIRT), The Persian Gulf Nuclear Medicine Research Center, Bushehr Medical University Hospital, School of Medicine, Bushehr University of Medical Sciences, Bushehr, Iran

FELIPE G. BARBOSA, MD
Department of Radiology, Hospital
Sirio-Libanes, Sao Paulo, Brazil

HANS-JÜRGEN BIERSACK, MD
Department of Nuclear Medicine, University
Hospital Bonn, Bonn, Germany

CARLOS A. BUCHPIGUEL, MD, PhD
Department of Radiology, Hospital Sirio-
Libanes, Department of Radiology and
Oncology, Hospital das Clinicas HCFMUSP,
Faculdade de Medicina, Universidade de Sao
Paulo, Sao Paulo, Brazil

JAVIER CARRASCOSO, MD
Department of Radiology, Quironsalud Madrid
University Hospital, Madrid, Spain

SARAH COHEN-GOGO, MD, PhD
Division of Haematology/Oncology,
Department of Paediatrics, The Hospital for
Sick Children, University of Toronto, Toronto,
Ontario, Canada

ARTUR M. COUTINHO, MD, PhD
Department of Radiology, Hospital
Sirio-Libanes, Department of Radiology and
Oncology, Hospital das Clinicas HCFMUSP,
Faculdade de Medicina, Universidade de Sao
Paulo, Sao Paulo, Brazil

HABIBOLLAH DADGAR, MSc
Cancer Research Center, RAZAVI Hospital,
Imam Reza International University, Mashhad,
Iran

KATHARINA DENDL, cand. med
Department of Nuclear Medicine, University
Hospital Heidelberg, Heidelberg, Germany

FRIEDERIKE EILSBERGER, MD
University Hospital Marburg, Department of
Nuclear Medicine, Baldingerstrasse, Marburg,
Germany.

ELISABETH EPPARD, PhD
Positronpharma SA, Santiago, Chile;
Department of Nuclear Medicine, University
Hospital Magdeburg, Germany

MARYAM FALLAHPOOR, MSc
Department of Nuclear Medicine, Vali-Asr
Hospital, Tehran University of Medical
Sciences, Tehran, Iran

SAEED FARZANEHFAR, MD
Department of Nuclear Medicine, Vali-Asr
Hospital, Tehran University of Medical
Sciences, Tehran, Iran

**ALI GHOLAMREZANEZHAD, MD, FEBNM,
DABR**
Assistant Professor of Clinical Radiology,
Department of Diagnostic Radiology, Keck
School of Medicine of USC, University of
Southern California, Los Angles, California, USA

FREDERIK L. GIESEL, MD, MBA
Professor, Department of Nuclear Medicine,
University Hospital Düsseldorf, Germany

UWE HABERKORN, MD
Professor, Department of Nuclear Medicine,
University Hospital Heidelberg, Clinical
Cooperation Unit Nuclear Medicine, German
Cancer Research Center (DKFZ), Translational
Lung Research Center Heidelberg, German
Center for Lung Research (DZL), Heidelberg,
Germany

MEREDITH S. IRWIN, MD
Division of Haematology/Oncology,
Department of Paediatrics, The Hospital for
Sick Children, University of Toronto, Toronto,
Ontario, Canada

ESMAIL JAFARI, MSc
Department of Molecular Imaging and
Radionuclide Therapy (MIRT), The Persian Gulf
Nuclear Medicine Research Center, Bushehr
Medical University Hospital, School of
Medicine, Bushehr University of Medical
Sciences, Bushehr, Iran

NARGES JOKAR, MSc
Department of Molecular Imaging and
Radionuclide Therapy (MIRT), The Persian Gulf
Nuclear Medicine Research Center, Bushehr
Medical University Hospital, School of
Medicine, Bushehr University of Medical
Sciences, Bushehr, Iran

SANAZ KATAL, MD, MPH
Department of Nuclear Medicine, Kowsar
Hospital, Shiraz, Iran

CLEMENS KRATOCHWIL, MD
Department of Nuclear Medicine,
University Hospital Heidelberg, Heidelberg,
Germany

MYKOL LARVIE, MD, PhD
Department of Radiology, Cleveland Clinic,
Cleveland, California, USA

ANTONIO MALDONADO, MD
Department of Nuclear Medicine,
Quironsalud Madrid University Hospital,
Madrid, Spain

JOSE FLAVIO G. MARIN, MD
Department of Radiology, Hospital
Sirio-Libanes, Department of Radiology and
Oncology, Hospital das Clinicas HCFMUSP,
Faculdade de Medicina, Universidade de Sao
Paulo, Sao Paulo, Brazil

UR METSER, MD
Joint Department Medical Imaging, University
Health Network, Mount Sinai Hospital and
Women's College Hospital, University of Toronto,
Ontario, Canada; Department of Medical
Imaging, Temerty Faculty of Medicine, University
of Toronto, Toronto, Canada

**DANIEL A. MORGENSTERN, MB, BChir,
PhD**
Division of Haematology/Oncology,
Department of Paediatrics, The Hospital for
Sick Children, University of Toronto, Toronto,
Ontario, Canada

IRAJ NABIPOUR, MD
Department of Internal Medicine (Division of
Endocrinology), Bushehr Medical University
Hospital, The Persian Gulf Tropical Medicine
Research Center, The Persian Gulf
Biomedical Sciences Research Institute,
Bushehr University of Medical Sciences,
Bushehr, Iran

REZA NEMATI, MD
Department of Neurology, Bushehr Medical
University Hospital, Bushehr University of
Medical Sciences, School of Medicine,
Bushehr, Iran

RAFAEL F. NUNES, MD
Department of Radiology, Hospital
Sirio-Libanes, Sao Paulo, Brazil

ANDREAS PFESTROFF, MD
University Hospital Marburg, Department of
Nuclear Medicine, Baldingerstrasse, Marburg,
Germany

MARGARIDA SIMAO RAFAEL, MD
Division of Haematology/Oncology,
Department of Paediatrics, The Hospital for
Sick Children, University of Toronto, Toronto,
Ontario, Canada

KAMBIZ RAHBAR, MD
Professor, Department of Nuclear Medicine,
University Hospital Münster, Münster,
Germany; West German Cancer Center (WTZ),
Universitätsklinikum Essen, Essen, Germany

MARGARIDA RODRIGUES, MD
Professor, Nuclear Medicine Physician,
Department of Nuclear Medicine, Medical
University of Innsbruck, Innsbruck, Austria

MARCELO T. SAPIENZA, MD, PhD
Department of Radiology and Oncology,
Hospital das Clinicas HCFMUSP, Faculdade
de Medicina, Universidade de Sao Paulo, Sao
Paulo, Brazil

JOEL SCHLITTENHARDT, MD
Department of Nuclear Medicine, University
Hospital Heidelberg, Heidelberg, Germany

ROBERT SEIFERT, MD
Department of Nuclear Medicine, University
Hospital Münster, Münster, Germany;
Department of Nuclear Medicine, University
Hospital Essen, West German Cancer Center
(WTZ), Universitätsklinikum Essen, Essen,
Germany; German Cancer Consortium (DKTK),
German Cancer Research Center, Heidelberg,
Germany

AMER SHAMMAS, MD
Division of Nuclear Medicine, Department of
Diagnostic Imaging, The Hospital for Sick
Children, University of Toronto, Toronto,
Ontario, Canada

HOSSEIN SHOOLI, MD
Department of Molecular Imaging and
Radionuclide Therapy (MIRT), The Persian Gulf
Nuclear Medicine Research Center, Bushehr
Medical University Hospital, School of
Medicine, Bushehr University of Medical
Sciences, Bushehr, Iran

FABIAN STAUDINGER, cand. med
Department of Nuclear Medicine, University
Hospital Heidelberg, Heidelberg, Germany

HANNA SVIRYDENKA, MD
Nuclear Medicine Physician, Department of
Nuclear Medicine, Medical University of
Innsbruck, Innsbruck, Austria

NASIM VAHIDFAR, PhD
Department of Nuclear Medicine, Vali-Asr
Hospital, Tehran University of Medical
Sciences, Tehran, Iran

REZA VALI, MD, MSc
Division of Nuclear Medicine, Department of
Diagnostic Imaging, The Hospital for Sick
Children, University of Toronto, Toronto,
Ontario, Canada

PATRICK VEIT-HAIBACH, MD
Joint Department Medical Imaging, University
Health Network, Mount Sinai Hospital and
Women's College Hospital, University of
Toronto, Ontario, Canada; Department of
Medical Imaging, Temerty Faculty of Medicine,
University of Toronto, Toronto, Canada

IRENE VIRGOLINI, MD
Professor, Director, Department of Nuclear
Medicine, Medical University of Innsbruck,
Innsbruck, Austria

REBECCA K.S. WONG, MSc, MBChB
Radiation Medicine Program, Princess
Margaret Cancer Center, University Health
Network, Department of Radiation Oncology,
Temerty Faculty of Medicine, University of
Toronto, Toronto, Canada

ANNA YORDANOVA, MD
Department of Nuclear Medicine, University
Hospital Bonn, Department of Radiology,
Marienhospital Bonn, Bonn, Germany

ROBERTA M.F. ZUPPANI, MD
Department of Radiology and Oncology,
Hospital das Clinicas HCFMUSP, Faculdade
de Medicina, Universidade de Sao Paulo, Sao
Paulo, Brazil

Contents

Theranostics describes the pairing of diagnostic biomarkers and therapeutic agents with common specific targets. Nuclear medicine is the greatest theranostics protagonist, relying on radioactive tracers for imaging biologic phenomena and delivering ionizing radiation to the tissues that take up those tracers. The concept has gained importance with the growth of personalized medicine, allowing customized management for diseases, refining patient selection, better predicting responses, reducing toxicity, and estimating prognosis. This work provides an overview of the general concepts of the theranostics approach in nuclear medicine discussing its background, features, and future directions in imaging and therapy.

Radiometal-based theranostics or theragnostics, first used in the early 2000s, is the combined application of diagnostic and therapeutic agents that target the same molecule, and represents a considerable advancement in nuclear medicine. One of the promising fields related to theranostics is radioligand therapy. For instance, the concepts of targeting the prostate-specific membrane antigen (PSMA) for imaging and therapy in prostate cancer, or somatostatin receptor targeted imaging and therapy in neuroendocrine tumors (NETs) are part of the field of theranostics. Combining targeted imaging and therapy can improve prognostication, therapeutic decision-making, and monitoring of the therapy.

Fibroblast activation protein inhibitor emerges as a novel and highly promising agent for diagnostic and possibly theranostic application in various malignant and non-malignant diseases. FAPI impresses with its selective expression in several pathologies, ligand induced internalization, and presence in a large variety of malignancies. Current studies indicate that FAPI is equal or even superior to the current standard oncological tracer fluorodeoxyglucose in several oncological diseases. It seems to present lower background activity, stronger uptake in tumorous lesions and thus sharper contrasts. For improved comprehension of fibroblast activation, protein expression and clinicopathologic conditions, further studies are of essence.

This article summarizes the role of PET imaging for detection, characterization, and theranostic/therapy planning for neuroendocrine tumors. Topics in this article span overall imaging accuracy with mostly 68Ga-DOTA-peptide imaging, basic principles of individualized dosimetry and specialized approaches in theranostics dosimetry. In addition, an overview of the literature on functional imaging in neuroendocrine tumors and the current understanding of imaging-derived clinical outcome prediction are presented.

Several studies have demonstrated the effectiveness of somatostatin receptor (SSTR)-targeted imaging for diagnosis, staging, evaluating the possibility of treatment with cold somatostatin analogs, as well peptide receptor radionuclide therapy (PRRT), and evaluation of treatment response. PET with ^{68}Ga-labeled somatostatin analogs provides excellent sensitivity and specificity for diagnosing and staging neuroendocrine tumors (NETs). Metabolic imaging with PET with fludeoxyglucose ^{18}F/computed tomography (CT) complements the molecular imaging with ^{68}Ga-SSTR PET/CT toward a personalized therapy in NET patients. The documented response rate of PRRT in NET summing up complete response, partial response, minor response, and stable disease is 70% to 80%.

The main targeting structure for theranostics in thyroid cancer is the sodium-iodine symporter (NIS), which has been used in clinical routine for the diagnosis and treatment of thyroid diseases for more than 70 years. Because the different iodine (I) nuclides (^{123}I, ^{124}I, ^{131}I) have the same kinetics, uniquely congruent theranostics are possible in differentiated thyroid cancer. Besides the NIS, there are further possibilities by using expression of somatostatin receptors or the expression of the prostate-specific membrane antigen, for example, in radioiodine-refractory differentiated thyroid cancer, medullary thyroid cancer, or anaplastic thyroid cancer.

Prostate-specific mebrane antigen postitron emission/computed tomographies (PSMA-PET/CT) is the investigation of choice for imaging prostate cancer. Demonstrating high diagnostic accuracy, PSMA-PET/CT detects disease at very early stages of recurrence where the chances of a definitive cure may be at their greatest. A number of PSMA-radioligands are in established clinical routine, for which there are currently only limited data and no single tracer can clearly be advocated over the others at present. Further clinical trial data, comparing and contrasting radiotracers and reporting outcome-based data are necessary to further increase the implementation of this very promising imaging modality.

Robert Seifert, Ian L. Alberts, Ali Afshar-Oromieh, and Kambiz Rahbar

Prostate-specific membrane antigen (PSMA) has been the subject of numerous studies within the last 3 decades. PSMA-targeted imaging and therapy have significantly changed the management of patients with prostate cancer in various disease stages, especially in advanced metastasized castration-resistant prostate cancer. Lutetium-177–conjugated PSMA-617 or PSMA-I&T (Lu-PSMA) has shown promising results in multicenter retrospective and monocenter prospective trials. The aim of this review is to provide an overview of the history and current and future developments of PSMA-targeted therapy. A special focus of this review is on PSMA PET–guided management of patients receiving PSMA-targeted radioligand therapy.

Hossein Shooli, Reza Nemati, Hojjat Ahmadzadehfar, Mariam Aboian, Esmail Jafari, Narges Jokar, Iraj Nabipour, Habibollah Dadgar, Ali Gholamrezanezhad, Mykol Larvie, and Majid Assadi

Theranostic nuclear oncology, mainly in neuro-oncology (neurotheranostics), aims to combine cancer imaging and therapy using the same targeting molecule. This approach tries to identify patients who are most likely to benefit from tumor molecular radionuclide therapy. The ability of radioneurotheranostic agents to interact with cancer cells at the molecular level with high specificity can significantly improve the effectiveness of cancer therapy. A variety of biologic targets are under investigation for treating brain tumors. PET-based precision imaging can substantially improve the therapeutic efficacy of radiotheranostic approach in brain tumors.

Margarida Simao Rafael, Sarah Cohen-Gogo, Meredith S. Irwin, Reza Vali, Amer Shammas, and Daniel A. Morgenstern

Theranostics combines diagnosis and targeted therapy, achieved by the use of the same or similar molecules labeled with different radiopharmaceuticals or identical with different dosages. One of the best examples is the use of metaiodobenzylguanidine (MIBG). In the management of neuroblastoma—the most common extracranial solid tumor in children. MIBG has utility not only for diagnosis, risk-stratification, and response monitoring but also for cancer therapy, particularly in the setting of relapsed/refractory disease. Improved techniques and new emerging radiopharmaceuticals likely will strengthen the role of nuclear medicine in the management of neuroblastoma.

Majid Assadi, Narges Jokar, Anna Yordanova, Ali Gholamrezanezhad, Abdullatif Amini, Farhad Abbasi, Hans-Jürgen Biersack, Azam Amini, Iraj Nabipour, and Hojjat Ahmadzadehfar

Studies in nuclear medicine have shed light on molecular imaging and therapeutic approaches for oncological and nononcological conditions. Using the same radiopharmaceuticals for diagnosis and therapeutics of malignancies, the theranostics approach, has improved clinical management of patients. Theranostic approaches for nononcological conditions are recognized as emerging topics of research. This review focuses on preclinical and clinical studies of nononcological disorders that include theranostic strategies. Theranostic approaches are demonstrated as possible in the clinical management of infections and inflammations. There is an

PET CLINICS

SERIES OF RELATED INTEREST

Advances in Clinical Radiology
Available at: Advancesinclinicalradiology.com
MRI Clinics of North America
Available at: MRI.theclinics.com
Neuroimaging Clinics of North America
Available at: Neuroimaging.theclinics.com
Radiologic Clinics of North America
Available at: Radiologic.theclinics.com

THE CLINICS ARE AVAILABLE ONLINE!
Access your subscription at:
www.theclinics.com

PROGRAM OBJECTIVE

The goal of the *PET Clinics* is to keep practicing radiologists and radiology residents up to date with current clinical practice in positron emission tomography by providing timely articles reviewing the state of the art in patient care.

TARGET AUDIENCE

Practicing radiologists, radiology residents, and other health care professionals who provide patient care utilizing radiologic findings.

LEARNING OBJECTIVES

Upon completion of this activity, participants will be able to:
1. Review the general concepts and basics of theranostics.
2. Discuss the role of theranostics in the management of various cancers.
3. Recognize non-cancer related applications of theranostics.

ACCREDITATION

The Elsevier Office of Continuing Medical Education (EOCME) is accredited by the Accreditation Council for Continuing Medical Education (ACCME) to provide continuing medical education for physicians.

The EOCME designates this journal-based CME activity for a maximum of 12 *AMA PRA Category 1 Credit*(s)™. Physicians should claim only the credit commensurate with the extent of their participation in the activity.

All other health care professionals requesting continuing education credit for this enduring material will be issued a certificate of participation.

DISCLOSURE OF CONFLICTS OF INTEREST

The EOCME assesses conflict of interest with its instructors, faculty, planners, and other individuals who are in a position to control the content of CME activities. All relevant conflicts of interest that are identified are thoroughly vetted by EOCME for fair balance, scientific objectivity, and patient care recommendations. EOCME is committed to providing its learners with CME activities that promote improvements or quality in healthcare and not a specific proprietary business or a commercial interest.

The planning committee, staff, authors, and editors listed below have identified no financial relationships or relationships to products or devices they or their spouse/life partner have with commercial interest related to the content of this CME activity:

Farhad Abbasi, MD; Mariam Aboian, MD, PhD; Ali Afshar-Oromieh, MD; Hojjat Ahmadzadehfar, MD, MSc; Ian L. Alberts, MD, MA; Anette Altmann, MD; Abdullatif Amini, MD; Azam Amini, MD; Majid Assadi, MD, FASNC; Felipe G. Barbosa, MD; Hans-Jürgen Biersack, MD; Carlos A. Buchpiguel, MD, PhD; Javier Carrascoso, MD; Regina Chavous-Gibson, MSN, RN; Sarah Cohen-Gogo, MD, PhD; Artur M. Coutinho, MD, PhD; Habibollah Dadgar, MSc; Katharina Dendl, cand. med; Friederike Eilsberger, MD; Elisabeth Eppard, PhD; Maryam Fallahpoor, MSc; Saeed Farzanehfar, MD; Ali Gholamrezanezhad, MD, FEBNM, DABR; Frederik L. Giesel MD, MBA; Uwe Haberkorn, MD; Meredith S. Irwin, MD; Esmail Jafari, MSc; Narges Jokar, MSc; Sanaz Katal, MD, MPH; Clemens Kratochwil, MD; Mykol Larvie, MD, PhD; Antonio Maldonado, MD; Jose Flavio G. Marin, MD; Ur Metser, MD; Iraj Nabipour, MD; Reza Nemati, MD; Rafael F. Nunes, MD; Andreas Pfestroff, MD; Margarida Simao Rafael, MD; Margarida Rodrigues, MD; Marcelo T. Sapienza, MD, PhD; Joel Schlittenhardt, MD; Robert Seifert, MD; Amer Shammas, MD; Hossein Shooli, MD; Fabian Staudinger, cand. med; Hanna Svirydenka, MD; Reni Thomas; Nasim Vahidfar, PhD; Reza Vali, MD, MSc; John Vassallo; Irene Virgolini, MD; Vignesh Viswanathan; Rebecca K.S. Wong, Sc, MBChB; Anna Yordanova, MD; Roberta M. F. Zuppani, MD

The planning committee, staff, authors, and editors listed below have identified financial relationships or relationships to products or devices they or their spouse/life partner have with commercial interest related to the content of this CME activity:

Daniel A. Morgenstern, MB, BChir, PhD: consultant/advisor: Clarity Pharmaceuticals and Y-mAbs Therapeutics, Inc, Kambiz Rahbar, MD: consultant/advisor: Bayer Ag and ABX advanced biochemical compounds GmbH; speakers bureau: AAA Pharmaceutical, Inc, Amgen Inc, Janssen Global Services, LLC, Siemens Healthcare GmbH, and Sirtex Medical, Patrick Veit-Haibach. MD: research support: Bayer AG, F. Hoffmann-La Roche Ltd, Siemens Healthcare GmbH, General Electric Company

UNAPPROVED/OFF-LABEL USE DISCLOSURE

The EOCME requires CME faculty to disclose to the participants:
1. When products or procedures being discussed are off-label, unlabelled, experimental, and/or investigational (not US Food and Drug Administration [FDA] approved); and
2. Any limitations on the information presented, such as data that are preliminary or that represent ongoing research, interim analyses, and/or unsupported opinions. Faculty may discuss information about pharmaceutical agents that is outside of FDA-approved labelling. This information is intended solely for CME and is not intended to promote off-label use of these medications. If you have any questions, contact the medical affairs department of the manufacturer for the most recent prescribing information.

TO ENROLL

To enroll in the *PET Clinics* Continuing Medical Education program, call customer service at 1-800-654-2452 or sign up online at http://www.theclinics.com/home/cme. The CME program is available to subscribers for an additional annual fee of USD 254.00

METHOD OF PARTICIPATION

In order to claim credit, participants must complete the following:

1. Complete enrolment as indicated above.
2. Read the activity.
3. Complete the CME Test and Evaluation. Participants must achieve a score of 70% on the test. All CME Tests and Evaluations must be completed online.

CME INQUIRIES/SPECIAL NEEDS

For all CME inquiries or special needs, please contact elsevierCME@elsevier.com

Preface
PET in the Era of Theranostics

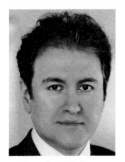
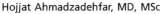
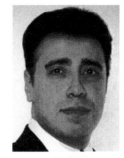

Hojjat Ahmadzadehfar, MD, MSc   Ali Gholamrezanezhad, MD, FEBNM, DABR

Editors

The heterogeneity of human malignancies has led the oncology community to the integration of modern imaging modalities into their management and the most critical components of treatment planning in this population. By providing accurate staging, molecular characterization, and accurate quantification of disease burden, clinicians are guided for optimal management of numerous cancers.

Combined diagnosis and therapy by radioactive agents originated with the groundbreaking initiative by Saul Hertz (1905-1950), who performed the first radioiodine therapy in 1941. This innovative approach started a new beginning in medical treatment and, over the last 2 decades, resulted in our growing knowledge about molecular oncology and tumor immunology. These developments together have generated the concept of theranostics, which bridges the gap between therapeutic interventions and diagnostics. In the field of molecular medicine, theranostics combines imaging and therapy techniques that use the same or similar molecules, either radiolabeled differently or administered with different dosages. This strategy makes it possible to select eligible patients for a specific therapy and, in turn, enhances response rate, and therefore, overall survival while minimizing side effects.

Adopting molecular imaging modalities, particularly PET, in treatment planning has shown significant benefits with regard to the outcomes, including progression-free and overall survival of patients with cancer. Furthermore, this approach has led to substantial improvement of clinical symptoms of the affected population. Most notably, personalized radionuclide therapy in the framework of theranostics provides promising outcomes and treatment responses with significantly decreased adverse effects, such as hematologic or nephrologic toxicity, resulting in improved quality of life for patients with various cancers.

The field of personalized medicine is rapidly adopting PET, single-photon emission computed tomography, optical imaging, and to some extent, MRI (including magnetic resonance [MR] fingerprinting and MR spectroscopy) to identify and visualize potential molecular targets and unmask the molecular phenotype of the neoplastic cells.

PET Clin 16 (2021) xv–xvi
https://doi.org/10.1016/j.cpet.2021.04.001
1556-8598/21/© 2021 Published by Elsevier Inc.

Numerous novel radiotracers are used as theranostic probes in clinical practice, among which ^{68}Ga-labeled somatostatin receptor agents, ^{177}Lu-based radiopharmaceuticals, and radiolabeled antibodies are especially noteworthy. This issue of *PET Clinics* aims to provide a summary of contextual knowledge and current clinical applications of theranostics in modern oncology. The comprehensive review articles of the subject selected for this issue of *PET Clinics* allow scientists, oncologists, and other specialists to realize the great potential of this innovative approach and encourage future studies in this expanding area of molecular imaging in medicine.

In this issue, Jose Flavio Marin and his colleagues outline the general concepts and basics of theranostics. Other articles cover the role of theranostics in the management of various cancers, including prostate, neuroendocrine, brain, and thyroid cancers and neuroblastoma. Non-cancer-related applications of theranostics are also discussed and include management of musculoskeletal diseases. We hope the articles in this issue compellingly illustrate what is known about theranostics, highlight gaps in current knowledge, and help point to promising opportunities for future research in this very exciting discipline in medicine.

Hojjat Ahmadzadehfar, MD, MSc
Department of Nuclear Medicine
Klinikum Westfalen
Am Knappschaftskrankenhaus 1
Dortmund 44301, Germany

Ali Gholamrezanezhad, MD, FEBNM, DABR
Department of Radiology-LAC+USC
1983 Marengo Street
Los Angeles, CA 90033, USA

E-mail addresses:
hojjat.ahmadzadehfar@ruhr-uni-bochum.de
(H. Ahmadzadehfar)
gholamre@usc.edu (A. Gholamrezanezhad)

General Concepts in Theranostics

Rafael F. Nunes, MD[a],*, Roberta M.F. Zuppani, MD[b], Artur M. Coutinho, MD, PhD[a,b], Felipe G. Barbosa, MD[a], Marcelo T. Sapienza, MD, PhD[b], Jose Flavio G. Marin, MD[a,b], Carlos A. Buchpiguel, MD, PhD[a,b]

KEYWORDS

• Theranostics • Nuclear medicine • Diagnosis • Therapy • Molecular imaging

KEY POINTS

• Molecular imaging is a modern and efficient modality capable of simultaneously depicting whole-body lesion burden and biologic characteristics of the disease.
• Treatment of those lesions is possible when α- or β-emitting radionuclides are bound to tracers addressing the targets depicted in imaging.
• Modern radionuclide therapies allow higher destructive effects to lesions while aiming to minimize toxicity to normal tissues.
• Substantial and growing data support the theranostics approach, demonstrating positive impact of the modality in the outcomes of the patients.

INTRODUCTION
Theranostics Concept

The term "theranostics" was conceived in 2002[1] with the acronym made by the fusion of the words "therapy" and "diagnostics." Simplistically, the terminology describes the combined use of one agent to diagnose a disease and the use of the same or a related agent to treat that condition. Although the term was recently adopted, the concept it represents has been continuously explored over the past decades,[2] and it has gained ground with remarkable progress in molecular biology, immunology, immunotherapy, and genomics, contributing to the emergence of personalized medicine.

Ultimately, theranostics empowers better selection of patients for treatment and allows prediction of outcomes, toxicity, and response evaluation. Correspondingly, the field has increasingly contributed to decision-making in patient-centered care by providing customized management of diseases and avoiding futile and costly diagnostic examinations and treatments.[3]

Bringing Theranostics to Nuclear Medicine

Radioisotopes may have imaging or therapeutic properties that are driven by the type of radiation emitted. Electromagnetic radiation (γ-rays) is detected by imaging systems, such as scintigraphy/single-photon emission computed tomography (SPECT) and PET, whereas particulate radiation promotes high transference of energy to tissues resulting in cell injury and DNA damage. The main types of particulate radiation used for therapeutic applications are α- and β-particles. α-Particles exhibit higher energy and much greater mass than β-particles, which in turn comprise high-energy, high-speed electrons, and are less ionizing than α-particles yet more ionizing than γ-rays. Therefore, diagnostic and therapeutic radiopharmaceuticals that address the same biologic process (ie, share the same target) are called theranostics pairs.

Nuclear theranostics encompass the combination of diagnostic imaging biomarkers with therapeutic radiopharmaceuticals that share a specific

[a] Department of Radiology, Hospital Sirio-Libanes, Sao Paulo, Brazil; [b] Department of Radiology and Oncology, Hospital das Clinicas HCFMUSP, Faculdade de Medicina, Universidade de Sao Paulo, Sao Paulo, Brazil
* Corresponding author. Rua Dona Adma Jafet, 115 – CEP 01308-060, Sao Paulo, Sao Paulo, Brazil.
E-mail address: rafaelskpk@gmail.com
Twitter: @rafaelskpk (R.F.N.)

PET Clin 16 (2021) 313–326
https://doi.org/10.1016/j.cpet.2021.03.010
1556-8598/21/© 2021 Elsevier Inc. All rights reserved.

pet.theclinics.com

target in cells or tissues. The expression of those specific targets, such as cell surface receptors or membrane transporters, allows imaging of the biologic phenomena of different disorders.[4] This way, different molecules are specifically designed to act in imaging or treatment of many diseases (**Fig. 1**).

This unique approach to evaluating a disease permits the assessment of key molecular phenotypes with increased sensitivity, specificity, and target-to-background ratio and translates into better diagnostic accuracy than preexisting options and better portrayal of total tumor burden, besides allowing to set up a baseline reference for future response assessment. These advantages might help providing new horizons of the disease spread.[5–9]

The investigation of theranostic agents in nuclear medicine began in the 1930s with Dr Saul Hertz, who postulated that radioactive isotopes of iodine could be used to evaluate iodine metabolism. The understanding of radioactive iodine mechanisms evolved and in the 1940s Dr Hertz began treating patients with hyperthyroid with radioiodine therapy.[10] Ever since, many other tracers have been used in clinical practice and remain important treatment modalities today.[10–12] More recent theranostic agents include tracers targeting bone lesions, prostate cancer, and neuroendocrine tumors. These newer agents leveraging advanced imaging technologies are influenced by molecular biology, are extensively evidence-based, and are based on a multidisciplinary approach to care.

Overview of Nuclear Theranostics Pairs

Radioiodine for differentiated thyroid cancer
A key constituent to triiodothyronine and thyroxine, iodide is taken up by thyroid follicular cells and differentiated neoplastic thyroid cells mainly through the sodium iodide membrane symporter (NIS) (**Table 1**). Therefore, iodine isotopes may be used as theranostic agents targeting NIS for imaging and treatment. The main radionuclides include iodine-131 (^{131}I), iodine-123 (^{123}I), and iodine-124 (^{124}I). Other radiopharmaceuticals (eg, ^{99m}Tc-pertechnetate) may also be taken up by thyroid cells and are able to generate imaging to pair with ^{131}I therapy.[11,13]

^{31}I-metaiodobenzylguanidine for neural crest–derived tumors
Metaiodobenzylguanidine (mIBG), an analogue of norepinephrine, is able to penetrate neuroendocrine cells of the sympathetic nervous system through endocytosis or diffusion. Afterward, those cells store mIBG in neurosecretory vesicles. Therefore, the agent is capable of identifying neural crest–derived tumors, especially neuroblastoma, pheochromocytoma, paraganglioma, and metastatic or recurrent medullary thyroid carcinoma. When labeled with ^{131}I, ^{131}I-mIBG is suitable to imaging and therapy.[11,14] The agent might be bound to imaging tracers, such as ^{123}I and ^{124}I, allowing for better imaging resolution, yet ^{123}I and ^{124}I-mIBG are not therapeutic agents.[15]

Bone-seeking agents for bone pain palliation
These agents comprise radiolabeled phosphonates, such as $^{186/188}$Re-HEDP and ^{153}Sm-EDTMP, and calcium analogues, such as ^{89}Sr (strontium chloride) and ^{223}Ra (radium-223 dichloride, Xofigo). All are taken up by areas of intense bone matrix formation, such as osteoblastic lesions, with the increased osseous turnover leading to higher affinity to these radiopharmaceuticals. The imaging component of the theranostics approach is often performed

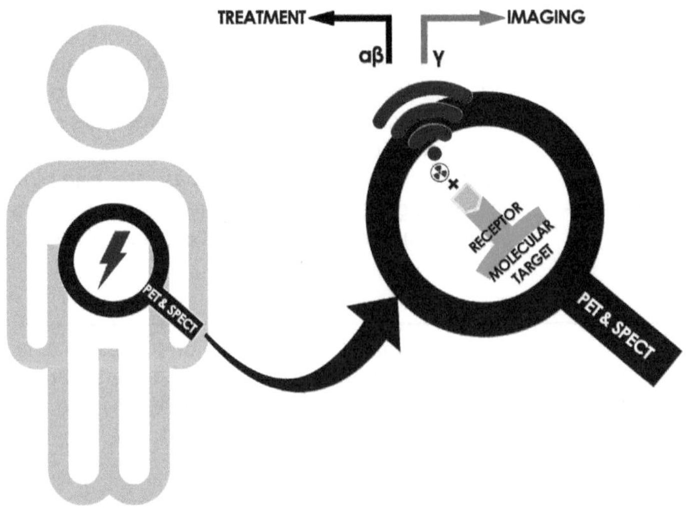

Fig. 1. Schematic representation of how nuclear theranostics works. Specific agents targeting biologic phenomena are called radiopharmaceuticals. They may be labeled with a γ-emitting radionuclide, which enables PET or SPECT imaging. When in combination with an α- or β-particle-emitting radionuclide, the agent is suitable for therapy.

Table 1
Examples of nuclear medicine theranostics pairs commonly used in clinical routines worldwide

Molecular Target	Diseases	Diagnostic	Therapy
Sodium/iodide symporter	Hyperthyroidism Differentiated thyroid cancer	^{123}I (NaI) ^{99m}Tc-pertechnetate	^{131}I (NaI)
Norepinephrine transporter	Neuroblastoma Pheochromocytoma Paraganglioma Medullary thyroid cancer	^{123}I-mIBG	^{131}I-mIBG
Hydroxyapatite in bones	Prostate cancer	^{99m}Tc-MDP ^{18}F-NaF	^{223}Ra
Somatostatin receptors	Neuroendocrine tumors	^{68}Ga-DOTA-peptides ^{99m}Tc/^{111}In-octreotate	^{177}Lu/^{90}Y-octreotate
PSMA	Prostate cancer	^{68}Ga/^{18}F-PSMA	^{177}Lu/^{225}Ac-PSMA
Hepatic microvasculature	Hepatocellular carcinoma Cholangiocarcinoma Liver metastases	^{99m}Tc-MAA	^{90}Y-microspheres
CD20 (B-lymphocyte antigen, expressed on the surface of B cells)	Non-Hodgkin lymphoma	Anti-CD20 immunohistochemistry	^{131}I/^{90}Y-anti-CD20

Abbreviations: MAA, macroaggregated albumin; MDP, methylene diphosphonate; mIBG, metaiodobenzylguanidine; PSMA, prostate-specific membrane antigen.

by bone scans with ^{99m}Tc–methylene diphosphonate or ^{99m}Tc-HEDP before the treatment.[11,12] Those agents are able to relieve bone pain caused by metastases and improve quality of life. Treatment with ^{223}Ra was more recently introduced, providing α emission with shorter range and much higher energy in comparison with the other, β-emitting radionuclides. As a result, ^{223}Ra has a proven impact on survival in patients with prostate cancer and is less toxic than the other bone-seeking agents, which fall into disuse.[12,16]

Somatostatin analogue radioligands
Somatostatin receptors are found on cells of neuroendocrine origin, including tumors,[17] enabling radiolabeled somatostatin analogue radioligands to be used in a theranostic approach. Although ^{68}Ga-DOTA-peptides and ^{99m}Tc/^{111}In-octreotate are used for imaging, ^{177}Lu or ^{90}Y-octreotate are used for therapy. The emergence of ^{68}Ga-DOTA-peptides (^{68}Ga-DOTATOC, ^{68}Ga-DOTATATE, and ^{68}Ga-DOTANOC) for PET imaging during the 2000s was a breakthrough for diagnosis, staging, and follow-up of neuroendocrine neoplasms[18] and these days, somatostatin receptor PET imaging is recommended by many guidelines and its use is considered appropriate from multidisciplinary panels.[19-21] In turn, peptide receptor radionuclide therapy procedures have become widely adopted around the world

because of the reduced risk of disease progression, prolonged maintenance of clinical performance status, longer time to deterioration of symptom, and longer time of functional health-related quality of life, as demonstrated by the phase 3 randomized, controlled trial NETTER-1 study.[22,23]

Prostate-specific membrane antigen radiopharmaceuticals for prostate cancer
Prostate-specific membrane antigen (PSMA) is a type II transmembrane glycoprotein highly expressed in prostate cancer cells, making it an excellent target for imaging because of the high detectability of prostate cancer lesions. PSMA PET provides higher sensitivity, specificity, and target-to-background ratio than other imaging methods, which leads to better diagnostic accuracy. This approach has revolutionized the evaluation of patients with prostate cancer and has even garnered new information about the way the disease spreads.[5-7] Furthermore, radionuclide therapy with PSMA-ligands is the subject of many studies around the world, and data supporting its use have soared during recent years. Many investigations have revealed the effectiveness of PSMA radioligand therapy (PRLT) for metastatic castration-resistant prostate cancer with ^{177}Lu-PSMA and its high response rates and low toxicity profile.[24-26]

Hepatic radioembolization

Hepatic radioembolization of primary or metastatic hepatic lesions is a multidisciplinary procedure comprising scintigraphy, SPECT/computed tomography (CT), CT, MRI, PET/CT/MRI, and arteriography. The procedure aims to deliver ionizing radiation to tumoral lesions by means of radiolabeled therapeutic microspheres that are introduced through the tumors' microvasculature system where they embolize those vessels and then promote a radioactive antineoplastic upshot. Most of the currently available microspheres are made of glass or resin and radiolabeled with ^{90}Y, a high-energy, β- and γ-emitting radioisotope with high potential for tissue damage.

In this scenario the target is mechanical and anatomic based, requiring an imaging component that simulates the microsphere distribution after arterial injection. Scintigraphy with ^{99m}Tc–macroaggregated albumin involves macroaggregated albumin particles with physical characteristics similar to those of microspheres, enabling the planning of the procedure and forecasting its outcome.[27,28]

Hybrid theragnostic pairs

Lastly, even though most nuclear theranostic pairs comprise radiopharmaceuticals in the diagnostic and therapeutic ends, hybrid pairs may be set by a radiopharmaceutical and a diagnostic or therapeutic component from other modalities, such as immunochemistry stains, antibodies, or tyrosine kinase inhibitors (**Table 2**).

DISCUSSION

Diagnostic Versus Theranostic: How Molecular Imaging Can Impact Outcomes

Following the acknowledged progress in molecular imaging and theranostics approach, new hope has rapidly emerged for patients with diseases, such as metastatic neuroendocrine and prostate tumors. Diseases with high radiotracer uptake mechanisms benefit from the effects of radioactive particles with shorter range and higher energy, enhancing the radiation dose delivered, thus increasing the destruction of lesions, while providing diminished radiation-induced normal tissue toxicity. Altogether, those treatments disrupt cancer cell survival and proliferation, yielding higher rates of partial response and stable disease and prolonging survival time in some types of cancers, especially those (eg, prostate and neuroendocrine) treated by novel radiopharmaceuticals.[12,16,29–33] Besides, most of the theranostic treatments provide positive impacts on symptom relief and quality of life for patients.

Several prospective studies have emerged supporting the use of novel therapies, such as ^{223}Ra, ^{177}Lu-DOTATATE, and ^{177}Lu-PSMA. These therapies have also helped shift the purpose of theranostic pairs from serving as palliative treatments aimed to only relieve symptoms and improve quality of life to serving as treatments that make a strong impact on survival and delay the course of diseases. More prospective studies are necessary encompassing broader and earlier scenarios. The main focus of current research in theranostics is finding new targets, polishing radiopharmaceutical dosimetry and regimens, and exploring the feasibility of combined multimodality therapies and treatments at earlier stages.

Theranostics in the Era of Evidence-Based Medicine

Until recently, targeted radionuclide therapy has been used clinically based on either empirical or long-term evidence of benefits in outcomes, after decades of treatments performed, as in the case of radioiodine therapy for thyroid diseases. Over the years, more radiopharmaceuticals with theranostic potential emerged, and their use was based on the same empiric criteria or, at most, justified by either compassionate use or right-to-try possibilities.[34,35] These efforts have served as therapeutic options to individuals with no other proven and/or safe alternative. However, although well-intentioned, they may become potentially misguided. Ultimately, this scenario no longer fits the current medical, evidence-based, and research practices. The most recent advances in nuclear medicine therapies have been based on robust clinical trials, with large cohorts and academic thoroughness, relying on industry support and inserted in multidisciplinary scenarios. This shift is in line with what is currently done in all areas of medicine, especially in oncology.

A randomized, controlled trial assessing the efficacy and safety of ^{177}Lu-DOTATATE treatment of patients with advanced, progressive, somatostatin-receptor–positive midgut neuroendocrine tumors explored a new approach for targeted radionuclide therapies.[22] Results of the study attracted industry leaders who purchased the rights to those molecules and subsequently, conducted clinical trials. Later, the development of PSMA-targeted therapeutics has led to even more attention to the field. The enthusiasm resulting from its development indirectly influenced the investigation of and emergence of several new radiolabeled, small α- or β-emitting molecules, which led to the expectation that many cancers might benefit from novel therapeutic avenues. Currently, many clinical trials are in course (**Table 3**) that bring hope of an unprecedented fast-growing progress in nuclear medicine.

Table 2
Examples of nuclear medicine theranostics pairs that are currently under investigation

Molecular Target	Diseases	Diagnostic	Therapy
CXCR4 chemokine receptor and CXCR4/CXCL12 signaling pathway	Multiples types of cancer, including: Multiple myeloma Lymphomas Leukemias Glioblastoma Head/neck cancer (larynx) Pancreatic cancer Melanoma Prostate cancer	^{68}Ga-CXCR4 ligand (eg, [8]Ga-pentixafor)	^{177}Lu-CXCR4 ligand
PD1/PD-L1	Multiple types of cancer, including: Lung cancer Melanoma Renal cancer Lymphomas	[89]Zr/^{18}F-anti-PD1/PD-L1	Anti-PD1/PD-L1 checkpoint inhibitors
HER2	Breast cancer	[89]Zr-anti-HER2 (eg, [89]Zr-trastuzumab)	Human epidermal growth factor receptor (HER2) inhibitors
Fibroblast activation protein	Multiple types of cancer, including Pancreatic cancer Sarcoma Head and neck cancer Ovarian cancer Gastrointestinal cancers	^{68}Ga-fibroblast activation protein inhibitor (FAPI)-04	^{90}Y-FAPI-04

Recent Advances in Nuclear Theranostics

Research on theranostics in nuclear medicine has been fruitful in the last years, with meaningful advances being made in identifying new agents and revisiting indications for established agents.

In regard to radionuclide treatment of neuroendocrine tumors, peptide receptor radionuclide therapy use has been seen in less-differentiated neuroendocrine tumors, such as grade 3 tumors, with reports of treatments used with Ki67 indexes of 20 to 50.[36] Also, the combination of ^{177}Lu-DOTA-TATE and ^{131}I-mIBG in treating tumors, such as metastatic neuroblastomas, that have been classically treated with only ^{131}I-mIBG, has been more intensively studied.[37] Earlier radionuclide regimens have been incorporated in the course of treatment of neuroblastoma, paraganglioma, and pheochromocytoma[38–41] and in less-established indications, such as medullary thyroid carcinoma, iodine-refractory thyroid carcinoma,[42,43] or even recurrent meningioma.[44]

New possibilities are also under investigation regarding [223]Ra in patients with metastatic castration-resistant prostate cancer. The ideal timepoint for using the therapy during the course

of the disease has been discussed, with some advocating an earlier use[45] or combining [223]Ra therapy with other therapies, such as enzalutamide, chemotherapy, and immunotherapy.[46] Conjugation with PSMA-based therapies is possible and potentially feasible, but requires further evaluation on safety, effectiveness, and impact on outcomes. Other tumors, such as breast cancer, could also benefit from its use.

Trials are also scrutinizing broader possibilities of PRLT of metastatic castration-resistant prostate cancer. Some aim to perform early treatment, such as before surgery. Other possibilities include PRLT used in different timepoints in the course of the disease, and in combination with other therapeutic agents. The relevance of this area in uro-oncology is substantial, and might lead to important changes in the way prostate cancer is diagnosed, managed, and understood.

Another topic that has been recently revived concerns the use of fluorodeoxyglucose (FDG)-PET as a gatekeeper for theranostics indication as evidenced by its combination with other agents (**Fig. 2**). Although ^{18}F-FDG uptake is not readily related to therapeutic success/failure of a radioisotope treatment, its uptake is usually associated with more

Table 3
Examples of ongoing clinical trials involving theranostics in nuclear medicine

Disease	Theranostics Approach	Clinical Trial[a]	Intervention	References
Differentiated thyroid cancer	^{123}I WBS/^{131}I RIT	ASTRA	Selumetinib in differentiated thyroid cancer at high risk of primary treatment failure ^{131}I	ClinicalTrials.gov Identifier: NCT01843062
		IoN	Disease-free survival rate for patients with low-risk differentiated thyroid cancer	ClinicalTrials.gov Identifier: NCT01398085
	^{124}I PET-CT/^{131}I RIT	CLERAD-PROBE	^{124}I PET/CT-based remnant radioiodine ablation decision	ClinicalTrials.gov Identifier: NCT01704586
Liver metastases	^{99m}Tc-MAA/^{90}Y-microspheres		TheraSphere for treatment of metastases in liver	ClinicalTrials.gov Identifier: NCT04517643
Neuroendocrine tumors	^{68}Ga/^{177}Lu-DOTATATE and ^{177}Lu-edotreotide	COMPETE NETTER-2	Everolimus vs ^{177}Lu-endocriteotide ^{177}Lu-DOTATATE vs long-acting octreotide in high doses	ClinicalTrials.gov Identifier: NCT03049189 ClinicalTrials.gov Identifier: NCT03972488
		CONTROL NETs	Chemotherapy and radiopeptide treatment combo vs standard therapy alone	ClinicalTrials.gov Identifier: NCT02358356
		LuPARP	^{177}Lu-DOTATATE and olaparib in somatostatin receptor–positive tumors	ClinicalTrials.gov Identifier: NCT04375267
		OCCLURANDOM	^{177}Lu-octreotate vs sunitinib in unresectable progressive well-differentiated neuroendocrine pancreatic tumor	ClinicalTrials.gov Identifier: NCT02230176
Neuroblastoma	^{123}I-mIBG WBS/^{131}I-mIBG therapy		^{131}I-mIBG therapy for relapsed/refractory neuroblastoma ^{131}I-mIBG therapy or crizotinib in high-risk neuroblastoma	ClinicalTrials.gov Identifier: NCT03649438 ClinicalTrials.gov Identifier: NCT03126916
Prostate cancer	^{225}Ac-PSMA		^{225}Ac-PSMA radioligand therapy of metastatic castration-resistant prostate cancer ^{225}Ac-PSMA617 in men with PSMA-positive prostate cancer	ClinicalTrials.gov Identifier: NCT04225910 ClinicalTrials.gov Identifier: NCT04597411

^{68}Ga/^{177}Lu-PSMA	VISION	^{177}Lu-PSMA vs best supportive care	ClinicalTrials.gov Identifier: NCT03511664
	LuTectomy	^{177}Lu-PSMA before prostatectomy	ClinicalTrials.gov Identifier: NCT04430192
	ENZA-p	Enzalutamide with ^{177}Lu-PSMA enzalutamide alone	ClinicalTrials.gov Identifier: NCT04419402
	PRINCE	PSMA-lutetium radionuclide therapy and immunotherapy pembrolizumab in prostate cancer	ClinicalTrials.gov Identifier: NCT03658447
	LuPARP	^{177}Lu-PSMA and olaparib	ClinicalTrials.gov Identifier: NCT04343885
	UpFrontPSMA	^{177}Lu-PSMA in addition to chemotherapy	ClinicalTrials.gov Identifier: NCT04343885

[a] Expansions of listed clinical trial abbreviations are found at ClinicalTrials.gov.

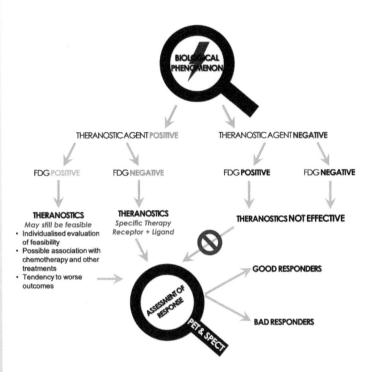

Fig. 2. Schematic diagram summarizes the rationale for indication and contraindication of radionuclide treatments. The approach is based on data on cell differentiation and aggressiveness. Those parameters are provided by PET and SPECT imaging with FDG and specific radiotracers.

aggressive and undifferentiated tumor phenotypes and is associated with a poorer prognosis for many neoplasms.[47] As by principle, theranostic procedures require a certain degree of differentiation to be successful. ^{18}F-FDG-PET might play a role as a gatekeeper for radionuclide therapy through identifying undifferentiated lesions prone to treatment failure (**Fig. 3**). This approach may enhance patient selection and prognostication while enabling the analysis of tumor heterogeneity in several

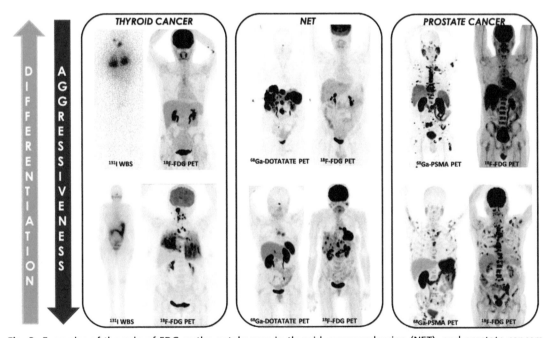

Fig. 3. Examples of the role of FDG as the gatekeeper in thyroid, neuroendocrine (NET), and prostate cancers. Images are depicted on anterior ^{131}I WBS and anterior maximum intensity projection PET scans. Tumor differentiation (*green*) and aggressiveness (*red*) are inversely proportional: the higher the FDG avidity, the less differentiated and more aggressive the tumor tends to be.

neoplasms, those currently treated with the theranostics model and those whose theranostics application is yet to emerge. Such an approach is already applied in treating prostatic cancer and neuroendocrine tumors.[48–50] It may also be a more suitable tool than other tracers to evaluate therapeutic response. The combination of ^{18}F-FDG and ^{68}Ga-DOTATATE to stratify neuroendocrine tumors and possibly improve theranostic selection is under active investigation.[47,48] Similar trials evaluate the combined use of ^{18}F-FDG and PSMA PET ligands in the evaluation and follow-up of prostatic cancer.[49,50] Both methods combined are used with in an off-label approach in many clinical centers, and data suggest that higher uptake of FDG than PSMA is indicative of poorer prognosis.[51]

When it comes to therapy response assessment, molecular imaging is likely more suitable than structural imaging, and there are several opportunities for research on this topic because there is little standardization of current evaluation methods, and traditional imaging methods are unsuitable for evaluating multimodal parameters including metabolic and multitracer data. As an example, PET response criteria in solid tumors (PERCIST) guidelines are designed for ^{18}F-FDG and are not easily applied to other tracers, such as PSMA.[52] As a result, questions arise regarding which tracer would be optimal or even suitable for this assessment. Radiomics and quantitative PET imaging techniques, such as metabolic tumor volume, may also be helpful in this regard.[53,54]

In terms of new avenues for novel tracers, basic nuclear medicine research is mostly comprised of exploring new theranostics agents. A wide variety of new ligands have emerged and are subject of investigation. Such molecules as C-X-C motif chemokine receptor-4 (CXCR4) ligands ([^{68}Ga] pentixafor) are promising and can probe new pathways not previously assessed in cancers, such as multiple myeloma.[55,56] Fibroblast activation protein inhibitor (FAPI) ligands are also potential theranostics agents; however, they are in an earlier phase of investigation (see **Table 2**).[57,58]

Lastly, the theranostics concept also refers to the integration between nuclear medicine and other diagnostic modalities, such as genetic tests, liquid biopsies, chemotherapies, and cancer treatments using drugs to target specific genes and proteins involved in the growth and survival of cancer cells. Good examples are the targeting of anti-PD1/PD-L1 checkpoint inhibitors for multiple types of cancer, using as theranostics pairs [89]Zr- or ^{18}F-anti-PD1/PD-L1 for imaging, and the anti-PD1/PD-L1 checkpoint inhibitors themselves as the therapeutic agent. The same rationale is seen with human epidermal growth factor receptor 2

(HER2/neu) in breast cancer. The theranostics pair includes [89]Zr-anti-HER2 (eg, [89]Zr-trastuzumab) for imaging and HER2 inhibitor drugs in the therapy end. Outside the oncology scope, opportunities emerge in the treatment of neurodegenerative diseases (ie, Alzheimer disease), where nuclear medicine can target specific protein aggregates in the cortex with PET being useful for diagnosis and possibly monitoring of treatment with antibodies (eg, ^{11}C and ^{18}F cortical amyloid ligands ^{11}C-PiB, ^{18}F-florbetapir, ^{18}F-flutemetamol, and ^{18}F-florbetaben; and cortical tau ligands ^{18}F-flortaucipir and ^{18}F-PI2620).[59,60] In conclusion, the future of nuclear medicine theranostics looks bright. Simply put, if a specific useful target molecule can be radiolabeled, it can be used in nuclear medicine theranostics.

CONTROVERSIES
Limitations of the Theranostics Model

More than a century ago the concept of a "magic bullet" was envisioned by the Nobel prize–winning German physician and scientist Paul Ehrlich.[61] The magic bullets were romanticized as drugs with chemical and biologic capabilities permitting them to accurately locate foci of disease and extinguish them while keeping nonaffected tissues immaculate.[3] Unfortunately, science has not evolved to the point of yielding perfect magic bullets and theranostics pairs in nuclear medicine have limitations, like all other diagnostic and treatment modalities.

The drawbacks related to sensitivity and specificity of the diagnostic tools that are based on imaging systems' parameters (eg, spatial and contrast resolution) may lead to imperfect selection of patients. Response assessment remains somewhat controversial because of the lack of established criteria for response assessment using the main modern theranostics imaging procedures.[62] A limitation of the therapeutic agent of the theranostics pairs is that it is not always feasible to offer radiation exclusively to the lesions while entirely avoiding irradiating adjacent nontarget tissues.

Lastly, the main potential limitations are questions related to availability of technology, regulatory approval, and financial sustainability. Solutions for those issues require joint effort by nuclear medicine specialists, referring specialties, academia, industry, regulatory agencies, and government policies and legislation.

Dosimetry: The Missing Link Between Imaging and Therapy

The application of dosimetric planning of radionuclide therapies is one of the stepping-stones to personalized medicine in theranostics. It is possible to predict the absorbed dose (ie, the amount of energy deposited in a certain tissue following an exposure to ionizing radiation) through pretreatment images, which reflect the distribution of the radiopharmaceutical within the lesions and physiologic organs of concentration and elimination for each tracer. In a more traditional and limited scenario, pretreatment images are often used to solely identify whether there is significant avidity of the tracer by the lesions. This way, they are part of a strictly binary decision on whether a particular therapy is feasible or not. Planning of radionuclide therapy may be used devoid of predicting therapeutic response, efficacy, or toxicity.[63–67]

The advantages of a dosimetric approach over an empirical method are not always obvious in clinical practice, because it is more laborious and requires multidisciplinary efforts. Lack of comprehensive clinical studies also hampers the degree of certainty on decision making. However, dosimetry studies can play a prominent role in phase 1 studies by determining the maximum tolerated dose and side effects recorded. In phase 2 studies, dosimetry studies can establish the threshold dose where clinically significant side effects occur and can establish the clinical relationship between dose-response in applying new therapies. Lastly, in phase 3 studies, dosimetry studies can elucidate efficacy and increasing survival rate.[63]

No consensual dosimetry practice is conclusively endorsed to calculate the absorbed dose to tumor targets or organs at risk. For this reason, in many centers protocols have been tailored based on experiences with small cohorts of patients receiving comparable administered activities. Such an empirical approach contrasts with the modern practice of external beam radiotherapy, whose calculations rely on structural images with well-defined disease volumes. Although the goal of radionuclide and external beam radiation therapies is to offer an absorbed radiation dose measured in Gray, the biology of radiation is not equivalent. In nuclear medicine, the absorbed dose depends on the biodistribution of the radiotracer, whereas external beam therapy revolves around physical specifications.[68,69] Other factors better established in external radiotherapy than in nuclide therapy are the foreseeable variation of the biologic effect according to different dose rates. The damage caused by radiation is not limited to DNA breakdown, but also changes the entire cellular microenvironment, which is influenced by intracellular and extracellular factors that extend the cellular response to other levels of the organism, mainly in relation to the stimulation of local immunologic reactions.[70] The use of ineffective doses allows the repair of tumor DNA, resulting in sublethal damage, allowing the selection of resistant tumor cells. Consequently, radioresistance is directly related to lower therapeutic efficacy and more side effects.

The ideal therapeutic dose is designed to achieve the therapeutic objective and avoid unnecessary side effects. Through individual dosimetry, it should be sufficient to promote therapeutic effects on the target but lower than levels that might lead to relevant adverse effects for nontarget organs. Estimating the clinically relevant absorbed doses by the tumor is challenging, especially in patients with multiple sites of disease and variable degrees of uptake and retention of the therapeutic agent.[71] Recent advances, such as voxel-based dosimetry methods using PET/CT and SPECT/CT, have helped with access to real and volumetric data of the patient.[72–74] The association among the predicted dose, therapeutic response, and normal tissue toxicity provides support for efforts in clinical validation of dosimetric methods. Ultimately, better prognosis and quality of life for patients are the outcomes expected.[74]

An important point brought by such advances is the shifting of the use of radionuclide therapies, moving from palliative treatment to earlier treatment scenarios ensuring safety profiles and less toxicity. As in frontline therapies, patients must keep renal and bone marrow status for further therapies.

Therefore, success in the dosimetric approach is linked to standardized and optimized internal dosimetry methods that are more compatible with clinical practice so that it might finally assume a more prominent role in treatment planning.[67]

PERSPECTIVES

After decades of development in theranostics, a variety of new agents to multiple targets are subject to investigation. Among the new emerging molecules that are being investigated in theranostics, CXCR4 ligands, glucagon-like peptides, and fibroblast activation protein ligands stand out as the most studied and potentially favorable, because their mechanisms are found in many cancer pathways, including multiple myeloma, insulinoma, and pancreatic cancer.[55,57] These developments and future perspectives require adjustments in the training model for nuclear medicine physicians, given the growing need to sharpen clinical skills. Foremost, the nuclear medicine specialist must strengthen his or her position as an active player in multidisciplinary clinical teams of radiologists, oncologists, endocrinologists, urologists, surgeons, pathologists, and radiation oncologists in making routine and patient care decisions. Joining efforts between academia and industry are expected to bolster, because theranostics has become an interesting business field for many companies. This cooperation may facilitate access to nuclear medicine therapies. Finally, regulatory agencies must re-evaluate barriers so that scientific advances can be integrated into practical clinical applications.

SUMMARY

Nuclear medicine evolved over the past decades since Dr Hertz's first seminal experiment with theranostics in the 1940s. Now the field is a major player in times of discoveries and developments allowing deeper comprehension of the complex biologic peculiarities of individuals and diseases, especially cancer. Some of the developments in nuclear theranostics are already being used worldwide in a clinical setting and many others are expected to flourish, following encouraging important results from research. The notable preclinical advances in molecular biology, immunology, immunotherapy, and genomics are expected to lead to more and more molecular targets with potential future theranostics applications. Molecular imaging and theranostics are likely to become a significant part of the routine of nuclear medicine physicians around the world and one must therefore be prepared for the many challenges and opportunities that will come.

CLINICS CARE POINTS

- Theranostics consists of coupling diagnostic/ predictive biomarkers and therapeutic agents that share an affinity for the same biologic target.

- Theranostic pairs (ie, diagnostic and therapeutic agents) can belong to different modalities and are potentially used in different human diseases.

- Nuclear medicine has materialized the concept of theranostics since its origins as a medical specialty. The development of nuclear theranostics continues to mainly focus on oncology. New possibilities for nononcologic theranostic procedures have emerged and are expected to be developed in the coming years.

- Recent advances in molecular imaging (PET and SPECT-based imaging) and in therapeutic isotopes technology and the emergence of high-impact clinical trials have made nuclear medicine reinforce its leading role in theranostics.

- Proper patient selection is one of the most important points of the theranostic approach. Patient selection is based not only on the diagnosis itself, but on the intensity of expression of the biologic target, on the prediction of response (and toxicity), and on the prognosis. In this scenario, molecular imaging, with its beyond diagnosis capabilities, has played a central role.

- Newer theranostic procedures, such as those for neuroendocrine tumors or prostate cancer, have been largely based on high-quality data provided by robust randomized clinical trials. This must be the path for the development and adoption of new theranostic procedures.

- Despite the great recent technological advancements, nuclear medicine physicians must be aware that the theranostic model still has imperfections to overcome. Examples are the sensitivity of the diagnostic component, differences in biodistribution between diagnostic and therapeutic radiopharmaceuticals, and unwanted affinity of radiopharmaceuticals for healthy tissues. These imperfections can lead to undesirable situations, such as potential exclusion of patients who would benefit from therapy and unforeseen and limiting toxicity.

- Dosimetry is one of the greatest opportunities for development in the theranostic field and its implementation can solve several current unmet needs. However, the wide adoption of dosimetry depends mainly on the migration from research environment to clinical practice, in addition to evidence of impact on outcomes in randomized clinical trials.

- Theranostics is an illustrative face of what has been called personalized or precision medicine. Increasingly individualized decisions at the patient level have been made in an increasingly shared (multidisciplinary) way at the care provider level.

- Considering all the challenging particularities of this field, regulatory and logistical issues can negatively impact the adoption of theranostic procedures worldwide. Nuclear medicine associations and societies should be prepared to assist regulatory authorities to deal with the assessment of new theranostic procedures.

DISCLOSURE

The authors have nothing to disclose.

REFERENCES

1. Funkhouser J. Reinventing pharma: the theranostic revolution. Curr Drug Discov 2002;2:17–9.
2. Denardo GL, Denardo SJ. Concepts, consequences, and implications of theranosis. Semin Nucl Med 2012;42(3):147–50.
3. Marin JFG, Nunes RF, Coutinho AM, et al. Theranostics in nuclear medicine: emerging and re-emerging integrated imaging and therapies in the era of precision oncology. Radiographics 2020;40(6):1715–40.
4. Hevesy G. The absorption and translocation of lead by plants: A contribution to the application of the method of radioactive indicators in the investigation of the change of substance in plants. In: Leicester HM, editor. A Source Book in Chemistry 1900–1950. Cambridge, Mass: Harvard University Press; 2014.
5. Afshar-Oromieh A, Zechmann CM, Malcher A, et al. The diagnostic value of PET/CT imaging with the 68Ga-labelled PSMA ligand HBED-CC in the diagnosis of recurrent prostate cancer. Eur J Nucl Med Mol Imaging 2015;42(1):197–209.
6. Hofman MS, Hicks RJ, Maurer T, et al. Prostate-specific membrane antigen PET: clinical utility in prostate cancer, normal patterns, pearls, and pitfalls. Radiographics 2018;38(1):200–17.
7. Eiber M, Maurer T, Souvatzoglou M, et al. Evaluation of hybrid 68Ga-PSMA ligand PET/CT in 248 patients with biochemical recurrence after radical prostatectomy. J Nucl Med 2015;56(5):668–74.
8. Kwekkeboom DJ. Hodgkin lymphoma. J Clin Oncol 2008;2124–30. https://doi.org/10.1016/B978-1-4557-2865-7.00105-3.
9. Barbosa FG, Queiroz MA, Nunes RF, et al. Revisiting prostate cancer recurrence with PSMA PET: atlas of typical and atypical patterns of spread. Radiographics 2019;39(1). https://doi.org/10.1148/rg.2019180079.
10. Silberstein EB, Alavi A, Balon HR, et al. The SNMMI practice guideline for therapy of thyroid disease with 131I 3.0. J Nucl Med 2012;53(10):1633–51.
11. Yordanova A, Eppard E, Kürpig S, et al. Theranostics in nuclear medicine practice. Onco Targets Ther 2017;10:4821–8.
12. Kratochwil C, Haberkorn U, Giesel FL. Radionuclide therapy of metastatic prostate cancer. Semin Nucl Med 2019;49(4):313–25.
13. Intenzo CM, Dam HQ, Manzone TA, et al. Imaging of the thyroid in benign and malignant disease. Semin Nucl Med 2012;42(1):49–61.
14. Drude N, Tienken L, Mottaghy FM. Theranostic and nanotheranostic probes in nuclear medicine. Methods 2017;130:14–22.
15. Sisson JC, Yanik GA. Theranostics: evolution of the radiopharmaceutical meta-iodobenzylguanidine in endocrine tumors. Semin Nucl Med 2012;42(3):171–84.
16. Parker C, Nilsson S, Heinrich D, et al. Alpha emitter radium-223 and survival in metastatic prostate cancer. N Engl J Med 2013;369(3):213–23.
17. Krenning EP, Breeman WAP, Kooij PPM, et al. Localisation of endocrine-related tumours with radioiodinated analogue of somatostatin. Lancet 1989;333(8632):242–4.
18. Hofmann M, Maecke H, Börner AR, et al. Biokinetics and imaging with the somatostatin receptor PET radioligand 68Ga-DOTATOC: preliminary data. Eur J Nucl Med 2001;28(12):1751–7.
19. Öberg K, Knigge U, Kwekkeboom D, et al. Neuroendocrine gastro-entero-pancreatic tumors: ESMO clinical practice guidelines for diagnosis, treatment and follow-up. Ann Oncol 2012;23(Suppl. 7). https://doi.org/10.1093/annonc/mds295.
20. Shah MH, Goldner WS, Halfdanarson TR, et al. NCCN guidelines insights: neuroendocrine and adrenal tumors, version 2.2018. J Natl Compr Cancer Netw 2018;16(6):693–702.
21. Hope TA, Bergsland EK, Bozkurt MF, et al. Appropriate use criteria for somatostatin receptor PET imaging in neuroendocrine tumors. J Nucl Med 2018;59(1):66–74.
22. Strosberg J, El-Haddad G, Wolin E, et al. Phase 3 trial of (177)Lu-Dotatate for Midgut neuroendocrine tumors. N Engl J Med 2017;376(2):125–35.
23. Strosberg J, Wolin E, Chasen B, et al. Health-related quality of life in patients with progressive midgut neuroendocrine tumors treated with 177 lu-dotatate in the phase III netter-1 trial. J Clin Oncol 2018;36(25):2578–84.
24. Fendler WP, Rahbar K, Herrmann K, et al. 177Lu-PSMA radioligand therapy for prostate cancer. J Nucl Med 2017;58(8):1196–200.
25. Rauscher I, Maurer T, Fendler WP, et al. 68Ga-PSMA ligand PET/CT in patients with prostate cancer: how we review and report. Cancer Imaging 2016;16(1):1–10.
26. Ballas LK, De Castro Abreu AL, QuINN DI. What medical, urologic, and radiation oncologists want from molecular imaging of prostate cancer. J Nucl Med 2016;57:6S–12S.
27. Murthy R, Nunez R, Szklaruk J, et al. Yttrium-90 microsphere therapy for hepatic malignancy: devices, indications, technical considerations, and potential complications. Radiographics 2005;25:41–56.
28. Sangro B, Iñarrairaegui M, Bilbao JI. Radioembolization for hepatocellular carcinoma. J Hepatol 2012;56(2):464–73.
29. Kratochwil C, Giesel FL, Stefanova M, et al. PSMA-targeted radionuclide therapy of metastatic castration-resistant prostate cancer with 177Lu-Labeled PSMA-617. J Nucl Med 2016;57(8):1170–6.

30. Hofman MS, Violet J, Hicks RJ, et al. 177 Lu]-PSMA-617 radionuclide treatment in patients with metastatic castration-resistant prostate cancer (LuPSMA trial): a single-centre, single-arm, phase 2 study. Lancet Oncol 2018;19(6):825–33.

31. Calopedos RJS, Chalasani V, Asher R, et al. Lutetium-177-labelled anti-prostate-specific membrane antigen antibody and ligands for the treatment of metastatic castrate-resistant prostate cancer: a systematic review and meta-analysis. Prostate Cancer Prostatic Dis 2017;20(3):352–60.

32. Rahbar K, Ahmadzadehfar H, Kratochwil C, et al. German multicenter study investigating 177 Lu-PSMA-617 radioligand therapy in advanced prostate cancer patients. J Nucl Med 2017;58(1):85–90.

33. Rahbar K, Bode A, Weckesser M, et al. Radioligand therapy with 177Lu-PSMA-617 as a novel therapeutic option in patients with metastatic castration resistant prostate cancer. Clin Nucl Med 2016;41(7):522–8.

34. Eiber M, Herrmann K. From NETTER to PETTER: PSMA-targeted radioligand therapy. J Nucl Med 2017. https://doi.org/10.2967/jnumed.116.184994.

35. Hope TA. From compassionate use to phase 3 trial: the impact of Germany's PSMA-617 literature. J Nucl Med 2020;61(Supplement 2):255S–6S.

36. Demirci E, Kabasakal L, Toklu T, et al. 177Lu-DOTATATE therapy in patients with neuroendocrine tumours including high-grade (WHO G3) neuroendocrine tumours. Nucl Med Commun 2018;39(8):789–96.

37. Gains JE, Bomanji JB, Fersht NL, et al. 177Lu-DOTATATE molecular radiotherapy for childhood neuroblastoma. J Nucl Med 2011;52(7):1041–7.

38. Taïeb D, Jha A, Treglia G, et al. Molecular imaging and radionuclide therapy of pheochromocytoma and paraganglioma in the era of genomic characterization of disease subgroups. Endocr Relat Cancer 2019;26(11):R627–52.

39. Kong G, Grozinsky-Glasberg S, Hofman MS, et al. Efficacy of peptide receptor radionuclide therapy for functional metastatic paraganglioma and pheochromocytoma. J Clin Endocrinol Metab 2017;102(9):3278–87.

40. Parisi MT, Eslamy H, Park JR, et al. 131I-metaiodobenzylguanidine theranostics in neuroblastoma: historical perspectives; practical applications. Semin Nucl Med 2016;46(3):184–202.

41. Carrasquillo JA, Pandit-Taskar N, Chen CC. I-131 metaiodobenzylguanidine therapy of pheochromocytoma and paraganglioma. Semin Nucl Med 2016;46(3):203–14.

42. Iten F, Muller B, Schindler C, et al. [90 Yttrium-DOTA]-TOC response is associated with survival benefit in iodine-refractory thyroid cancer. Cancer 2009;115(10):2052–62.

43. Iten F, Muller B, Schindler C, et al. Response to [90Yttrium-DOTA]-TOC treatment is associated with long-term survival benefit in metastasized medullary thyroid cancer: a phase II clinical trial. Clin Cancer Res 2007;13(22):6696–702.

44. Bartolomei M, Bodei L, De Cicco C, et al. Peptide receptor radionuclide therapy with 90Y-DOTATOC in recurrent meningioma. Eur J Nucl Med Mol Imaging 2009;36(9):1407–16.

45. Rizzini EL, Dionisi V, Ghedini P, et al. Clinical aspects of mCRPC management in patients treated with radium-223. Sci Rep 2020;10:6681. https://doi.org/10.1038/s41598-020-63302-2.

46. Heinrich D, Bektic J, Bergman AM, et al. The contemporary use of radium-223 in metastatic castration-resistant prostate cancer. Clin Genitourin Cancer 2018;16(1):e223–31.

47. Bahri H, Laurence L, Edeline J, et al. High prognostic value of 18F-FDG PET for metastatic gastroenteropancreatic neuroendocrine tumors: a long-term evaluation. J Nucl Med 2014;55(11):1786–90.

48. Sansovini M, Severi S, Ianniello A, et al. Long-term follow-up and role of FDG PET in advanced pancreatic neuroendocrine patients treated with 177Lu-DOTATATE. Eur J Nucl Med Mol Imaging 2017;44(3):490–9.

49. Suman S, Parghane RV, Joshi A, et al. Therapeutic efficacy, prognostic variables and clinical outcome of 177 Lu-PSMA-617 PRLT in progressive mCRPC following multiple lines of treatment: prognostic implications of high FDG uptake on dual tracer PET-CT vis-à-vis Gleason score in such cohort. Br J Radiol 2019;92(1104):20190380.

50. Perez PM, Hope TA, Behr SC, et al. Intertumoral heterogeneity of 18F-FDG and 68Ga-PSMA uptake in prostate cancer pulmonary metastases. Clin Nucl Med 2019;44(1):e28–32.

51. Michalski K, Ruf J, Goetz C, et al. Prognostic implications of dual tracer PET/CT: PSMA ligand and [18F]FDG PET/CT in patients undergoing [177Lu]PSMA radioligand therapy. Eur J Nucl Med Mol Imaging 2020. https://doi.org/10.1007/s00259-020-05160-8.

52. Wahl RL, Jacene H, Kasamon Y, et al. From RECIST to PERCIST: evolving considerations for PET response criteria in solid tumors. J Nucl Med 2009;50(Suppl_1):122S–50S.

53. Schöder H, Moskowitz C. Metabolic tumor volume in lymphoma: hype or hope? J Clin Oncol 2016;34(30):3591–4.

54. Winther-Larsen A, Fledelius J, Sorensen BS, et al. Metabolic tumor burden as marker of outcome in advanced EGFR wild-type NSCLC patients treated with erlotinib. Lung Cancer 2016;94:81–7.

55. Walenkamp AME, Lapa C, Herrmann K, et al. CXCR4 ligands: the next big hit? J Nucl Med 2017;58:77S–82S.

56. Kircher M, Herhaus P, Schottelius M, et al. CXCR4-directed theranostics in oncology and inflammation. Ann Nucl Med 2018;32(8):503–11.

57. Watabe T, Liu Y, Kaneda-Nakashima K, et al. Theranostics targeting fibroblast activation protein in the tumor stroma: 64Cu- and 225Ac-Labeled FAPI-04 in pancreatic cancer xenograft mouse models. J Nucl Med 2020;61(4):563–9.

58. Sharma P, Singh SS, Gayana S. Fibroblast activation protein inhibitor PET/CT. Clin Nucl Med 2020. https://doi.org/10.1097/RLU.0000000000003489.

59. Congdon EE, Sigurdsson EM. Tau-targeting therapies for Alzheimer disease. Nat Rev Neurol 2018; 14(7):399–415.

60. van Dyck CH. Anti-Amyloid-β monoclonal antibodies for Alzheimer's disease: pitfalls and promise. Biol Psychiatry 2018;83(4):311–9.

61. Valent P, Groner B, Schumacher U, et al. Paul Ehrlich (1854-1915) and his contributions to the foundation and birth of translational medicine. J Innate Immun 2016;8(2):111–20.

62. Barbosa FG, Queiroz MA, Ferraro DA, et al. Prostate-specific membrane antigen pet: therapy response assessment in metastatic prostate cancer. Radiographics 2020;40(5):1412–30.

63. Brans B, Bodei L, Giammarile F, et al. Clinical radionuclide therapy dosimetry: the quest for the "Holy Gray". Eur J Nucl Med Mol Imaging 2007;34(5): 772–86.

64. Bodei L, Cremonesi M, Ferrari M, et al. Long-term evaluation of renal toxicity after peptide receptor radionuclide therapy with 90Y-DOTATOC and 177Lu-DOTATATE: the role of associated risk factors. Eur J Nucl Med Mol Imaging 2008;35(10):1847–56.

65. Bander NH, Milowsky MI, Nanus DM, et al. Phase I trial of [177] Lutetium-Labeled J591, a monoclonal antibody to prostate-specific membrane antigen, in patients with androgen-independent prostate cancer. J Clin Oncol 2005. https://doi.org/10.1200/JCO.2005.05.160.

66. Fendler WP, Reinhardt S, Ilhan H, et al. Preliminary experience with dosimetry, response and patient reported outcome after (177)Lu-PSMA-617 therapy for metastatic castration-resistant prostate cancer. Oncotarget 2017;8(2):3581–90.

67. Eberlein U, Cremonesi M, Lassmann M. Individualized dosimetry for theranostics: necessary, nice to have, or counterproductive? J Nucl Med 2017; 58(Supplement 2):97S–103S.

68. Turner JH. An introduction to the clinical practice of theranostics in oncology. Br J Radiol 2018;91(1091): 1–9.

69. Turner JH. Recent advances in theranostics and challenges for the future. Br J Radiol 2018;91(1091): 20170893. https://doi.org/10.1259/bjr.20170893.

70. Kumar C, Shetake N, Desai S, et al. Relevance of radiobiological concepts in radionuclide therapy of cancer. Int J Radiat Biol 2016;92(4):173–86.

71. Violet J, Jackson P, Ferdinandus J, et al. Dosimetry of 177 Lu-PSMA-617 in metastatic castration-resistant prostate cancer: correlations between pretherapeutic imaging and whole-body tumor dosimetry with treatment outcomes. J Nucl Med 2019; 60(4):517–23.

72. Sgouros G, Kolbert KS, Sheikh A, et al. Patient-specific dosimetry for 131I thyroid cancer therapy using 124I PET and 3-Dimensional-Internal Dosimetry (3D-ID) software. J Nucl Med 2004;45(8):1366–72.

73. Jentzen W, Weise R, Kupferschläger J, et al. Iodine-124 PET dosimetry in differentiated thyroid cancer: recovery coefficient in 2D and 3D modes for PET(/CT) systems. Eur J Nucl Med Mol Imaging 2008; 35(3):611–23.

74. Sapienza MT, Willegaignon J. Radionuclide therapy: current status and prospects for internal dosimetry in individualized therapeutic planning. Clinics (Sao Paulo) 2019;74. https://doi.org/10.6061/clinics/2019/e835.

An Impressive Approach in Nuclear Medicine
Theranostics

Nasim Vahidfar, PhD[a], Elisabeth Eppard, PhD[b,c], Saeed Farzanehfar, MD[a],
Anna Yordanova, MD[d], Maryam Fallahpoor, MSc[a],
Hojjat Ahmadzadehfar, MD, MSc[e,*]

KEYWORDS

• Prostate cancer • PSMA • Theranostics • Radionuclide therapy • Neuroendocrine tumor

KEY POINTS

- The application of theranostics is considered a success story in nuclear medicine.
- The initial step in therapeutic treatment using a theranostic agent is the evaluation of radioligand affinity to the target by diagnostic imaging.
- By using PRRT for the treatment of neuroendocrine tumors a significantly increased median survival of over 40 months could be reached.
- PSMA based imaging and therapy has revolutionary changed the prognosis of prostate cancer patients.
- Fibroblast activation protein is a new promising target for doing imaging and therapy of different types of aggressive tumors.

INTRODUCTION

One of the most common cancers among men worldwide (**Fig. 1**) is prostate cancer (PCa).[1] Prostate-specific membrane antigen (PSMA) is a valuable target for the diagnosis of PCa and for therapeutic purposes, because PSMA is overexpressed in many PCas.[1] In the past decade, various studies[2,3] have demonstrated the advantage of theranostics in comparison to traditional methods in metastatic, multiple pretreated PCa. Similarly, peptide receptor radionuclide therapy (PRRT), which targets well-differentiated neuroendocrine tumors (NETs) with high expression of somatostatin receptors (SSTR), is one of the most effective therapeutic methods for treating advanced NET to date.[4]

The initial step in therapeutic treatment using a theranostic agent is the evaluation of radioligand affinity to the target by diagnostic imaging. The superiority of this method over conventional treatment is the lower amount of radioactivity to which patients may subsequently be exposed during the therapy. Basically, depending on radiopharmaceutical uptake in the diagnostic stages, the introduction of a related therapeutic protocol can be logically determined.

This review provides an overview of theranostics by presenting practical examples of their routine applications in daily nuclear medicine practice. The principle behind the use of theranostics, that is combining imaging and therapy, is "to see what we treat and treat what we see." Using a combination of imaging and therapy can improve the specificity and potency of therapeutic protocols and result in improved, personalized patient management/care. This article outlines the most

[a] Department of Nuclear Medicine, Vali-Asr Hospital, Tehran University of Medical Sciences, Tehran, Iran; [b] Positronpharma SA, Santiago, Chile; [c] Department of Nuclear Medicine, University Hospital Magdeburg, Germany; [d] Department of Radiology, Marienhospital Bonn, Bonn; [e] Department of Nuclear Medicine, Klinikum Westfalen, Dortmund, Germany
* Corresponding author.
E-mail address: Hojjat.ahmadzadehfar@ruhr-uni-bochum.de

PET Clin 16 (2021) 327–340
https://doi.org/10.1016/j.cpet.2021.03.011
1556-8598/21/

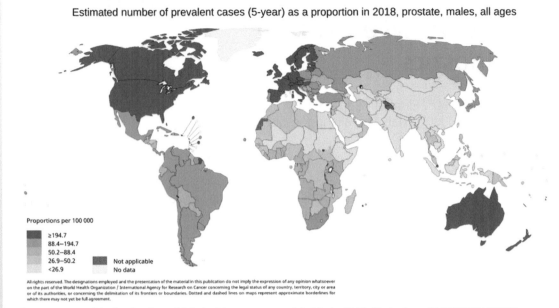

Estimated number of prevalent cases (5-year) as a proportion in 2018, prostate, males, all ages

Proportions per 100 000

≥194.7
88.4–194.7
50.2–88.4
26.9–50.2
<26.9
Not applicable
No data

Fig. 1. Geographic distribution of PCa incidence rate worldwide in 2018. (*Data from* GLOBOCAN 2018.)

promising theranostic agent applications for the management of different medical conditions.

TREATMENT OF HYPERPARATHYROIDISM AND THYROID CANCER IN NUCLEAR MEDICINE

The most striking concern with regard to endocrine tumors is thyroid cancer.[5] The theranostic radioiodine, Iodine-131 (^{131}I), has been widely used as a gold standard for the management of differentiated types of thyroid cancers in recent years.[5] Sodium iodide symporters (NIS), key plasma glycoproteins with 13 transmembrane domains, are responsible for the intracellular transfer of iodide ions simultaneously with 2 sodium ions into follicular thyroid cells.[6] Although Iodine-131 has been used as a therapeutic agent for hyperparathyroidism since the 1940s,[7] its mechanism of uptake was not clear until 1960, when Carrasco and colleagues defined the details.[8] Given its proven efficacy in these applications, the prospective application of Iodine-131 postoperation to evaluate the possibility of recurrence is inevitable.[9,10] The physical characteristics of Iodine-131, including its 8-day half-life, average range in tissue of 0.4 mm, beta emission with a maximum energy of 0.61 MeV and principle gamma radiation of 364 keV, make it appropriate for therapy and follow-up diagnosis. In the choice between capsule and liquid administrations, capsule application is preferred due to the lower possibility of contamination.[7] However, liquid formulation or even intravenous application is

used for patients with severe swelling complications.[7] Due to the aforementioned advantages, radioiodine therapy (RIT) using Iodine-131 has been applied for the imaging and treatment of differentiated thyroid cancers (DTC) for more than 70 years, long before the concept of theranostics, as it is known today, was defined.[6] However, soon after the first experiences with RIT, Seidlin and colleagues[11] reported the first cases of acute myeloid leukemia after repeated treatment with radioiodine. These and other cases of radiation-induced cancer demonstrate the importance of optimization of the treatment dose to avoid unnecessary radiation. Thus, one of the advantages of theranostics is pretreatment and posttreatment imaging, which enables proper treatment planning and dosimetry to adjust the treatment dose to the tumor.[12]

Currently, RIT is still a gold standard for the diagnosis and therapy of DTC.[13] The application of molecular imaging in nuclear medicine is an impressive, key technology, making semiquantitative and quantitative follow-up of the therapy in molecular stages feasible. These evaluations are important in the management of treatment approaches, particularly for residual thyroid cancers, as well as their recurrence and metastases.[5]

TREATMENT OF NEUROENDOCRINE TUMOR IN NUCLEAR MEDICINE

Somatostatin receptors, which belong to G protein transmembrane receptors, are normally overexpressed in NETs.[14] It has been demonstrated that among the 5 known subtypes of somatostatin receptors (SSTR1, SSTR2, SSTR3, SSTR4, and SSTR5), somatostatin receptor subtype-2 (SSTR2) is the most important,[15,16] because it is overexpressed in most gastropancreatic NETs.[17,18] PRRT was applied as early as 1994, when ^{111}In-octreotide was first used as a therapeutic agent for gastrointestinal NETs.[19] As a consequence of the satisfactory results gained from therapeutic trials, widespread series of radiolabeled octreotide derivatives found their way into clinics. Nowadays, imaging with ^{68}Ga-labeled 1,4,7,10-tetraazacyclododecane-N,N',N'',N'''-tetraacetic acid-d-Phe(1)-Tyr(3)-octreotide/-octreotate ([68 Ga]Ga-DOTA-TOC/-TATE) before therapy is routinely used to evaluate the rate of receptors' expression.[20,21] The mechanism of internalization includes endocytosis of the somatostatin receptor and the radiolabeled receptor agonist analogue, which releases the radiation near the cell nucleus and induces DNA strand breaks. Within 24 hours, the cell surface receptor has been replaced via endosome recycling.[22] Due to differences in the chemical structure of the various derivatives, affinity to the SSTR subtypes differs to some extent. For example, DOTA-TATE shows a high affinity to SSTR2 and SSTR5, and DOTATOC predominantly to SSTR2.[4]

NET-specific radiotracers frequently used in clinics for therapy are Yttrium-90 (^{90}Y) or Lutetium-177 (^{177}Lu) labeled octreotide or octreotate analogues. These 2 radionuclides have appropriate physical properties for therapy.

Table 1 presents the main physical properties of the common radionuclides used for theranostic purposes. Most of them emit beta particles that induce DNA damage and, because of the small tissue penetration and relatively short half-life of these radionuclides, the exposure to nontarget tissue is very limited.[4] Lutetium-177 has an advantage over Ytrriuim-90 because of the lower energy and smaller tissue penetration of its beta emissions, as well as its accompanying gamma radiation, which is suitable for imaging and dosimetry.[4] [177Lu]Lu-DOTA-TATE was approved by the US Food and Drug Administration for adult patients with somatostatin receptor–positive gastroenteropancreatic NETs after the NETTER-1 prospective phase III trial showed the advantages of PRRT over octreotide (Sandostatin LAR) in patients with midgut NET, and the positive experience of a single site study in the Netherlands with 1214 GEP-NET patients treated with PRRT.[21,23,24] A clinical trial of pancreatic NETs (pNETs) and non-pNETs with progressive disease demonstrated partial remission in 48% of the patients with non-pNETs and 52% with pNETs after 3 cycles of [177Lu]Lu-DOTA-TATE.[20] Another study reported a clinical response with symptom improvement in 93% of treated patients.[25] Furthermore, with PRRT, a significantly increased median survival of more than 40 months could be reached.[26,27] As long as renal protection agents are coinjected, the adverse effects of PRRT are negligible and transient. However, in rare cases, it may induce delayed, noticeable side effects, including renal failure, myelodysplastic syndrome and leukemia.[26]

Table 1
Main physical characteristics of radionuclides

Radionuclide	Physical Half-Life	Decay Mode	Maximal Range in Soft Tissue	Availability
Iodine-131	8.0 d	β⁻	2.3 mm	Reactor
Samarium-153	46 h	β⁻	4 mm	Reactor
Strontium-89	50.6 d	β⁻	8 mm	Reactor
Holmium-166	27 h	β⁻	9 mm	Reactor/Generator
Lutetium-177	6.7 d	β⁻	2 mm	Reactor
Rhenium-186	89 h	β⁻	5 mm	Reactor/Cyclotron
Rhenium-188	17 h	β⁻	10 mm	Generator
Radium-223	11.4 d	α	100 μm	Generator
Actinium-225	10.0 d	α	<100 μm	Generator/Reactor
Yttrium-90	64.2 h	β⁻	2.5 mm	Generator
Bismuth-213	0.75 h	α/β⁻	<100 μm	Generator/Reactor
Lead-212	10.64 h	α	<100 μm	Generator/Reactor

TREATMENT OF PROSTATE CANCER IN NUCLEAR MEDICINE

PSMA is a type II glycoprotein, overexpressed in prostatic adenocarcinoma,[28] which makes it a suitable target for theranostics of PCa. In the past decade, optimistic results with different PSMA derivatives have supported further clinical evaluation.[29–31] To evaluate the risk-benefit of therapeutic applications for potential patients, pretreatment imaging with PSMA derivatives should be performed.[32] Initial attempts to use PSMA imaging in PET go back to 2002[3]; however, the clinical imaging evolution associated with these trials is attributable to [^{68}Ga]Ga-PSMA-11 (also called HBED-CC, HBED, PSMA-HBED, or Prostamedix) introduced in 2012.[3] ^{68}Ga-PSMA-derivatives demonstrated desirable pharmacokinetic parameters, including stability, fast blood clearance, low liver uptake and high uptake in PSMA-expressing tissues.[33] However, Seifert and colleagues[34] reported that ^{18}F-PSMA-1007 is a superior diagnostic agent, particularly in pelvic lesions. This case report compared ^{68}Ga-PSMA-11 and ^{18}F-PSMA-1007 images; encouragingly, increased uptake with ^{18}F-PSMA-1007 was demonstrated.[34] These PSMA-targeting PET tracers can be combined PSMA-targeting therapeutic radiopharmaceuticals with beta or alpha emitters as theranostic pairs.

[^{177}Lu]Lu-PSMA-617 is a well-tolerated theranostic agent with negligible side effects in clinical assessments. Insignificant and temporary changes in hematological and renal functions, as well as xerostomia and other probable toxicities have been reported.[27,35–37]

We discussed other radiopharmaceuticals for detection and treatment of PCa in our previous work.[1] Among the mentioned instances, ^{177}Lu-PSMA-617 was reported as a superior agent for therapeutic purpose of treating PCa.[1] Favorable response to therapy was reported in clinical trials, including significant decline in prostate-specific antigen (PSA) level and improved long-term survival after repeated cycles with ^{177}Lu-PSMA-617.[3,38]

Imaging simultaneity with therapy is beneficial; however, the physical characteristics of the specific radionuclides are strongly determinative. Accordingly, ^{177}Lu-PSMA derivatives are superior to ^{131}I-PSMA derivatives, beccause Iodine-131 is not appropriate for therapy due to its higher range of gamma radiation compared with lutetium-177.[3] For this reason, ^{177}Lu-PSMA derivatives can be used as an efficient and effectual tracer in patients with progressive metastatic PCa, because the therapeutic responses were significantly conclusive.[39] In addition to beta-emitting radionuclides, alpha emitters are also suitable for therapeutic applications. Targeted alpha therapy (TAT) is a significant development in nuclear medicine. Therefore Bismuth-213 (^{213}Bi), Lead-212 (^{212}Pb) and Actinium-225 (^{225}Ac) were considered radionuclides for labeling in therapeutic procedures. Preliminary clinical trials have been done with [^{225}Ac]Ac-PSMA-617 in patients with no/low outcome of [^{177}Lu]Lu-PSMA-617 therapy.[40] Actinium-225 is an alpha emitter (5.8 Mev) with a physical half-life of 238 hours, and seems to be an appropriate radionuclide for therapy (**Table 1**). Furthermore, PSMA-TAT showed an efficient decline in PSA level and positive tumor response in clinical trials.[41,42]

Given the respectable clinical results to date, increasing applications of theranostic agents in PCa are expectable. In this case, the diagnosis of specific target regions using ^{68}Ga-/^{18}F-PSMA derivatives should be performed before therapy. The following figures depict the pretreatment, therapy and follow-up of a patient suffering from PCa undergoing ^{177}Lu-PSMA therapy based on ^{68}Ga-PSMA-PET/computed tomography (CT). **Fig. 2** represents pretreatment [^{68}Ga]Ga-PSMA-11 whole-body PET/CT scans (Department of Nuclear Medicine, Vali-Asr Hospital, Tehran University of Medical Sciences, Tehran, Iran). **Fig. 3** shows representative post-therapy single-photon emission CT (SPECT)/CT images after the first, third and last cycle of the ^{177}Lu-dose. After 6 cycles of therapy with [^{177}Lu] Lu-PSMA-617, excellent response to treatment with significant reduction in size and avidity of multiple lesions could be observed. These impressive results were verified by a follow-up diagnostic PET/CT with [^{68}Ga] Ga-PSMA-11, shown in **Fig. 4** that revealed a significant decrease of uptake compared with the baseline diagnostic study.

TREATMENT OF BONE METASTASES IN NUCLEAR MEDICINE

Considering the increased rate of bone metastases in almost all cancers, particularly prostate, breast, lung, kidney, and thyroid cancers, diagnosis and pain palliation of spreading bone metastases would be a desirable approach in nuclear medicine.[43] Skeletal metastases often cause severe pain, pathologic fractures, nerve compression syndromes, and hypercalcemia, significantly reducing patients' quality of life.[44–46] Furthermore, incurable skeletal metastases considerably contribute to increased morbidity as well as mortality.[47–49]

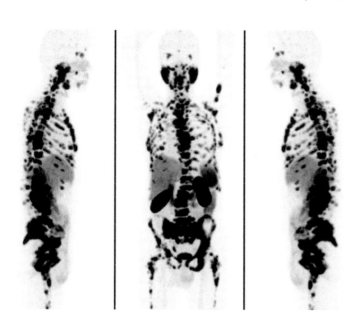

Fig. 2. Pretreatment [^{68}Ga] Ga-PSMA-11 whole-body PET/CT scans in a 78-year-old patient. Active and viable primary prostate tumors, multiple retroperitoneal and pelvic lymph node metastases, and widespread bone metastases are visible. (*Courtesy of* Department of Nuclear Medicine, Vali-Asr Hospital, Tehran University of Medical Sciences, Tehran, Iran.)

Two groups of bone-seeking radiopharmaceuticals can be distinguished, calcimimetic and phosphonate-based radiopharmaceuticals. Calcimimetic agents (eg, Phosphorus-32; Strontium-89, Radium-223) are the most common bone-seeking radiopharmaceuticals used for palliative treatment. Their accumulation is based on the same metabolic mechanism as calcium and may therefore be variable and unpredictable[50] with wide distribution through bone.[43]

To overcome this disadvantage, great efforts have been made to enhance target accumulation through the introduction and further development of phosphonate-based radiopharmaceuticals. Non-hydrolysable phosphonates are analogues of naturally occurring pyrophosphates, which have a high affinity for bone mineral and regulate bone mineralization.[50] A well-known group of phosphonates, used for treatment of bone disease for many years, are bisphosphonates (also known as diphosphonates). Several studies have proven the ability of bisphosphonates to inhibit osteoclast-mediated bone resorption in vitro and in vivo.[51–56] Furthermore, bisphosphonates suppress bone resorption, induced by multiple other agents (eg, vitamin D), and are effective in preventing bone destruction.[57] Due to their high bone adsorption and their chelating properties, early research focused on labeling bisphosphonates directly with radionuclides for therapeutic purposes.

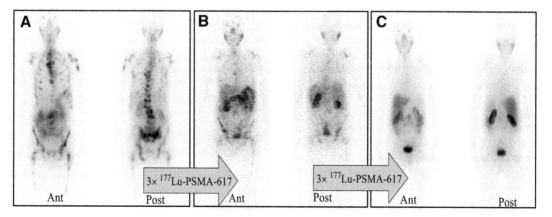

Fig. 3. The same patient underwent therapy with 6 cycles of [^{177}Lu] Lu-PSMA-617. Post-therapy images after (*A*) the first cycle of [^{177}Lu] Lu-PSMA-617, (*B*) the third cycle, and (*C*) the sixth/last, show an excellent response to treatment with significant reduction in size and avidity in multiple lesions. (*Courtesy of* Department of Nuclear Medicine, Vali-Asr Hospital, Tehran University of Medical Sciences, Tehran, Iran.)

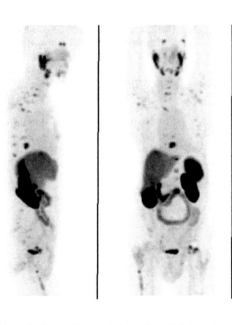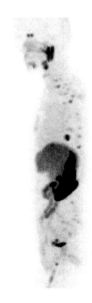

Fig. 4. Follow-up [^{68}Ga] Ga-PSMA-11 whole-body PET/CT scan after 6 cycles of [^{177}Lu] Lu-PSMA-617 showed significant decrease in uptake compared with the baseline diagnostic study. (*Courtesy of* Department of Nuclear Medicine, Vali-Asr Hospital, Tehran University of Medical Sciences, Tehran, Iran.)

Nevertheless, the uptake of radiolabeled phosphates is dependent on the osseous involvement expanses.[58]

A list of radionuclides clinically tested for the treatment of bone pain and their main physical characteristics are presented in **Table 1**.

Samarium-153 (^{153}Sm) is a radionuclide with a convenient half-life (1.9 d) for imaging and therapy with a gamma energy of 103 keV and beta emissions of (0.81 MeV (20%), 0.71 MeV (30%) and 0.64 MeV (50%)). Compared with other therapeutic radionuclides such as Phosphourus-32 (^{32}P) with a mean beta range of 0.695 MeV and a 14.3 d half-life, probably leading to higher bone marrow suppression, Samarium-153 seems to be a more appropriate radionuclide for bone pain palliation.[43,59] Based on that assessment, it can be concluded that Samarium-153 can be applied for both diagnosis and therapeutic indications.[60] Clinical trials utilizing ethylene diamine tetramethylene phosphonate (EDTMP) chelating Samarium-153 proved its suitability as a theranostic agent for the diagnosis and treatment of bone metastases.[59] Similarly, Lutetium-177, also emitting beta particles (0.176 MeV [12.2%], 0.385 MeV [9.1%], 0.498 MeV [78.6%]) as well as gamma rays (208 keV [11%] and 113 keV [(6.4%]) with a half-life of 6.73 d, is appropriate for simultaneous imaging and therapy. Several studies investigated ^{177}Lu-labeled bisphosphonates, for example, [^{177}Lu]Lu-EDTMP,[61–63] [^{177}Lu]Lu-BPAMD[44,64,65] or [^{177}Lu]Lu-DOTMP.[66–69] Although [^{177}Lu]Lu-EDTMP proved to have high potential for pain palliation in phase I and II studies,[59,70–73] as well as favorable radiation dose characteristics compared with other bone targeting drugs,[74–76] its ^{68}Ga-

labeled-analogue, with lower accumulation in bone, is not suitable as a diagnostic pair.[75] In contrast, the DOTA-conjugated bisphosphonate BPAMD showed excellent results when labeled with Lutetium-177 as well as with Gallium-68, enabling individualized patient treatment.[2,33,43,67]

Holmium-166 emits beta particles (1.774 MeV [48.8%] and 1.854 MeV [49.9%]) as well as gamma rays (80.57 keV [6.7%] and 1379.40 keV [0.9%]) and has a half-life of 26.8 h.[77] ^{166}Ho-labeled bone-seeking agents, including 1,4,7,10-tetraazacyclododecane-1,4,7,10-tetramethylene-phosphonate (^{166}Ho-DOTMP),[78,79] EDTMP[60,78] and N,N-dimethylenephosphonate-1-hydroxy-4-aminopropylidene-diphosphonate (APDDMP),[80,81] have been reported previously. Clinical phase I/II studies with ^{166}Ho-DOTMP resulted in remarkable and high bone uptake, fast clearance with low and negligible adverse toxicities and soft tissue uptake.[82,83] In a comparative study of Holmium-166, Lutetium-177 and Samarium-153 conjugated with EDTMP, the preclinical scintigraphic images of all 3 agents revealed the lowest bone uptake for the ^{166}Ho-labeled compound, indicating that it is a relatively inferior bone-seeking tracer.[60]

THERANOSTICS APPLICATIONS IN NEUROBLASTOMA

Norepinephrine transporter (NET) is a remarkable target for the imaging and treatment of a variety of physiologic problems, particularly in neuroblastoma, paraganglioma and pheochromocytoma.[84]

^{123}I/^{131}I-labeled metaiodobenzylguanidine ([^{123}I/^{131}I] MIBG) can be transferred through norepinephrine channels into the cytoplasm and mitochondria of tumors for diagnostic or therapeutic purposes.[85,86] Specific accumulation with significant tracer uptake in tumors with overexpression of NETs in soft tissue, bone or red marrow has been proven.[87] [^{123}I]MIBG has shown high sensitivities in the range 88% to 92% and specificities in the range 83% to 92% for the diagnosis of neuroblastoma.[88] Thus, patients with MIBG-avid tumors might be good candidates for the therapeutic application of [^{131}I] MIBG.

Initial palliative therapy using [^{131}I]MIBG was attempted along with development of this tracer in 1980.[89] Clinical trials in phase I/II, in chemo refractory patients demonstrated a 10% to 60% response rate.[90–92] This receptor targeting agent could be an effective therapeutic tool for those with high risk and remarkable avidity to [^{123}I] MIBG.[93] Recently, by developing the PRRT concept and the amendable application of related tracers, it seems that the replacement of radiolabeled guanidine derivatives would be more desirable, because the sensitivity of radiolabeled octreotide (^{68}Ga-DOTA-peptides) is higher compared with [^{123}I]MIBG[94] and the necessity of thyroid blockade is eliminated. According to these safety and feasibility considerations, it can be concluded that PRRT would be a potential field for the detection and treatment of NETs.[94]

TREATMENT OF MELANOMA IN NUCLEAR MEDICINE

In vitro investigations to find theranostic agents for melanoma led to [^{64}Cu]Cu-B16F10 and [^{64}Cu]Cu-A375 M.[95] These tracers have been proven to be promising agents, because they specifically target the copper transport protein CTR1, which is overexpressed in both melanotic and amelanotic melanoma abnormalities.[95] Recently, another preclinical study demonstrated promising results for the detection and therapy of metastatic melanomas. [^{131}I]I-Ixolaris, which targets tissue factor (TF), is stable for at least 24 hours in plasma and saline and maintains its inhibitory characteristic activity in blood coagulation.[96] TF has a very remarkable role in tumor growth, metastases, and invasions, as it promotes tumor cell proliferation through different mechanisms. Preclinical scintigraphy studies showed specific accumulation of [^{131}I]I-Ixolaris in pulmonary topography and reduction of metastatic nodules, providing a proof for the therapeutic efficacy of this tracer.[97]

Finally, [^{123}I]I-/[^{131}I]I-BA52 and [^{18}F]F-/[^{131}I]I-ICF15002 are expected to find widespread use in the future for the targeting of melanin.[12] A clinical study has been done with [^{123}I] I-BA52 and [^{18}F]F-ICF15002, aiming to evaluate the specificity of the tracers in melanin. The efficacy of [^{123}I] I-BA52 in detection and its therapeutic ^{131}I-counterpart has been proven in a pilot study.[12] The most important concern regarding these tracers is dosimetry, because a 30% decrease of retinal thickness was reported after 2 cycles of therapeutic doses of [^{131}I]I-ICF15002.[12]

THERANOSTICS APPLICATIONS IN MULTIPLE MYELOMA

Chemokine receptor 4 (CXCR4) can provide a considerable target for the diagnosis and treatment of multiple myeloma (MM). CXCR4 is overexpressed in tumor cells and has a significant role in tumor growth, progression and invasion. ^{68}Ga-Pentixafor is a new CXCR4 ligand that has been radiolabeled with ^{68}Ga.[98] Clinical trials showed substantial detection capability in atherosclerotic lesions with high reproducibility over time.[98]

A NEW HORIZON FOR TUMOR TARGETING AND THERAPY: FIBROBLAST ACTIVATION PROTEIN INHIBITOR

Fibroblast activation protein (FAP), a serine protease, is expressed in many cells of stroma with malignant origin (**Table 2**). It is proven that more than 90% of epithelial tumors, especially in colon, breast, and pancreatic cancer, are associated with FAP overexpression.[99] This tumoral stroma or microenvironment represents a potential, specific target for the development of diagnostic and therapeutic agents in nuclear medicine. Efforts to radiolabel FAP-specific enzyme inhibitors (FAPIs) coupled with 1,4,7,10-tetraazacyclododecane-1,4,7,10-tetraacetic acid (DOTA) or other chelators with diagnostic (gallium-68) radionuclides or theranostics (Lutetium-177/Yttrium-90) have been successfully accomplished.[100] Since specific targeted therapy based on specific targeted diagnostic agents (theranostics) have made a significant contribution in nuclear medicine,[1] designing FAPIs based on those diagnostic/therapeutic pairs has received a lot of attention.[101] A vast series of these promising low molecular weight inhibitors have been investigated. Among almost 55 derivatives of FAPIs studied to date, some have outstanding preclinical and clinical specificities.[100] To have a significant pronounced effect, including the time-dependent deiodination of the final tracer by enzymatic systems, initially developed radiolabeled FAPI ([^{125}I]-FAPI-01), led to the introduction of other promising derivatives of FAPIs.[100,102] Loktev and colleagues[100] reported FAPI-02, a non-halogen compound with enhanced uptake in FAP

Table 2
Chemical structures and modifications leading to the most important FAPIs[101,102]

FAPI Derivatives	R	R'	R"	Preclinical/ Clinical Studies	Base Chemical Structure
FAPI-01	H	H	H	[125]I[100,102]	
FAPI-02	DOTA-piperazine-(O)3	H	H	[68]Ga, [177]Lu[102]	
FAPI-03	DOTA-piperazine-(O)4	H	H	-	
FAPI-04: FAPI-20	DOTA-NH-propyl-O	H	F	[68]Ga, ^{177}Lu, [90]Y[102]	
	DOTA-piperazine-(O)1-4	DOTA-piperazine-(O)3	H		
	DOTA-piperazine-(O)3				
FAPI-21: FAPI-55	H DOTA-N-bicyclic-N-propyl-O	F	F	[68]Ga, ^{177}Lu, [90]Y[101–103]	
	DOTA-piperazine-(O)3				

overexpressing cells. It was demonstrated that [^{68}Ga]Ga-FAPI-02 accumulates specifically in protein expressing tissues in metastasized breast, lung and pancreatic cancer.[100] According to the mentioned attempts,[100,102,103] FAPI-02 was introduced as an ideal candidate appropriate for therapeutic purposes. Eligible pharmacokinetic aspects, including high target affinity, rapid tumor internalization, and fast body clearance were driving factors toward the development of therapeutic analogues with Lutetium-177 or Yttrium-90.[100] Chemical structure modifications led to FAPI-04, which proved to have more stable tumor accumulation compared with FAPI-02.[103] Although FAPI-02 showed a washout of 75% within 3 hours, FAPI-04 provided higher tumor retention and a slower washout of about 50%.[103]

In addition, radiolabeled FAPI-04 was demonstrated to have a significantly increased binding ratio compared with previous derivatives.[102] Cell culture studies in human FAP-expressing HT-1080 cells have been conducted to investigate the accumulation ratios of several FAPI derivatives. The internalization ratios of FAPI-21, -35, -46, and -55 was comparable to the results of FAPI-04 or even better.[103] Based on clinical imaging studies, the previously mentioned derivatives were selected for extended trials as theranostic agents. For this purpose, biodistribution studies of ^{177}Lu-radiolabeled tracers have been performed over a period of 1 week.[103] Among these tracers, FAPI-21 and -46 showed the highest accumulations; FAPI-21, followed by FAPI-35 and -46, showed the longest retention in tumors. With

Table 3
Summary of current theranostics

Indication	Target	Theranostics/Radiopharmaceuticals
Differentiated thyroid cancer	Na^+/I^- symporter	^{131}I
Prostate cancer	PSMA	$[^{68}Ga]Ga$-PSMA-11 $[^{177}Lu]Lu$-PSMA-617 ^{225}Ac-PSMA $[^{18}F]$PSMA-1007
Neuroendocrine tumor	SSTR	$[^{68}Ga]Ga$-DOTA-TATE $[^{68}Ga]Ga$-DOTA-TOC $[^{177}Lu]Lu$-DOTA-TATE
Melanoma	CXCR4 CTR1	$[^{68}Ga]Ga$-Pentixafor $[^{177}Lu]Lu$-Pentixafor $[^{64}Cu]Cu$-B16F10 $[^{64}Cu]Cu$-A375 M $[^{131}I]$-Ixolaris $[^{123}I/^{131}I]$-BA52 $[^{18}F/^{131}I]$-ICF15002
Tumors	FAP	$[^{68}Ga]Ga$-FAPI $[^{177}Lu]Lu$-FAPI
Neuroblastoma, Paraganglioma, Pheochromocytoma	NET	$[^{131}I]$-MIBG
Bone metastases	Bone compartments	$[^{153}Sm]Sm$-EDTMP $[^{166}Ho]Ho$-HEDP $[^{166}Ho]Ho$-EDTMP $[^{177}Lu]Lu$-EDTMP $[^{166}Ho]Ho$-DOTMP $[^{166}Ho]Ho$-APDDMP

Abbreviations: CD20, B-lymphocyte antigen; CTR1, Human copper transporter 1; CXCR4, chemokine receptor 4; FAP, fibroblast activation protein; NET, norepinephrine transporter; PSMA, prostate-specific membrane antigen; SSTR, somatostatin receptor.

the exception of FAPI-46, all of the tracers presented higher liver uptake compared with FAPI-04. Renal activity uptake studies demonstrated comparable results for FAPI-04, -21, and -35. Activity accumulation in kidneys was considerably decreased for FAPI-46 and -55 at any point of time in contrast to FAPI-21 and -35, which showed comparable results to FAPI-04.[103]

Given the epidemiologic proof of the remarkable accumulation of FAPIs in tumors (specifically pancreatic, head, neck, colon, lung, and breast cancer), implementation of noninvasive diagnosis and therapy in nuclear medicine based on radiolabeled FAPIs would be predictable. Although application of FAPIs is beneficial in various nonmalignant diseases like myocardial infarction, sarcoidosis, chronic or acute inflammation, lung, liver and kidney fibrosis, and rheumatoid arthritis, as well as atherosclerosis, which is detectable as tissue remodeling patterns.[102]

The pharmacologic specifications of the new radiolabeled FAPI tracers compared with the standard $[^{18}F]$ FDG, seem to be equal or even superior in treating tumor accumulation. Faster tracer uptake and clearance, negligible uptake in the liver, oral pharyngeal mucosa and brain, as well as independency from blood sugar are the major benefits of radiolabeled FAPIs cited in various clinical investigations.[100,104] Future studies will focus on the quantification of FAPI accumulation based on FAP overexpression in tumors[104,105] **(Table 3)**.

SUMMARY

The application of theranostics is considered a success story in nuclear medicine. The estimation and planning of a therapy is indebted to certainty of significant avidity to the involved target organs. To achieve such a goal, it is essential to have pretreatment diagnostic methods to evaluate radiolabeled tracer intensity and accumulation in target organs and, building on this, thoroughly planned therapeutic procedures.

This review provided a proof of concept for the advantages of theranostics in regular nuclear medicine applications. Among the many promising theranostics approaches, a revolutionary new method, PRRT, has been developed. It includes a broad spectrum of radiopharmaceuticals with a chemical structure based on peptides. Octreotide-based radiopharmaceuticals, such as DOTA-TATE, DOTA-TOC or DOTA-NOC, as well as PSMA derivatives, including PSMA-11, PSMA-617, PSMA-I&T, and PSMA-1007, for diagnosis and therapy of neuroendocrine tumors and prostate cancer, respectively, are very attractive tracers. Studies are continuously ongoing to develop and enhance the most appropriate derivatives. Future studies will focus on randomized trials to identify more specific and appropriate radiotracers for diagnostic and therapeutic purposes.

DISCLOSURE

The authors have nothing to disclose.

REFERENCES

1. Vahidfar N, Fallahpoor M, Farzanehfar S, et al. Historical review of pharmacological development and dosimetry of PSMA-based theranostics for prostate cancer. J Radioanal Nucl Chem 2019;322(2): 237–48.
2. Ahmadzadehfar H, Rahbar K, Essler M, et al. PSMA-based theranostics: a step-by-step practical approach to diagnosis and therapy for mCRPC patients. Semin Nucl Med 2020;50(1): 98–109.
3. Rahbar K, Afshar-Oromieh A, Jadvar H, et al. PSMA theranostics: current status and future directions. Mol Imaging 2018;17. 1536012118776068.
4. Pencharz D, Gnanasegaran G, Navalkissoor S. Theranostics in neuroendocrine tumours: somatostatin receptor imaging and therapy. Br J Radiol 2018;91(1091):20180108.
5. Liu H, Wang X, Yang R, et al. Recent development of nuclear molecular imaging in thyroid cancer. Biomed Res Int 2018;2018:2149532.
6. Ahn B-C. Personalized medicine based on theranostic radioiodine molecular imaging for differentiated thyroid cancer. Biomed Res Int 2016;2016: 1680464.
7. Stokkel MP, Handkiewicz Junak D, Lassmann M, et al. EANM procedure guidelines for therapy of benign thyroid disease. Eur J Nucl Med Mol Imaging 2010;37(11):2218–28.
8. Dai G, Levy O, Carrasco N. Cloning and characterization of the thyroid iodide transporter. Nature 1996;379(6564):458–60.
9. Cooper DS, Doherty GM, Haugen BR, et al. Management guidelines for patients with thyroid nodules and differentiated thyroid cancer. Thyroid 2006;16(2):109–42.
10. Haugen BR, Alexander EK, Bible KC, et al. 2016 2015 American Thyroid Association management guidelines for adult patients with thyroid nodules and differentiated thyroid cancer: the American thyroid association guidelines Task Force on thyroid nodules and differentiated thyroid cancer. Thyroid 2016;26(1):1–133.
11. Seidlin S, Siegel E, Yalow AA, et al. Acute myeloid leukemia following prolonged iodine-131 therapy for metastatic thyroid carcinoma. Science 1956; 123(3201):800–1.
12. Yordanova A, Eppard E, Kürpig S, et al. Theranostics in nuclear medicine practice. Onco Targets Ther 2017;10:4821.
13. Luster M, Clarke SE, Dietlein M, et al. Guidelines for radioiodine therapy of differentiated thyroid cancer. Eur J Nucl Med Mol Imaging 2008;35(10):1941.
14. Refardt J, Hofland J, Kwadwo A, et al. Theranostics in neuroendocrine tumors: an overview of current approaches and future challenges. Rev Endocr Metab Disord 2020. https://doi.org/10.1007/s11154-020-09552-x.
15. Gatto F, Hofland LJ. The role of somatostatin and dopamine D2 receptors in endocrine tumors. Endocr Relat Cancer 2011;18(6):R233.
16. Reubi J, Waser B, Schaer JC, et al. Erratum to: somatostatin receptor sst1-sst5 expression in normal and neoplastic human tissues using receptor autoradiography with subtype-selective ligands. Eur J Nucl Med 2001;28(9):1433–846.
17. Reubi JC, Waser B, Liu Q, et al. Subcellular distribution of somatostatin sst2A receptors in human tumors of the nervous and neuroendocrine systems: membranous versus intracellular location. J Clin Endocrinol Metab 2000;85(10): 3882–91.
18. Reubi JC. Peptide receptor expression in GEP-NET. Virchows Arch 2007;451:S47–50. Suppl 1(1).
19. Severi S, Grassi I, Nicolini S, et al. Peptide receptor radionuclide therapy in the management of gastrointestinal neuroendocrine tumors: efficacy profile, safety, and quality of life. Onco Targets Ther 2017;10:551.
20. Lee ST, Kulkarni HR, Singh A, et al. Theranostics of neuroendocrine tumors. Visc Med 2017;33(5):358–66.
21. Mittra ES. Neuroendocrine tumor therapy: 177Lu-DOTATATE. AJR Am J Roentgenol 2018;211(2): 278–85.
22. Werner RA, Weich A, Kircher M, et al. The theranostic promise for Neuroendocrine Tumors in the late 2010s - where do we stand, where do we go? Theranostics 2018;8(22):6088.
23. Strosberg J, El-Haddad G, Wolin E, et al. Phase 3 Trial of 177Lu-Dotatate for Midgut Neuroendocrine Tumors. N Engl J Med 2017;376(2):125–35.
24. Brabander T, van der Zwan WA, Teunissen JJM, et al. Long-term efficacy, survival, and safety of

[177Lu-DOTA0,Tyr3]octreotate in patients with gastroenteropancreatic and bronchial neuroendocrine tumors. Clin Cancer Res 2017;23(16): 4617–24.

25. Baum RP, Kulkarni HR, Carreras C. Peptides and receptors in image-guided therapy: theranostics for neuroendocrine neoplasms. Semin Nucl Med 2012;42(3):190.

26. Öberg K. Molecular imaging and radiotherapy: theranostics for personalized patient management. Theranostics 2012;2(5):424.

27. Yordanova A, Wicharz MM, Mayer K, et al. The role of adding somatostatin analogues to peptide receptor radionuclide therapy as a combination and maintenance therapy. Clin Cancer Res 2018; 24(19):4672–9.

28. Rizvi T, Deng C, Rehm PK. Indium-111 capromab Pendetide (ProstaScint®) demonstrates renal cell carcinoma and aortocaval nodal metastases from prostate adenocarcinoma. World J Nucl Med 2015;14(3):209.

29. Ebenhan T, Vorster M, Marjanovic-Painter B, et al. Development of a single vial kit solution for radiolabeling of 68Ga-DKFZ-PSMA-11 and its performance in prostate cancer patients. Molecules 2015;20(8):14860–78.

30. Eder M, Eisenhut M, Babich J, et al. PSMA as a target for radiolabelled small molecules. Eur J Nucl Med Mol Imaging 2013;40(6):819–23.

31. Barrett JA, Coleman RE, Goldsmith SJ, et al. First-in-man evaluation of 2 high-affinity PSMA-avid small molecules for imaging prostate cancer. J Nucl Med 2013;54(3):380–7.

32. Lenzo N, Meyrick D, Turner J. Review of gallium-68 PSMA PET/CT imaging in the management of prostate cancer. Diagnostics 2018;8(1):16.

33. Van Dongen G, Huisman MC, Boellaard R, et al. 89Zr-immuno-PET for imaging of long circulating drugs and disease targets: why, how and when to be applied. Q J Nucl Med Mol Imaging 2015; 59(1):18–38.

34. Seifert R, Schafigh D, Bögemann M, et al. Detection of local relapse of prostate cancer with 18F-PSMA-1007. Clin Nucl Med 2019;44(6):e394–5.

35. Ahmadzadehfar H, Rahbar K, Kürpig S, et al. Early side effects and first results of radioligand therapy with (177)Lu-DKFZ-617 PSMA of castrate-resistant metastatic prostate cancer: a two-centre study. EJNMMI Res 2015;5(1):114.

36. Ahmadzadehfar H, Eppard E, Kürpig S, et al. Therapeutic response and side effects of repeated radioligand therapy with 177Lu-PSMA-DKFZ-617 of castrate-resistant metastatic prostate cancer. Oncotarget 2016;7(11):12477.

37. Ahmadzadehfar H, Wegen S, Yordanova A, et al. Overall survival and response pattern of castration-resistant metastatic prostate cancer to multiple cycles of radioligand therapy using [177Lu]Lu-PSMA-617. Eur J Nucl Med Mol Imaging 2017;44(9):1448–54.

38. Roll W, Bräuer A, Weckesser M, et al. Long-term survival and excellent response to repeated 177Lu-prostate-specific membrane antigen 617 radioligand therapy in a patient with advanced metastatic castration-resistant prostate cancer. Clin Nucl Med 2018;43(10):755–6.

39. Sun M, Niaz MO, Nelson A, et al. Review of 177Lu-PSMA-617 in patients with metastatic castration-resistant prostate cancer. Cureus 2020;12(6): e8921.

40. Kratochwil C, Haberkorn U, Giesel FL. ^{225}Ac-PSMA-617 for therapy of prostate cancer. Semin Nucl Med 2020;50(2):133–40.

41. Kratochwil C, Bruchertseifer F, Rathke H, et al. Targeted α-therapy of metastatic castration-resistant prostate cancer with 225Ac-PSMA-617: dosimetry estimate and empiric dose finding. J Nucl Med 2017;58(10):1624–31.

42. Kratochwil C, Bruchertseifer F, Giesel FL, et al. 225Ac-PSMA-617 for PSMA-targeted α-radiation therapy of metastatic castration-resistant prostate cancer. J Nucl Med 2016;57(12):1941–4.

43. Pandit-Taskar N, Batraki M, Divgi CR. Radiopharmaceutical therapy for palliation of bone pain from osseous metastases. J Nucl Med 2004; 45(8):1358–65.

44. Pfannkuchen N, Meckel M, Bergmann R, et al. Novel radiolabeled bisphosphonates for PET diagnosis and endoradiotherapy of bone metastases. Pharmaceuticals (Basel) 2017;10(2):45.

45. Ye L, Kynaston HG, Jiang WG. Bone metastasis in prostate cancer: molecular and cellular mechanisms (Review). Int J Mol Med 2007;20(1): 103–11.

46. Hensel J, Thalmann GN. Biology of bone metastases in prostate cancer. Urology 2016;92:6–13.

47. Agarwal MG, Nayak P. Management of skeletal metastases: an orthopaedic surgeon's guide. Indian J Orthop 2015;49(1):83–100.

48. González-Sistal À, et al. Advances in medical imaging applied to bone metastases. Vol. 16. 2011.

49. Ulmert D, Solnes L, Thorek DLj. Contemporary approaches for imaging skeletal metastasis. Bone Res 2015;3:15024.

50. Lange R, Ter Heine R, Knapp RF, et al. Pharmaceutical and clinical development of phosphonate-based radiopharmaceuticals for the targeted treatment of bone metastases. Bone 2016;91:159–79.

51. Fleisch H, Russell RG, Francis MD. Diphosphonates inhibit hydroxyapatite dissolution in vitro and bone resorption in tissue culture and in vivo. Science 1969;165(3899):1262–4.

52. Gasser AB, Morgan DB, Fleisch HA, et al. The influence of two diphosphonates on calcium metabolism in the rat. Clin Sci 1972;43(1):31–45.

53. Luckman SP, Hughes DE, Coxon FP, et al. Nitrogen-containing biphosphonates inhibit the mevalonate pathway and prevent post-translational prenylation of GTP-binding proteins, including Ras. J Bone Miner Res 2005;20(7):1265–74.

54. Schenk R, Eggli P, Fleisch H, et al. Quantitative morphometric evaluation of the inhibitory activity of new aminobisphosphonates on bone resorption in the rat. Calcif Tissue Int 1986;38(6):342–9.

55. Schenk R, Merz WA, Mühlbauer R, et al. Effect of ethane-1-hydroxy-1,1-diphosphonate (EHDP) and dichloromethylene diphosphonate (Cl 2 MDP) on the calcification and resorption of cartilage and bone in the tibial epiphysis and metaphysis of rats. Calcif Tissue Res 1973;11(3):196–214.

56. Russell RG, Mühlbauer RC, Bisaz S, et al. The influence of pyrophosphate, condensed phosphates, phosphonates and other phosphate compounds on the dissolution of hydroxyapatite in vitro and on bone resorption induced by parathyroid hormone in tissue culture and in thyroparathyroidectomised rats. Calcif Tissue Res 1970;6(3):183–96.

57. Russell RGG. Bisphosphonates: the first 40 years. Bone 2011;49(1):2–19.

58. Ahmadzadehfar H. Targeted therapy for metastatic prostate cancer with radionuclides. In: Hojjat Ahmadzadehfar H, editor. Prostate cancer-leading-edge diagnostic procedures and treatments. Croatia: InTech; 2016. p. 60–4.

59. Thapa P, Nikam D, Das T, et al. Clinical efficacy and safety comparison of 177Lu-EDTMP with 153Sm-EDTMP on an equidose basis in patients with painful skeletal metastases. J Nucl Med 2015;56(10):1513–9.

60. Sohaib M, Ahmad M, Jehangir M, et al. Ethylene diamine tetramethylene phosphonic acid labeled with various β–-Emitting radiometals: labeling optimization and animal biodistribution. Cancer Biother Radiopharm 2011;26(2):159–64.

61. Chakraborty S, Das T, Unni PR, et al. 177Lu labelled polyaminophosphonates as potential agents for bone pain palliation. Nucl Med Commun 2002;23(1):67–74.

62. Chakraborty S, Das T, Banerjee S, et al. 177Lu-EDTMP: a viable bone pain palliative in skeletal metastasis. Cancer Biother Radiopharm 2008;23(2):202–13.

63. Máthé D, Balogh L, Polyák A, et al. Multispecies animal investigation on biodistribution, pharmacokinetics and toxicity of 177Lu-EDTMP, a potential bone pain palliation agent. Nucl Med Biol 2010;37(2):215–26.

64. Passah A, Tripathi M, Ballal S, et al. Evaluation of bone-seeking novel radiotracer 68Ga-NO2AP-Bisphosphonate for the detection of skeletal metastases in carcinoma breast. Eur J Nucl Med Mol Imaging 2017;44(1):41–9.

65. Rösch F, Baum RP. Generator-based PET radiopharmaceuticals for molecular imaging of tumours: on the way to THERANOSTICS. Dalton Trans 2011;40(23):6104–11.

66. Das T, Chakraborty S, Unni PR, et al. 177Lu-labeled cyclic polyaminophosphonates as potential agents for bone pain palliation. Appl Radiat Isot 2002;57(2):177–84.

67. Das T, Shinto A, Karuppuswamy Kamaleshwaran K, et al. Theranostic treatment of metastatic bone pain with 177Lu-DOTMP. Clin Nucl Med 2016;41(12):966–7.

68. Meckel M, Nauth A, Timpe J, et al. Development of a [177Lu]BPAMD labeling kit and an automated synthesis module for routine bone targeted endoradiotherapy. Cancer Biother Radiopharm 2015;30(2):94–9.

69. Chakraborty S, Das T, Sarma HD, et al. Comparative studies of 177Lu–EDTMP and 177Lu–DOTMP as potential agents for palliative radiotherapy of bone metastasis. Appl Radiat Isot 2008;66(9):1196–205.

70. Agarwal KK, Singla S, Arora G, et al. (177)Lu-EDTMP for palliation of pain from bone metastases in patients with prostate and breast cancer: a phase II study. Eur J Nucl Med Mol Imaging 2015;42(1):79–88.

71. Alavi M, Omidvari S, Mehdizadeh A, et al. Metastatic bone pain palliation using 177Lu-ethylenediaminetetramethylene phosphonic acid. World J Nucl Med 2015;14(2):109.

72. Yuan J, Liu C, Liu X, et al. Efficacy and safety of 177Lu-EDTMP in bone metastatic pain palliation in breast cancer and hormone refractory prostate cancer: a phase II study. Clin Nucl Med 2013;38(2):88–92.

73. Mazzarri S, Guidoccio F, Mariani G. The emerging potential of 177Lu-EDTMP: an attractive novel option for radiometabolic therapy of skeletal metastases. Clin Transl Imaging 2015;3(2):167–8.

74. Balter H, Victoria T, Mariella T, et al. 177Lu-Labeled agents for neuroendocrine tumor therapy and bone pain palliation in Uruguay. Curr Radiopharm 2016;9(1):85–93.

75. Mirzaei A, Jalilian AR, Badbarin A, et al. Optimized production and quality control of (68)Ga-EDTMP for small clinical trials. Ann Nucl Med 2015;29(6):506–11.

76. Meckel M, Bergmann R, Miederer M, et al. Bone targeting compounds for radiotherapy and

imaging: *Me(III)-DOTA conjugates of bisphosphonic acid, pamidronic acid and zoledronic acid. EJNMMI Radiopharm Chem 2017;1(1):14.

77. Nijsen JF, van het Schip AD, Hennink WE, et al. Advances in nuclear oncology: microspheres for internal radionuclide therapy of liver tumours. Curr Med Chem 2002;9(1):73–82.

78. Louw WK, Dormehl IC, van Rensburg AJ, et al. Evaluation of samarium-153 and holmium-166-EDTMP in the normal baboon model. Nucl Med Biol 1996;23(8):935–40.

79. Breitz HB, Wendt RE, Stabin MS, et al. 166Ho-DOTMP radiation-absorbed dose estimation for skeletal targeted radiotherapy. J Nucl Med 2006; 47(3):534–42.

80. Marques F, Gano L, Paula Campello M, et al. 13- and 14-membered macrocyclic ligands containing methylcarboxylate or methylphosphonate pendant arms: chemical and biological evaluation of their (153)Sm and (166)Ho complexes as potential agents for therapy or bone pain palliation. J Inorg Biochem 2006;100(2):270–80.

81. Zeevaart JR, Jarvis NV, Louw WK, et al. Metal-ion speciation in blood plasma incorporating the tetraphosphonate, N,N-dimethylenephosphonate-1-hydroxy-4-aminopropilydenediphosphonate (APDDMP), in therapeutic radiopharmaceuticals. J Inorg Biochem 2001;83(1):57–65.

82. Giralt S, Bensinger W, Goodman M, et al. 166Ho-DOTMP plus melphalan followed by peripheral blood stem cell transplantation in patients with multiple myeloma: results of two phase 1/2 trials. Blood 2003;102(7):2684–91.

83. Rajendran JG, Eary JF, Bensinger W, et al. High-dose 166Ho-DOTMP in myeloablative treatment of multiple myeloma: pharmacokinetics, biodistribution, and absorbed dose estimation. J Nucl Med 2002;43(10):1383–90.

84. Pandit-Taskar N, Modak S. Norepinephrine transporter as a target for imaging and therapy. J Nucl Med 2017;58(Suppl 2):39S.

85. Gaze MN, Chang YC, Flux GD, et al. Feasibility of dosimetry-based high-dose 131I-meta-iodobenzylguanidine with topotecan as a radiosensitizer in children with metastatic neuroblastoma. Cancer Biother Radiopharm 2005;20(2):195–9.

86. Lashford LS, Hancock JP, Kemshead JT. Meta-iodobenzylguanidine (mIBG) uptake and storage in the human neuroblastoma cell line SK-N-BE(2C). Int J Cancer 1991;47(1):105–9.

87. Matthay KK, Shulkin B, Ladenstein R, et al. Criteria for evaluation of disease extent by (123)I-metaiodobenzylguanidine scans in neuroblastoma: a report for the International neuroblastoma risk group (INRG) Task Force. Br J Cancer 2010; 102(9):1319–26.

88. Bar-Sever Z, Biassoni L, Shulkin B, et al. Guidelines on nuclear medicine imaging in neuroblastoma. Eur J Nucl Med Mol Imaging 2018;45(11):2009–24.

89. Yanik GA, Villablanca JG, Maris JM, et al. 131I-metaiodobenzylguanidine with intensive chemotherapy and autologous stem cell transplantation for high-risk neuroblastoma. A new approaches to neuroblastoma therapy (NANT) phase II study. Biol Blood Marrow Transplant 2015;21(4):673–81.

90. Hutchinson RJ, Sisson JC, Miser JS, et al. Long-term results of [131I]metaiodobenzylguanidine treatment of refractory advanced neuroblastoma. J Nucl Biol Med 1991;35(4):237–40.

91. Matthay KK, DeSantes K, Hasegawa B, et al. Phase I dose escalation of 131I-metaiodobenzylguanidine with autologous bone marrow support in refractory neuroblastoma. J Clin Oncol 1998; 16(1):229–36.

92. Yanik GA, Levine JE, Matthay KK, et al. Pilot study of iodine-131–metaiodobenzylguanidine in combination with myeloablative chemotherapy and autologous stem-cell support for the treatment of neuroblastoma. J Clin Oncol 2002;20(8):2142–9.

93. Parisi MT, Eslamy H, Park JR, et al. 131I-metaiodobenzylguanidine theranostics in neuroblastoma: historical perspectives; practical applications. Semin Nucl Med 2016;46(3):184–202.

94. Kroiss A, Putzer D, Uprimny C, et al. Functional imaging in phaeochromocytoma and neuroblastoma with 68Ga-DOTA-Tyr 3-octreotide positron emission tomography and 123I-metaiodobenzylguanidine. Eur J Nucl Med Mol Imaging 2011;38(5):865–73.

95. Qin C, Liu H, Chen K, et al. Theranostics of malignant melanoma with 64CuCl2. J Nucl Med 2014; 55(5):812–7.

96. Barboza T, Gomes T, da Costa Medeiros P, et al. Development of 131I-ixolaris as a theranostic agent: metastatic melanoma preclinical studies. Clin Exp Metastasis 2020;37(4):489–97.

97. Barboza A, et al. Utopie. J Nucl Med 2019; 60(supplement 1):348–53.

98. Lapa C, Schreder M, Schirbel A, et al. [68Ga]Pentixafor-PET/CT for imaging of chemokine receptor CXCR4 expression in multiple myeloma - comparison to [18F]FDG and laboratory values. Theranostics 2017;7(1):205.

99. Langbein T, Weber WA, Eiber M. Future of theranostics: an outlook on precision oncology in nuclear medicine. J Nucl Med 2019;60(Suppl 2): 13S–9S.

100. Loktev A, Lindner T, Mier W, et al. A tumor-imaging method targeting cancer-associated fibroblasts. J Nucl Med 2018;59(9):1423–9.

101. Lindner T, Loktev A, Altmann A, et al. Development of quinoline-based theranostic ligands for the

targeting of fibroblast activation protein. J Nucl Med 2018;59(9):1415–22.

102. Lindner T, Loktev A, Giesel F, et al. Targeting of activated fibroblasts for imaging and therapy. EJNMMI Radiopharm Chem 2019;4(1):16.

103. Loktev A, Lindner T, Burger EM, et al. Development of fibroblast activation protein–targeted radiotracers with improved tumor retention. J Nucl Med 2019;60(10):1421–9.

104. Giesel FL, Kratochwil C, Lindner T, et al. 68Ga-FAPI PET/CT: biodistribution and preliminary dosimetry estimate of 2 DOTA-containing FAP-targeting agents in patients with various cancers. J Nucl Med 2019;60(3):386–92.

105. Kratochwil C, Flechsig P, Lindner T, et al. 68Ga-FAPI PET/CT: tracer uptake in 28 different kinds of cancer. J Nucl Med 2019;60(6):801–5.

The Role of Fibroblast Activation Protein Ligands in Oncologic PET Imaging

Katharina Dendl, cand. med[a], Joel Schlittenhardt, MD[a],
Fabian Staudinger, cand. med[a], Clemens Kratochwil, MD[a],
Anette Altmann, MD[a,b,c], Uwe Haberkorn, MD[a,b,c],
Frederik L. Giesel, MD, MBA[d,*]

KEYWORDS

- Fibroblast activation protein • FAP • FAPI PET/CT • Cancer-associated fibroblasts
- Small molecule inhibitors

KEY POINTS

- Fibroblast activation protein (FAP) is expressed by cancer-associated fibroblasts which are a key element for tumor growth and yet present in non-malignant diseases as well.
- FAP crystallizes as a diagnostic and possible therapeutic agent in one molecule, enabling theranostic application.
- Fibroblast activation protein inhibitor (FAPI) emerges as a powerful imaging tool demonstrating high uptake in primary and metastatic lesions in various tumor entities.
- Current studies indicate that FAPI is equal or even superior to the current oncologic standard tracer FDG in several tumor entities. It seems to impress with lower background activity, stronger uptake of tumorous lesions and thus sharper contrasts.

INTRODUCTION

Fibroblast activation protein (FAP) is an atypical type II transmembrane serine protease with post proline dipeptidyl-peptidase and endopeptidase activity.[1] FAP is expressed by many cancer-associated fibroblasts (CAFs), which are a key element for tumor growth and correlate with poor prognosis.[2] Fibroblasts are ubiquitous in the body, yet resting fibroblasts in healthy tissue have no or very slight FAP expression. In contrast, activated fibroblasts, such as CAFs, are characterized by high numbers of FAP, promoting tumor cell migration, invasion, and tumor angiogenesis.[3–5] However, nonmalignant FAP expression can also be found in wound healing and chronic inflammatory processes and particularly in fibrosis or liver cirrhosis.[1,6] Based on its dual enzymatic ability,[1] FAP can be targeted by small molecule FAP inhibitors (FAPIs), which have been developed recently as novel diagnostic probes for imaging of cancer, chronic inflammation, and myocardial scare.[7–9] Because of its selective expression in several pathologies, ligand-induced internalization, and presence in a large variety of malignancies, FAPI represents a unique and promising target for molecular imaging techniques and possibly enables theranostic application.

TUMOR STROMA

Tumor growth and spread is not only determined by neoplastic cells but also various nonmalignant constituents shaping the tumor microenvironment,

[a] Department of Nuclear Medicine, University Hospital Heidelberg, INF 400, 69120 Heidelberg, Germany; [b] Clinical Cooperation Unit Nuclear Medicine, German Cancer Research Center (DKFZ), INF280, 69120 Heidelberg, Germany; [c] Translational Lung Research Center Heidelberg, German Center for Lung Research (DZL), 69120 Heidelberg, Germany; [d] Department of Nuclear Medicine, University Hospital Düsseldorf, Germany
* Corresponding author.
E-mail address: frederik@egiesel.com

PET Clin 16 (2021) 341–351
https://doi.org/10.1016/j.cpet.2021.03.012
1556-8598/21/© 2021 Elsevier Inc. All rights reserved.

defined as tumor stroma. Furthermore, the stroma can account for up to 90% of the mass in common malignancies, such as breast, colon, and pancreatic cancer,[10] including endothelial cells, the basement membrane, extracellular matrix, immune cells, and fibroblast-like cells subsumed as CAFs (**Fig. 1**). These noncancerous stromal cells may contribute with the help of various growth factors, chemokines, and cytokines to tumor progression, growth, drug resistance, and generation of metastasis.[11–13]

Cancer-Associated Fibroblasts

Previous studies have shown that CAFs emerge from a variety of different cell types, including resident fibroblasts, endothelial and epithelial cells,[13] and mesenchymal bone marrow–derived precursor cells.[14,15] Growth factors, such as the transforming growth factor-β (TGF-β), induce several protumoral effects, such as the activation of local fibroblasts to form CAFs.[16] Moreover, further messenger substances that are activating additional cell types are released by these stimulated CAFs. This leads to crosstalk of CAFs with the surrounding extracellular matrix, stromal cells, immune cells, and tumor-cells, resulting in cancer-promoting effects, such as cancer cell invasion, migration and growth, metabolic reprogramming, immunosuppression, angiogenesis, and drug resistance (**Fig. 2**). In addition to reactive CAFs, activated endothelial cells and pericytes are important factors in the process of tumor progression. Growing to a size of 1 to 2 mm, malignant tumors require their own vascular connection for progressive growth.[17] The release of angiogenic factors can be caused by a hypoxic environment. Vascular endothelial growth factor (VEGF), for example, is important for angiogenesis.[18] VEGF and TGF-β stimulate the endothelial cell-pericyte network and promote procancerous angiogenesis.[19] Consequently, the signaling pathway of VEGF may present a promising target for novel and current tumor therapies.

Fibroblast Activation Protein

The type II serine protease FAP is a 760 amino acid membrane-bound glycoprotein belonging to the dipeptidyl peptidase 4 (DPP4) family with dipeptidyl-peptidase and endopeptidase activity. The latter predominates in its activity and distinguishes FAP from other members of the DPP4 family.[1] FAP is an integral protein that is overexpressed in more than 90% of all epithelial carcinomas and in addition selectively in benign diseases and normal tissue during remodeling. Under physiologic conditions FAP plays a significant role during embryogenesis[20] and is coexpressed with DPP4 in the alpha cells of Langerhans-islets and moreover expressed in multipotent bone marrow stromal cells.[21,22] Furthermore, FAP is also slightly present in the cervix and uterine stroma reaching the peak during the proliferative cycle.[23] FAP is also associated with several nonmalignant conditions, including chronic inflammatory processes, such as wound healing, arthritis, atherosclerotic plaques, and fibrosis, and its expression in ischemic heart tissue after myocardial infarction.[24–29] To our knowledge several malignancies overexpress FAP and it might be present in other cellular components of the tumor microenvironment. For example, it has been detected in osteoclasts in multiple myeloma,[30] endothelial cells,[31–36] and macrophages.[37,38] Moreover, FAP is involved in several hallmarks of malignancies, such as contribution to tumor cell adhesion and invasion.[39] Furthermore,

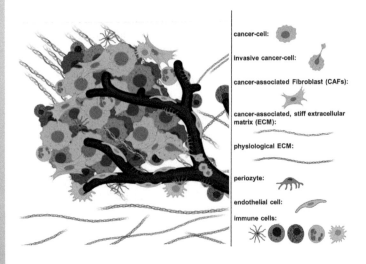

cancer-cell:

invasive cancer-cell:

cancer-associated Fibroblast (CAFs):

cancer-associated, stiff extracellular matrix (ECM):

physiological ECM:

periozyte:

endothelial cell:

immune cells:

Fig. 1. Malignant tumors are not only determined by cancer cells. When growing to a size of 2 mm, the tumor-associated stroma is essential for tumor progression, growth, and metastases. This stroma consists of basement membrane, extracellular matrix, immune cells, and CAFs. (Modified with Biorender.)

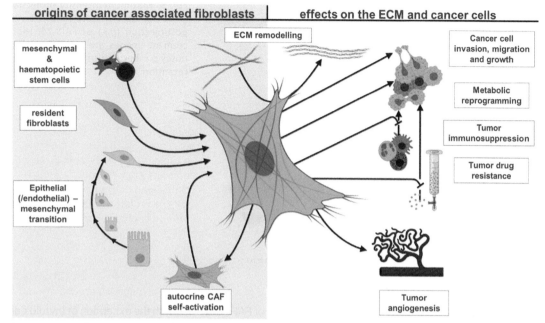

| origins of cancer associated fibroblasts | effects on the ECM and cancer cells |

Fig. 2. CAFs are known to be the decisive cell type regarding tumor-promoting changes of the extracellular matrix (ECM). Crosstalk of CAFs with the surrounding ECM, stromal cells, immune cells, and tumor cells results in cancer-promoting effects, as shown on the *right side*. (Modified with Biorender.)

FAP is able to build complexes with other DPP4s, influencing tumor cell growth and dedifferentiation.[5] The protease complexes are localized at extensions of the cell surface, defining them as key structures for tumor progression.[40] Remodeling of substrates of the protease, such as collagen-I, antitrypsin, and neuropeptide-Y, leads to protumoral modifications regarding the extracellular matrix.[41–43] The FAP substrate neuropeptide-Y contributes to extracellular matrix remodeling processes associated with neovascularization of the tumor stroma and inducing angiogenesis in ischemic tissue.[44] The enzymatic product NPY3-36 is active with angiogenic Y2/Y5 receptors of endothelial cells and acts as a vascular growth factor.[45] Thus, FAP-expressing tumors present a higher microvascular density and accelerated growth. In contrast, in animal models of pancreatic and lung cancer, tumors with deactivated FAP-expressing cells showed a lower vascular density.[46] Overexpression of FAP in CAFs correlate in several tumor entities, such as colon, pancreatic, ovarian, and hepatocellular carcinomas with worse prognosis and rapid progression.[47–50]

FIBROBLAST ACTIVATION PROTEIN LIGANDS IN PET IMAGING

Evolution of FAP-ligand labeling into clinical translation started with the use of FAPI-02 and FAPI-04. Recently FAPI-46 was developed for theranostic

purposes presenting longer tumor residence time.[51] The derivates FAPI-02, -04, and -46 are loaded with the radionuclide ^{68}Ga. However, for different imaging modalities and institutional infrastructures, FAPI-34 is labeled with ^{99m}Tc (gamma camera) and FAPI-74 enables ^{68}Ga and ^{18}F (PET scanner).[28,52,53]

Fibroblast Activation Protein Inhibitor Versus Fluorodeoxyglucose

The objective of this novel tracer is to be equal or even superior to previously existing nuclear tracers regarding diagnostic sensitivity, specificity, and additionally possible theranostic application. Therefore, FAPI has to be compared with the oncologic standard tracer fluorodeoxyglucose (FDG). Primarily the application of FAPI is not in need of special preparation in contrast with ^{18}F-FDG, whose accumulation is influenced by nutrition and blood glucose levels. Furthermore, a PET/computed tomography (CT) scan with FAPI seems to already provide adequate images 10 minutes postinjection resulting in significantly reduced radiation doses (**Fig. 3**).[28,53–55] Additionally, FAP-uptake in the brain is low in comparison with FDG facilitating diagnostics of brain tumors and metastases. Remarkably, the FAPI is a diagnostic and possible therapeutic agent in one molecule, enabling theranostic application. Loktev and colleagues[28] reported a first intraindividual

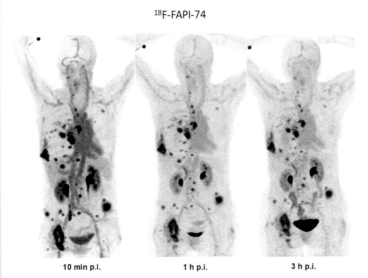

¹⁸F-FAPI-74

10 min p.i.   1 h p.i.   3 h p.i.

Fig. 3. Maximum intensity projection at 10 minutes, 1 hour, and 3 hours postinjection (p.i.) of FAPI-74. High-contrast images are possible 10 minutes p.i. because of fast uptake and retention.

comparative single case study between ¹⁸F-FDG and ⁶⁸Ga-FAPI-02, describing a patient with locally advanced lung adenocarcinoma (**Fig. 4**). In this case FAPI presented a better tumor-to-background ratio (TBR) and a lower background activity particularly in brain, liver, and spleen.[28] Furthermore, another study compared ⁶⁸Ga-FAPI-02 and ¹⁸F-FDG in six different tumor entities (n = 6 patients; esophageal, colon, lung, pancreatic, and thyroid cancer). Five out of six tumors showed no significant difference in accumulation of FAPI and FDG, with the exception of thyroid carcinoma with no FAPI-uptake. Background activity was significantly lower for FAPI in brain, oral mucosa, and liver, leading to improved detection of metastases.[54] A recently conducted intraindividual study reported the efficacy of ⁶⁸Ga-FAPI-04 versus ¹⁸F-FDG regarding the diagnosis of primary tumors and metastases. The examination and analysis of 75 oncologic patients presented equal to superior findings for ⁶⁸Ga-FAPI-04 in terms of tracer accumulation and sensitivity of detecting

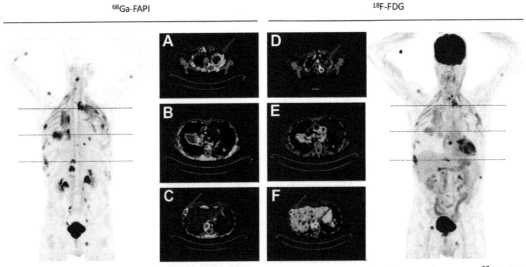

⁶⁸Ga-FAPI   ¹⁸F-FDG

Fig. 4. A 60-year-old patient with a histologically confirmed adenocarcinoma of the lung underwent a ⁶⁸Ga-FAPI-PET/CT for restaging showing strong FAP uptake in both lobes of the lung with a maximum standardized uptake value (SUVmax) of 8.3 (*A*) and 12.7 (*B*), respectively. ¹⁸F-FDG-PET/CT demonstrated low tracer accumulation with an SUVmax of 2.2 (*D*) and 3.7 (*E*), respectively. Tracer uptake in the exemplary bone lesions was slightly higher for ⁶⁸Ga-FAPI (*C*) compared to 18F-FDG (*F*). The arrows are placed in order to help the reader identify the lesions.

primary tumor and metastases (**Fig. 5**).[56] These current studies indicate that FAPI may be an equal or even superior tracer over FDG in many indications.

Brain, Head, and Neck

Because ^{18}F-FDG shows a high physiologic uptake in the brain, reliable diagnoses of malignancies located in the brain are challenging to derive. A potential solution might arise with the novel tracer FAPI. FAPI, in contrast to FDG, impresses with a significant lower background accumulation favoring improved detection of primary and secondary malignancies in the brain (**Fig. 6**). Fu and colleagues and Giesel and colleagues reported improved uptake in brain metastasis in two individual case studies of patients with the diagnosis of lung cancer.[57,58] Additionally, Röhrich and colleagues[59] conducted an in vitro, in vivo, and clinical study, using FAP-specific PET imaging, regarding isocitrate dehydrogenase (IDH) mutant gliomas and IDH wild-type glioblastomas. The clinical part of this study included 18 glioma patients (5 IDH mutant glioma, 13 IDH wild-type glioblastomas) and was performed with ^{68}Ga-labeled FAPI-02/04. IDH wild-type glioblastomas and high-grade IDH mutant astrozytomas presented elevated tracer uptake. In diffuse astrozytomas, no increased uptake and low TBRs were measured, possibly providing a noninvasive differentiation between low-grade IDH mutant and high-grade gliomas.[59] Furthermore, Windisch and colleagues[60] analyzed the same 13 glioblastoma patients evaluating the potential of FAPI-PET/CT or PET/MRI in terms of radiotherapy planning. The previously mentioned comparison of FAPI and FDG by Chen and colleagues[56] included four glioma patients presenting a lower total FAP uptake, yet a higher TBR. Regarding head and neck cancers Syed and colleagues[61] analyzed 14 patients (1 mucoepidermoid carcinoma, 1 undifferentiated, 12 squamous cell carcinoma) with a FAPI-PET/CT and CT used for radiotherapy planning, using four different thresholds.[3,5,7,10] Regarding these patients, the three-fold threshold seemed to be most advantageous for target volume delineation. Thus, the FAPI-PET/CT may provide a new and low-risk imaging modality leading to possibly improved target volume delineation in head and neck cancers for enhanced radiotherapy planning.[61]

Lung and Cardiac

Lung cancer is, with approximately 25% of all cancer deaths (men and women) in 2020, the most frequent cause in the United States.[62] Therefore, a precise and reliable imaging modality regarding diagnostics and therapy is extremely relevant. A recent study analyzed 10 FAPI-74-PET/CT scans of patients with lung cancer, labeled with ^{18}F-AlF

^{18}F-FDG

^{68}Ga-FAPI

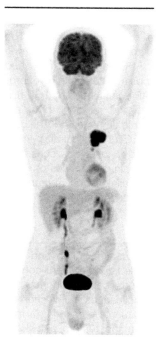 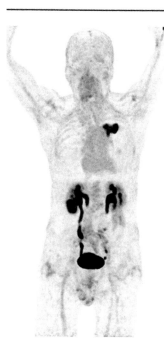

Fig. 5. A patient initially staged per FDG presented with poorly adjustable blood sugar after neoadjuvant chemotherapy and FAPI-PET/CT was performed before radiotherapy. Because of similar tumor-to-background contrast, it seems reasonable that the proposed segmentation cutoffs for FAPI are in similar range than for FDG.

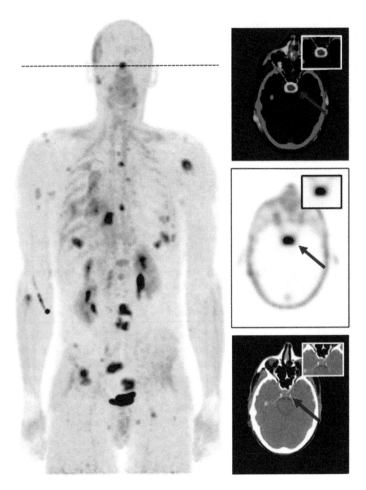

Fig. 6. A 48-year-old man with a tumor in the pituitary underwent a ^{68}Ga-FAPI-PET/CT for evaluation of radioligand ^{90}Y-FAPI-therapy. The tumoral lesion presented an FAPI uptake of 7.3. The arrows are placed in order to help the reader identify the lesions.

or ^{68}Ga in terms of biodistribution, radiation dosimetry, and tumor delineation. The evaluation revealed a high contrast, represented by a maximum standardized uptake value (SUVmax) of 10 and higher, respectively, in primary tumors, lymph nodes, and metastases. Reduced radiation burden enables even further clinical use.[52] Two individual patients with adenocarcinoma of the lung underwent a FAPI-PET/CT showing high TBRs and the detection of a cerebral metastasis[58] (see **Fig. 4**) and leptomeningeal disease.[63]

A further relevant topic is cardiac disease. After myocardial infarction the presence of activated fibroblasts expressing FAP is upregulated anticipating the quality of remodeling. These remodeling processes were experimentally analyzed by Varasteh and colleagues[9] in rats after sham-operation and coronary ligation leading to myocardial infarction. The FAPI-04 uptake in the damaged myocardium peaked at 6 days after coronary litigation. It was predominantly expressed at the border zone of infarction, visualized by autoradiography and common staining. The myocardial infarction zone presented a strong FAPI-positive, FDG-negative and immunofluorescence-positive uptake in myofibroblasts. Furthermore, FAP is influenced by TGF-ß, a growth factor during tissue remodeling in the myocardium after ischemic damage.[24,25] The clinical potential of FAPI-PET/CT visualizing these processes has already been successfully assessed.[64,65] These noninvasive findings may contribute significantly to clinical patient management regarding diagnostics and prognosis.

Upper Abdomen

In terms of esophageal cancer, Chen and colleagues[56] investigated the largest patient cohort, highlighting five squamous cell carcinomas. In addition, Ristau and colleagues[66] investigated seven treatment-naive patients presenting a median SUVmax of 17.2 in the tumorous lesions, respectively. The high TBR led to precise target volume delineation and improved detection of regional lymph node metastases.[66] These findings are in concordance with further conducted studies regarding esophageal cancer.[67–69]

For gastric cancer the same publication described 12 patients (four signet ring cell carcinomas, eight adenocarcinomas) presenting a higher FAP-uptake in comparison with FDG.[69] Furthermore, Pang and colleagues[70] conducted a study with 35 patients evaluating the uptake of ^{68}Ga-FAPI versus ^{18}F-FDG in gastric, duodenal, and colorectal cancers. The measured results indicate that ^{68}Ga-FAPI-PET/CT has a higher sensitivity than ^{18}F-FDG-PET/CT regarding the detection of primary tumors and metastatic lesions, such as bone and visceral metastases leading to upstaging of TNM classification in 21% of all patients.[70] In pancreatic cancer FAP expression or upregulation is connected to desmoplasia and poor prognosis (**Fig. 7**).[47,71] Röhrich and colleagues[72] analyzed the influence of ^{68}Ga-FAPI-PET/CT on oncologic management in 19 patients with pancreatic ductal adenocarcinomas. TNM classification was defined previously by contrast-enhanced CT for each patient. The additional FAPI-PET/CT led to changes in TNM classification in 10 out of 19 patients and therapeutic changes in seven patients.[72] Shi and colleagues[73] conducted a pilot study of 25 patients with hepatic carcinoma analyzing the diagnostic performance of ^{68}Ga-FAPI-04-PET/CT, which presented a high sensitivity in detecting hepatic malignancies. In a further prospective pilot study, Shi and colleagues[74] assessed the potential of ^{68}Ga-FAPI-PET/CT compared with ^{18}F-FDG-PET/CT in 20 patients with suspected hepatic malignancies. The results indicated FAPI to be the superior tracer in detecting primary hepatic lesions.[74] These findings are in concordance with an additional retrospective analysis comparing FAPI, MRI, and FDG in liver cancer conducted by Guo and colleagues.[75] In summary, ^{68}Ga-FAPI-PET/CT might improve tumor staging, relapse detection, and oncologic management in patients with hepatic cancer.

Lower Abdomen

Reporting more than 148,000 estimated new diagnoses of colorectal cancer in the United States in 2020, it presents the third most frequent cancer in terms of incidence and mortality.[62] Multiple studies suggest that CAFs are commonly harbored in malignancies of the lower gastrointestinal tract (**Fig. 8**).[48,76–79] A first study including 28 different kinds of cancer presented promising results regarding colorectal and anal cancer.[80] A further clinical study analyzed 22 patients with malignancies in the lower gastrointestinal tract regarding the role of ^{68}Ga-FAPI-PET/CT. The cohort consisted of six treatment-naive patients, 16 for restaging, and one with possible recurrence presenting a high TBR of more than 3 in most tumor lesions. More specific, colorectal cancer (n = 16) and anal cancer (n = 6) showed an SUVmax of 8.6 and 13.9, respectively. The median SUVmax of all metastases was 7.95. The highest SUVmax uptake was determined in the liver with 9.1, respectively, explained by low background uptake of healthy liver tissue (SUVmax 1.5). In 47% of the patients with metastases (n = 15) new lesions were observed and TNM classification was changed in 50% of all treatment-naive patients leading to high, medium, and low therapeutic modifications in 19%, 33%, and 29% of the patients, respectively. Also, target volume delineation using the ^{68}Ga-FAPI-PET/CT was improved for almost all patients.[81]

Prostate cancer represents the most frequent malignancy in men worldwide. Nevertheless, experiences of FAPI-PET/CT and prostate cancer are still limited, whereas PSMA, another novel radiopharmaceutical, seems to be highly reliable and precise. However, there are indications, such as high-grade prostate cancer with a Gleason score of 8 and higher, where FAP expression

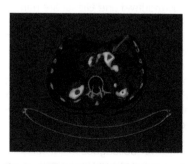
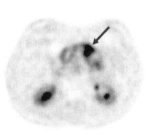
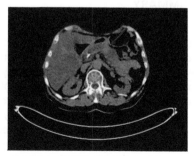

Fig. 7. A 78-year-old man with intraductal papillary mucinous neoplasm underwent a ^{68}Ga-FAPI-PET/CT because of a suspicious lesion in the pancreas, which showed a moderate accumulation of 5.85. The arrows are placed in order to help the reader identify the lesions.

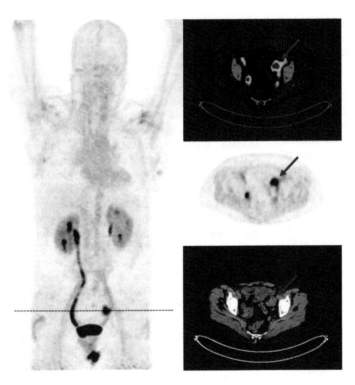

Fig. 8. Because of a suspicious sigmoidal lesion a 59-year-old woman underwent a ^{68}Ga-FAPI-PET/CT. The investigation presented a strong FAP uptake in the sigmoid with an SUV-max of 10.65. In the following surgery the diagnosis was histologically confirmed. The arrows are placed in order to help the reader identify the lesions.

might add value to standard diagnostic imaging. Case studies described a positive FAPI-PET/CT in PSMA-negative tumor phenotype and high interlesional or intralesional heterogeneity.[82,83] However, the experience of FAP-ligands in prostate cancer is still limited and needs further clinical exploration.

In terms of gynecologic tumors, highly promising results were determined in first studies regarding breast, ovarian, and cervical cancer.[80] These initial findings are in concordance with further conducted studies regarding gynecologic malignancies.[55,56,69,84] Two additional individual case studies are describing the influence of external and internal hormones on increased FAP-uptake in breasts and uterus.[85,86]

SUMMARY

FAPI is a novel and highly promising agent for diagnostics and possible theranostic application for various tumor entities and nononcologic diseases. High-contrast images already 10 minutes postinjection are possible because of fast uptake and rapid clearance out of the circulation with reduced radiation doses. Moreover, it seems to be equal or even superior to the current oncologic standard FDG in several malignancies and benign pathologies. For improved comprehension of FAP expression and clinicopathologic conditions, further studies are required.

CLINICS CARE POINTS

- FAPI-PET/CT enhances standard diagnostic imaging and staging and therefore influences therapeutic implications in several tumor entities.
- Non-malignant uptake is encountered exemplary in wound healing, inflammation, hormone-sensitive-tissue and fibrosis.
- Knowledge of causes for uptake and potential pitfalls is thus of essence.

DISCLOSURE

Drs. Haberkorn, Kratochwil and Giesel are named in a patent application (EP 18155420.5) for quinolone-based FAP-targeting agents for imaging and therapy in nuclear medicine. Drs. Kratochwil, Haberkorn and Giesel also have shares of a consultancy group for iTheranostics. Dr. Giesel is also advisor for ABX, SOFIE Biosciences and Telix pharmaceuticals. The other authors declare no potential conflict of interests.

REFERENCES

1. Hamson EJ, Keane FM, Tholen S, et al. Understanding fibroblast activation protein (FAP): substrates,

activities, expression and targeting for cancer therapy. Proteomics Clin Appl 2014;8(5–6):454–63.

2. Cirri P, Chiarugi P. Cancer associated fibroblasts: the dark side of the coin. Am J Cancer Res 2011; 1(4):482–97.

3. Chen WT, Kelly T. Seprase complexes in cellular invasiveness. Cancer Metastasis Rev 2003;22(2–3):259–69.

4. Huang Y, Wang S, Kelly T. Seprase promotes rapid tumor growth and increased microvessel density in a mouse model of human breast cancer. Cancer Res 2004;64(8):2712–6.

5. Kelly T. Fibroblast activation protein-alpha and dipeptidyl peptidase IV (CD26): cell-surface proteases that activate cell signaling and are potential targets for cancer therapy. Drug Resist Updat 2005;8(1–2):51–8.

6. Schmidkonz C, Rauber S, Atzinger A, et al. Disentangling inflammatory from fibrotic disease activity by fibroblast activation protein imaging. Ann Rheum Dis 2020;79(11):1485–91.

7. Jansen K, Heirbaut L, Cheng JD, et al. Selective inhibitors of fibroblast activation protein (FAP) with a (4-quinolinoyl)-glycyl-2-cyanopyrrolidine scaffold. ACS Med Chem Lett 2013;4(5):491–6.

8. Poplawski SE, Lai JH, Li Y, et al. Identification of selective and potent inhibitors of fibroblast activation protein and prolyl oligopeptidase. J Med Chem 2013;56(9):3467–77.

9. Varasteh Z, Mohanta S, Robu S, et al. Molecular imaging of fibroblast activity after myocardial infarction using a 68Ga-labeled fibroblast activation protein inhibitor, FAPI-04. J Nucl Med 2019; 60(12):1743–9.

10. Zi F, He J, He D, et al. Fibroblast activation protein α in tumor microenvironment: recent progression and implications. Mol Med Rep 2015;11:3203–11.

11. Bussard KM, Mutkus L, Stumpf K, et al. Tumor-associated stromal cells as key contributors to the tumor microenvironment. Breast Cancer Res 2016;18(1):84.

12. An Y, Liu F, Chen Y, et al. Crosstalk between cancer-associated fibroblasts and immune cells in cancer. J Cell Mol Med 2020;24(1):13–24.

13. Erdogan B, Webb DJ. Cancer-associated fibroblasts modulate growth factor signaling and extracellular matrix remodeling to regulate tumor metastasis. Biochem Soc Trans 2017;45(1):229–36.

14. Karnoub AE, Dash AB, Vo AP, et al. Mesenchymal stem cells within tumour stroma promote breast cancer metastasis. Nature 2007;449(7162):557–63.

15. Ishii G, Sangai T, Oda T, et al. Bone-marrow-derived myofibroblasts contribute to the cancer-induced stromal reaction. Biochem Biophys Res Commun 2003;309(1):232–40.

16. Blobe GC, Schiemann WP, Lodish HF. Role of transforming growth factor beta in human disease. N Engl J Med 2000;342(18):1350–8.

17. Davidson B, Goldberg I, Kopolovic J. Angiogenesis in uterine cervical intraepithelial neoplasia and squamous cell carcinoma: an immunohistochemical study. Int J Gynecol Pathol 1997;16(4):335–8.

18. Welti J, Loges S, Dimmeler S, et al. Recent molecular discoveries in angiogenesis and antiangiogenic therapies in cancer. J Clin Invest 2013;123(8):3190–200.

19. Zonneville J, Safina A, Truskinovsky AM, et al. TGF-β signaling promotes tumor vasculature by enhancing the pericyte-endothelium association. BMC cancer 2018;18(1):670.

20. Rettig G. Development of retinofugal neuropil areas in the brain of the alpine newt, Triturus alpestris. II. Topographic organization and formation of projections. Anat Embryol 1988;177(3):257–65.

21. Busek P, Hrabal P, Fric P, et al. Co-expression of the homologous proteases fibroblast activation protein and dipeptidyl peptidase-IV in the adult human Langerhans islets. Histochem Cell Biol 2015;143(5):497–504.

22. Bae S, Park CW, Son HK, et al. Fibroblast activation protein alpha identifies mesenchymal stromal cells from human bone marrow. Br J Haematol 2008; 142(5):827–30.

23. Schuberth PC, Hagedorn C, Jensen SM, et al. Treatment of malignant pleural mesothelioma by fibroblast activation protein-specific re-directed T cells. J translational Med 2013;11:187.

24. Tillmanns J, Hoffmann D, Habbaba Y, et al. Fibroblast activation protein alpha expression identifies activated fibroblasts after myocardial infarction. J Mol Cell Cardiol 2015;87:194–203.

25. Nagaraju CK, Dries E, Popovic N, et al. Global fibroblast activation throughout the left ventricle but localized fibrosis after myocardial infarction. Sci Rep 2017;7:10801.

26. Bauer S, Jendro MC, Wadle A, et al. Fibroblast activation protein is expressed by rheumatoid myofibroblast-like synoviocytes. Arthritis Res Ther 2006;8(6):R171.

27. Garin-Chesa P, Old LJ, Rettig WJ. Cell surface glycoprotein of reactive stromal fibroblasts as a potential antibody target in human epithelial cancers. Proc Natl Acad Sci U S A 1990;87(18):7235–9.

28. Loktev A, Lindner T, Mier W, et al. A tumor-imaging method targeting cancer-associated fibroblasts. J Nucl Med 2018;59(9):1423–9.

29. Rettig WJ, Garin-Chesa P, Beresford HR, et al. Cell-surface glycoproteins of human sarcomas: differential expression in normal and malignant tissues and cultured cells. Proc Natl Acad Sci U S A 1988;85(9):3110–4.

30. Ge Y, Zhan F, Barlogie B, et al. Fibroblast activation protein (FAP) is upregulated in myelomatous bone and supports myeloma cell survival. Br J Haematol 2006;133(1):83–92.

31. Aimes RT, Zijlstra A, Hooper JD, et al. Endothelial cell serine proteases expressed during vascular morphogenesis and angiogenesis. Thromb Haemost 2003;89(3):561–72.

32. Bhati R, Patterson C, Livasy CA, et al. Molecular characterization of human breast tumor vascular cells. Am J Pathol 2008;172(5):1381–90.

33. Mori Y, Kono K, Matsumoto Y, et al. The expression of a type II transmembrane serine protease (seprase) in human gastric carcinoma. Oncology 2004;67(5–6):411–9.

34. Okada K, Chen WT, Iwasa S, et al. Seprase, a membrane-type serine protease, has different expression patterns in intestinal- and diffuse-type gastric cancer. Oncology 2003;65(4):363–70.

35. Iwasa S, Okada K, Chen WT, et al. Increased expression of seprase, a membrane-type serine protease, is associated with lymph node metastasis in human colorectal cancer. Cancer Lett 2005;227(2):229–36.

36. Saigusa S, Toiyama Y, Tanaka K, et al. Cancer-associated fibroblasts correlate with poor prognosis in rectal cancer after chemoradiotherapy. Int J Oncol 2011;38(3):655–63.

37. Tchou J, Zhang PJ, Bi Y, et al. Fibroblast activation protein expression by stromal cells and tumor-associated macrophages in human breast cancer. Hum Pathol 2013;44(11):2549–57.

38. Arnold JN, Magiera L, Kraman M, et al. Tumoral immune suppression by macrophages expressing fibroblast activation protein-α and heme oxygenase-1. Cancer Immunol Res 2014;2(2):121–6.

39. Mueller SC, Ghersi G, Akiyama SK, et al. A novel protease-docking function of integrin at invadopodia. J Biol Chem 1999;274(35):24947–52.

40. Chen WT, Kelly T, Ghersi G. DPPIV, seprase, and related serine peptidases in multiple cellular functions. Curr Top Dev Biol 2003;54:207–32.

41. Keane FM, Nadvi NA, Yao TW, et al. Neuropeptide Y, B-type natriuretic peptide, substance P and peptide YY are novel substrates of fibroblast activation protein-α. FEBS J 2011;278(8):1316–32.

42. Park JE, Lenter MC, Zimmermann RN, et al. Fibroblast activation protein, a dual specificity serine protease expressed in reactive human tumor stromal fibroblasts. J Biol Chem 1999;274(51):36505–12.

43. Lee EW, Michalkiewicz M, Kitlinska J, et al. Neuropeptide Y induces ischemic angiogenesis and restores function of ischemic skeletal muscles. J Clin Invest 2003;111(12):1853–62.

44. Zukowska Z, Pons J, Lee EW, et al. Neuropeptide Y: a new mediator linking sympathetic nerves, blood vessels and immune system? Can J Physiol Pharmacol 2003;81(2):89–94.

45. Lo A, Wang LS, Scholler J, et al. Tumor-promoting desmoplasia is disrupted by depleting FAP-expressing stromal cells. Cancer Res 2015;75(14):2800–10.

46. Busek P, Mateu R, Zubal M, et al. Targeting fibroblast activation protein in cancer: prospects and caveats. Front Biosci (Landmark Ed) 2018;23:1933–68.

47. Cohen SJ, Alpaugh RK, Palazzo I, et al. Fibroblast activation protein and its relationship to clinical outcome in pancreatic adenocarcinoma. Pancreas 2008;37(2):154–8.

48. Henry LR, Lee HO, Lee JS, et al. Clinical implications of fibroblast activation protein in patients with colon cancer. Clin Cancer Res 2007;13(6):1736–41.

49. Ju MJ, Qiu SJ, Fan J, et al. Peritumoral activated hepatic stellate cells predict poor clinical outcome in hepatocellular carcinoma after curative resection. Am J Clin Pathol 2009;131(4):498–510.

50. Zhang Y, Tang H, Cai J, et al. Ovarian cancer-associated fibroblasts contribute to epithelial ovarian carcinoma metastasis by promoting angiogenesis, lymphangiogenesis and tumor cell invasion. Cancer Lett 2011;303(1):47–55.

51. Loktev A, Lindner T, Burger EM, et al. Development of fibroblast activation protein-targeted radiotracers with improved tumor retention. J Nucl Med 2019; 60(10):1421–9.

52. Giesel F, Adeberg S, Syed M, et al. FAPI-74 PET/CT using either 18F-AlF or cold-kit 68Ga-labeling: biodistribution, radiation dosimetry and tumor delineation in lung cancer patients. J Nucl Med 2020;62(2):201–7.

53. Lindner T, Loktev A, Altmann A, et al. Development of quinoline-based theranostic ligands for the targeting of fibroblast activation protein. J Nucl Med 2018; 59(9):1415–22.

54. Giesel FL, Kratochwil C, Lindner T, et al. 68Ga-FAPI PET/CT: biodistribution and preliminary dosimetry estimate of 2 DOTA-containing FAP-targeting agents in patients with various cancers. J Nucl Med 2019; 60(3):386–92.

55. Meyer C, Dahlbom M, Lindner T, et al. Radiation dosimetry and biodistribution of 68Ga-FAPI-46 PET imaging in cancer patients. J Nucl Med 2020;61(8):1171–7.

56. Chen H, Pang Y, Wu J, et al. Comparison of [68Ga] Ga-DOTA-FAPI-04 and [18F] FDG PET/CT for the diagnosis of primary and metastatic lesions in patients with various types of cancer. Eur J Nucl Med Mol Imaging 2020;47(8):1820–32.

57. Fu W, Liu L, Liu H, et al. Increased FAPI uptake in brain metastasis from lung cancer on 68Ga-FAPI PET/CT. Clin Nucl Med 2021;46(1):e1–2.

58. Giesel FL, Heussel CP, Lindner T, et al. FAPI-PET/CT improves staging in a lung cancer patient with cerebral metastasis. Eur J Nucl Med Mol Imaging 2019; 46(8):1754–5.

59. Röhrich M, Loktev A, Wefers AK, et al. IDH-wildtype glioblastomas and grade III/IV IDH-mutant gliomas show elevated tracer uptake in fibroblast activation protein-specific PET/CT. Eur J Nucl Med Mol Imaging 2019;46(12):2569–80.

60. Windisch P, Röhrich M, Regnery S, et al. Fibroblast activation protein (FAP) specific PET for advanced target volume delineation in glioblastoma. Radiother Oncol 2020;150:159–63.

61. Syed M, Flechsig P, Liermann J, et al. Fibroblast activation protein inhibitor (FAPI) PET for diagnostics

and advanced targeted radiotherapy in head and neck cancers. Eur J Nucl Med Mol Imaging 2020; 47(12):2836–45.

62. Siegel RL, Miller KD, Jemal A. Cancer statistics, 2020. CA Cancer J Clin 2020;70(1):7–30.

63. Hao B, Wu J, Pang Y, et al. 68Ga-FAPI PET/CT in assessment of leptomeningeal metastases in a patient with lung adenocarcinoma. Clin Nucl Med 2020;45(10):784–6.

64. Heckmann MB, Reinhardt F, Finke D, et al. Relationship between cardiac fibroblast activation protein activity by positron emission tomography and cardiovascular disease. Circ Cardiovasc Imaging 2020;13(9):e010628.

65. Siebermair J, Köhler MI, Kupusovic J, et al. Cardiac fibroblast activation detected by Ga-68 FAPI PET imaging as a potential novel biomarker of cardiac injury/remodeling. J Nucl Cardiol 2020. https://doi. org/10.1007/s12350-020-02307-w.

66. Ristau J, Giesel FL, Haefner MF, et al. Impact of primary staging with fibroblast activation protein specific Enzyme inhibitor (FAPI)-PET/CT on radio-oncologic treatment planning of patients with esophageal cancer. Mol Imaging Biol 2020;22(6):1495–500.

67. Liu Q, Shi S, Xu X, et al. The superiority of [68Ga]-FAPI-04 over [18F]-FDG PET/CT in imaging metastatic esophageal squamous cell carcinoma. Eur J Nucl Med Mol Imaging 2020. https://doi.org/10.1007/ s00259-020-04997-3.

68. Zhao L, Chen S, Lin L, et al. [68Ga]Ga-DOTA-FAPI-04 improves tumor staging and monitors early response to chemoradiotherapy in a patient with esophageal cancer. Eur J Nucl Med Mol Imaging 2020;47(13):3188–9.

69. Chen H, Zhao L, Ruan D, et al. Usefulness of [68Ga] Ga-DOTA-FAPI-04 PET/CT in patients presenting with inconclusive [18F]FDG PET/CT findings. Eur J Nucl Med Mol Imaging 2020. https://doi.org/10. 1007/s00259-020-04940-6.

70. Pang Y, Zhao L, Luo Z, et al. Comparison of 68Ga-FAPI and 18F-FDG uptake in gastric, duodenal, and colorectal cancers. Radiology 2020;298(2): 393–402.

71. Shi M, Yu DH, Chen Y, et al. Expression of fibroblast activation protein in human pancreatic adenocarcinoma and its clinicopathological significance. World J Gastroenterol 2012;18(8):840–6.

72. Röhrich M, Naumann P, Giesel FL, et al. Impact of 68Ga-FAPI-PET/CT imaging on the therapeutic management of primary and recurrent pancreatic ductal adenocarcinomas. J Nucl Med 2020. https://doi.org/ 10.2967/jnumed.120.253062.

73. Shi X, Xing H, Yang X, et al. Fibroblast imaging of hepatic carcinoma with 68Ga-FAPI-04 PET/CT: a pilot study in patients with suspected hepatic nodules. Eur J Nucl Med Mol Imaging 2020. https://doi.org/ 10.1007/s00259-020-04882-z.

74. Shi X, Xing H, Yang X, et al. Comparison of PET imaging of activated fibroblasts and 18F-FDG for diagnosis of primary hepatic tumours: a prospective pilot study. Eur J Nucl Med Mol Imaging 2020. https://doi. org/10.1007/s00259-020-05070-9.

75. Guo W, Pang Y, Yao L, et al. Imaging fibroblast activation protein in liver cancer: a single-center post hoc retrospective analysis to compare [68Ga]Ga-FAPI-04 PET/CT versus MRI and [18F]-FDG PET/ CT. Eur J Nucl Med Mol Imaging 2020. https://doi. org/10.1007/s00259-020-05095-0.

76. Henriksson ML, Edin S, Dahlin AM, et al. Colorectal cancer cells activate adjacent fibroblasts resulting in FGF1/FGFR3 signaling and increased invasion. Am J Pathol 2011;178(3):1387–94.

77. Lotti F, Jarrar AM, Pai RK, et al. Chemotherapy activates cancer-associated fibroblasts to maintain colorectal cancer-initiating cells by IL-17A. J Exp Med 2013;210(13):2851–72.

78. Tommelein J, Verset L, Boterberg T, et al. Cancer-associated fibroblasts connect metastasis-promoting communication in colorectal cancer. Front Oncol 2015;5:63.

79. Wikberg ML, Edin S, Lundberg IV, et al. High intratumoral expression of fibroblast activation protein (FAP) in colon cancer is associated with poorer patient prognosis. Tumour Biol 2013;34(2):1013–20.

80. Kratochwil C, Flechsig P, Lindner T, et al. 68Ga-FAPI PET/CT: tracer uptake in 28 different kinds of cancer. J Nucl Med 2019;60(6):801–5.

81. Koerber SA, Staudinger F, Kratochwil C, et al. The role of 68Ga-FAPI PET/CT for patients with malignancies of the lower gastrointestinal tract: first clinical experience. J Nucl Med 2020;61(9):1331–6.

82. Khreish F, Rosar F, Kratochwil C, et al. Positive FAPI-PET/CT in a metastatic castration-resistant prostate cancer patient with PSMA-negative/FDG-positive disease. Eur J Nucl Med Mol Imaging 2020;47(8):2040–1.

83. Xu T, Zhao Y, Ding H, et al. [68Ga]Ga-DOTA-FAPI-04 PET/CT imaging in a case of prostate cancer with shoulder arthritis. Eur J Nucl Med Mol Imaging 2020. https://doi.org/10.1007/s00259-020-05028-x.

84. Pang Y, Zhao L, Chen H. 68Ga-FAPI Outperforms 18F-FDG PET/CT in identifying bone metastasis and peritoneal carcinomatosis in a patient with metastatic breast cancer. Clin Nucl Med 2020;45(11):913–5.

85. Sonni I, Lee-Felker S, Memarzadeh S, et al. 68Ga-FAPi-46 diffuse bilateral breast uptake in a patient with cervical cancer after hormonal stimulation. Eur J Nucl Med Mol Imaging 2020. https://doi.org/10. 1007/s00259-020-04947-z.

86. Dendl K, Koerber SA, Adeberg S, Röhrich M, Kratochwil C, Haberkorn U, Giesel FL. Physiological FAP-activation in a postpartum woman observed in oncological FAPI-PET/CT. Eur J Nucl Med Mol Imaging. 2021 Feb 4. https://doi.org/10.1007/s00259-021-05203-8. Epub ahead of print.

Neuroendocrine Tumors
Imaging Perspective

Rebecca K.S. Wong, MSc, MBChB[a,b], Ur Metser, MD[c,d], Patrick Veit-Haibach, MD[c,d,*]

KEYWORDS

• PET imaging • 68-Gallium DOTA-peptides • Neuroendocrine tumors • Theranostic • Dosimetry
• Outcome prediction

KEY POINTS

• 68-Gallium PET imaging identifies neuroendocrine tumors with high accuracy depending on grading.
• A standardized individualized dosimetry process is feasible in a multicenter setting. It is expected to be the cornerstone for improving the therapeutic ratio of theranostics in NET.
• On pretreatment ^{68}Ga-DOTA-peptide PET, tumor maximal standardized uptake value correlates with therapy response and tumor heterogeneity correlates inversely with time to progression and overall survival.

INTRODUCTION

Neuroendocrine tumor (NET) is an orphan disease and is increasing in incidence. Part of that trend is attributed to better, earlier, and more sensitive detection methods, including imaging. These tumors have several different biological features and are thus considered clinically a very heterogeneous group. In general, there are the well-differentiated grade 1 and 2 tumors. There is also a group of slow-growing and still well-differentiated grade 3 tumors. However, within the grade 3 tumor groups, there are also aggressive and poorly differentiated grade 3 tumors. Also, NETs show a wide range of clinical presentation and behavior, partly based on whether they are hormone secreting or not. Because this inhomogeneous group of tumors is increasing in incidence, there has also been an increasing interest in exploring therapy options for patients. Although there has been steady development of therapies

for patients with different stages of NETs, in patients who do not respond to standard therapy there is now an additional option available.

Especially in well-differentiated (G1/2) NET, peptide radionuclide receptor therapy (PRRT) has now been shown to be effective in prolonging progression-free survival with trends toward survival benefits in patients with metastatic gastroenteropancreatic (GEP) tumors. The hallmark of overexpression of somatostatin receptors (SSRs) in well-differentiated tumors meant that imaging plays a critical role in the entire patient journey. Molecular imaging has become an integral part of understanding the full extent of disease, tumoral heterogeneity, and patient selection for radionuclide therapy. Patients now undergo hybrid molecular imaging at different stages of their disease: for initial detection of the primary tumors in the correct clinical setting; for restaging in case of clinical suspicion of recurrence; for evaluation of NET-suggestive findings on computed tomography (CT)

[a] Radiation Medicine Program, Princess Margaret Cancer Center, University Health Network, 610 University Ave, Toronto, ON M5G 2M9, Canada; [b] Department of Radiation Oncology Temerty Faculty of Medicine, University of Toronto, 149 College Street, Suite 504, Toronto, ON M5T 1P5, Canada; [c] Joint Department Medical Imaging, University Health Network, Mount Sinai Hospital & Women's College Hospital, University of Toronto, 610 University Ave, Suite 3-920, Toronto, ON M5G 2M9, Canada; [d] Department of Medical Imaging, University of Toronto, 263 McCaul Street, 4th Floor, Toronto, ON M5T 1W7, Canada
* Corresponding author. Toronto General Hospital, 1 PMB-275, 585 University Avenue, Toronto, ON M5G 2N2.
E-mail address: Patrick.Veit-Haibach@uhn.ca

PET Clin 16 (2021) 353–364
https://doi.org/10.1016/j.cpet.2021.03.002
1556-8598/21/© 2021 Elsevier Inc. All rights reserved.

or magnetic resonance (MR) imaging; or, in the context of PRRT, for evaluation of qualification of patients for PRRT therapies. It has been shown that the imaging of NETs with somatostatin analogues in the adequate clinical context is not only the most sensitive and specific method compared with the previously used octreotide scan, CT, or MR but also has a significant clinical impact on decision making in conventional therapies, let alone the implications for PRRT itself. In the context of PRRT, it has been used to quantify the radiation dose absorbed, enabling individualized dosimetry. Widespread use of individualized dosimetry has the potential of improving safety, although standardization of process needs to be established to ensure data generated across centers are comparable. The same mechanism can be used to individualize the dose absorbed by tumors with the potential for increased efficacy. Tumor image characteristics and response to treatment are expected to have the potential of predicting clinical outcomes. Several approaches are currently being investigated in research studies addressing the question of tumor/imaging heterogeneity, possible dual-tracer studies, accurate quantification for small lesions, as well as technical questions such as motion correction. This article discusses the state-of-the-art and emerging trends in molecular imaging for diagnosis, treatment individualization, and prognostication as it relates to the use of PRRT. It is anticipated that the optimal and future innovative use of imaging tools will be the cornerstone of improving survival and quality of life for patients with NETs.

ROLE OF PET IMAGING TO IDENTIFY PATIENTS WITH SOMATOSTATIN RECEPTOR POSITIVITY

In the past, NET have been imaged with standard cross-sectional imaging such as multiphase CT or multiparametric MR imaging. Early on, nuclear medicine techniques such as octreotide-based imaging complimented these cross-sectional imaging modalities. However, with the introduction of the radiolabeled somatostatin analogues ^{68}Ga-DOTATATE [DOTA, Tyr(3)-octreotate], ^{68}Ga-DOTANOC [DOTA,1-Nal(3)-octreotide], and ^{68}Ga-DOTATOC [DOTA, D-Phe1, Tyr(3)-octreotide], PET imaging has become the main imaging modality in staging and therapy follow-up after PET/CT or PET/MR in many jurisdictions. At present, molecular imaging with the named peptides is already integrated in the diagnostic part of clinical care guidelines.[1] There are a few summarizing meta-analyses available on the use of PET imaging using DOTA-peptides, and, overall, multiple studies have shown the value of DOTA-TATE/DOTATOC/DOTANOC PET imaging in patients with different types of NETs.[2,3]

A recent, relatively specific meta-analysis was performed on the detection and staging of pancreatic-only NET, with 18 studies being evaluated overall, comprising 1143 patients. Several studies focusing on specific indications were included (namely insulinomas, von Hippel-Lindau, and multiple endocrine neoplasia type 1). Overall, satisfying results were found for the sensitivity and tumor detection, with excellent results for specificity.

The study reported a pooled sensitivity of SSR-PET/CT for the assessment of primary pancreatic NET of 79.6% (95% confidence interval [CI], 70.5%–87%) and specificity of 95% (75%–100%). A heterogeneity of 59.6% and 51.5%, respectively (both P = nonsignificant) was found. In addition, the pooled diagnostic odds ratio was 35.579 (95% CI, 4.673–270.90), with a heterogeneity of 21% concerning the detection rates for primary pancreatic NET.

Pooled detection rates for the primary tumors in the patient-based analysis were 81% (95% CI, 65%–90%) and 92% (95% CI, 80%–97%) for the lesion-based analysis.

More importantly, the influence on and change in patient management compared with standard work-up was found to be up to 39%. Although these are compelling results, there are several aspects that need to be considered. Many studies reported in this overview did not include histopathology as the standard of reference; however, demanding a clinical biopsy for every lesion is not possible for technical and ethical reasons, especially in patients with disseminated metastases. Also, although most studies reported on diagnostic accuracy, only a few studies evaluated prognostication of ^{68}Ga-DOTA-peptide PET. Also, there were differences seen in detection of primary tumors versus metastases. This finding can be explained by technical reasons (size of lung lesions, smearing artifacts) as well as pathophysiologic reasons such as varying degree of SSR density in primary tumor and/or metastases.

A more overarching meta-analysis, of GEP NET in general, found an even higher diagnostic accuracy for DOTA-peptide PET imaging[3] (example are shown in **Figs. 1**A and B) After evaluation of 22 articles and with overall 2105 patients included, there was a pooled sensitivity of 93% (95% CI, 91%–94%). The specificity was similar at 96% (95% CI, 95%–98%). Accordingly, the area under the summary receiver operating characteristic curve was 0.98 (95% CI, 0.95–1.0).

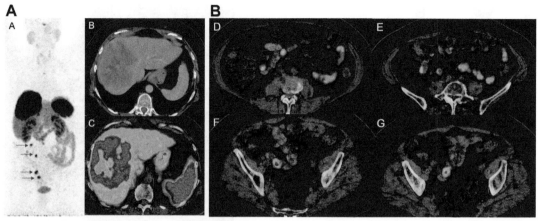

Fig. 1. A 59-year-old woman with large necrotic liver mass and increased cromogranin A level (151 ng/mL). Patient underwent extended right hepatectomy with histology showing well-differentiated NET (Ki-67, 2%); unknown primary tumor. Maximum intensity projection (MIP) (*A*) images and axial CT (*B*) and PET/CT (*C*) images. Ga-DOTATATE PET-CT shows somatostatin receptor overexpression in the large hepatic mass with central photopenia secondary to necrosis. The MIP image shows multiple foci of DOTATATE uptake in the right abdomen (*red arrows*). (*B*) Axial coregistered PET-CT image shows multiple DOTATATE avid lesions in loops of small bowel (*D, F, G*) and in small mesenteric lymph nodes (*E*) in keeping with multifocal NET.

These impactful findings show again the value of PET imaging in staging, therapy response, and thereby also for definition and selection of patients for PRRT.

JOINT ¹⁸F-FLUORODEOXYGLUCOSE AND ⁶⁸GA-DOTA-PEPTIDE PET/COMPUTED TOMOGRAPHY USE IN THE EVALUATION OF NEUROENDOCRINE TUMOR

Several studies evaluated the diagnostic accuracy and, hence, the usefulness of ^{18}F-fluorodeoxyglucose (FDG) PET/CT versus ^{68}Ga-DOTA-peptide PET/CT for therapy planning. In a large comparison including 30 studies with overall 3401 evaluated patients, it was shown on a per-patient basis that the overall sensitivity for DOTA-peptide PET/CT versus FDG-PET/CT was as high as 0.92 (95% CI, 0.89–0.95) versus 0.70 (95% CI, 0.41–0.89).[4] However, the specificity was similar: 0.91 (95% CI, 0.83–0.95) versus 0.97 (95% CI, 0.70–1.00). The diagnostic odds ratio of the two methods were 119 (95% CI, 51–282) versus 119 (95% CI, 51–282), and the overall areas under the curves (AUCs) were 0.96 (0.94–0.98) and 0.94 (0.92–0.96). However, significant differences were found in terms of grading and Ki-67 index. Although well-differentiated tumors (G1) showed higher sensitivity when imaging with SSR-PET/CT, FDG-PET/CT showed similar higher detection rates in moderately and poorly differentiated tumors. Additional studies summarizing articles that directly compared results of FDG-PET/CT and ^{68}Ga-DOTA-peptide PET imaging showed

similar results. In 1 analysis, 7 studies with overall 236 patients were evaluated, including a significant number of neuroendocrine lung tumors.[5] Here, both examinations might reveal complementary information concerning the underlying biological behavior, predominantly in moderately and poorly differentiated tumors. In many tumor types, FDG-PET/CT is known to correlate with viability, aggressiveness, and even hypoxia and can provide prognostication. Similarly in this patient cohort, it was described that FDG avidity was associated with a worse prognosis (progression-free survival or overall survival). It was also pointed out that the combination of ^{68}Ga-DOTA-peptide imaging and FDG imaging showed the highest sensitivity in primary tumor detection. In contrast, imaging derived from ^{68}Ga-DOTA-peptide PET/CT provided the information on SSR density and expression of tumors, which in turn offers evaluation of tumor differentiation and guidance for targeted PRRT (see also the example in **Fig. 2**).

OUTSTANDING QUESTIONS IN IMAGING OF NEUROENDOCRINE TUMORS FOR PEPTIDE RADIONUCLIDE RECEPTOR THERAPY PLANNING

Although there is a solid body of literature underlining the value of ^{68}Ga-DOTA-peptide PET/CT and FDG imaging for characterization, prognostication, and targeted therapy planning, there are still many aspects to be evaluated. Many of the cited studies had varying clinical and imaging reference standards, and histopathology was only available

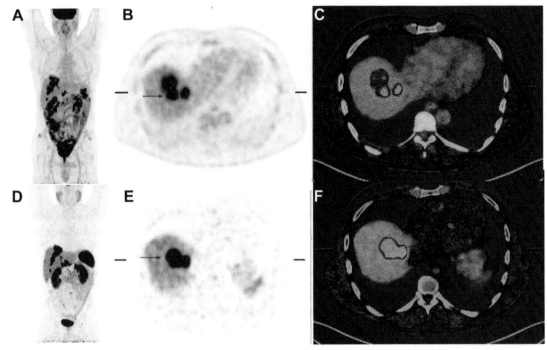

Fig. 2. Patient with a primary NET in the pancreatic neck with liver metastases. FDG-PET/CT (*top row*) shows partly different tracer distribution compared with the DOTATATE PET/CT (*bottom row*). FDG-PET/CT MIP (*A*), axial PET (*B*), and PET/CT (*C*) images show 2 discrete foci of uptake in the metastases in the liver dome (*red arrows in B*). The DOTATATE PET/CT MIP (*D*), axial PET (*E*), and PET/CT (*F*) show more homogeneous uptake in this metastases. The findings of both imaging methods complement information concerning tumor heterogeneity and differentiation.

in a minority of patients. Although it is ethically challenging in clinical routine to obtain biopsies from many tumors lesions, it leaves some uncertainty about the overall accuracy of those studies. Furthermore, there is currently no agreement on the value of standardized uptake value (SUV) measurements or ratios for tumor characterization, and especially not for PRRT planning. Although Krenning score is one measure that is documented and that is adopted by many centers, no further validation has been published.

There are also several logistical issues that are left unanswered: although the value of both FDG-PET/CT and ^{68}Ga-DOTA-peptide PET/CT is widely documented and was discussed earlier, it is not known when exactly is the best time point to use one or the other imaging methods. There are arguments to use them both in the beginning/at the time point of the initial diagnosis to have a full baseline tumor and tumor spread characterization. Also, serial additional FDG imaging might be beneficial later during the course of the patient's disease, especially when there are signs of progression. There is no consensus on the degree of disease progression that would trigger

additional FDG imaging or whether additional FDG imaging should always be used for follow-up after documented progression. In addition, the role of PET/MR versus PET/CT is not entirely clear either.[6,7] Although ^{68}Ga-DOTA-peptide–based PET/MR is already mentioned in the National Comprehensive Cancer Network (NCCN) guidelines for diagnosis, only a few studies have imaged patients with NETs with PET/MR in a systematic way. The role in primary staging of gastroentero-NETs is understandable, given the higher diagnostic accuracy of the MR component in detection of pancreatic, bowel, or lever lesions compared with PET/CT. However, the role in follow-up imaging, especially in a metastatic setting is unclear.

IMAGING TO QUANTIFY DOSE

Peptide receptor radionuclide therapy, a molecular guided form of radiotherapy, exerts its therapeutic effect on cancer through depositing radiation dose to cancer cells. The degree of cellular injury achievable is a function of radiation dose deposited. In contrast with external beam radiotherapy, the energy deposited across tumors is heterogeneous, being a function of the degree of molecular target overexpression, distribution of cancer deposits, the particle travel length, physical half-life, and the biological half-life of the isotope. Being able to quantify the radiation dose absorbed is critical to designing ways to augment the therapeutic effect of radiopharmaceuticals.

CAN DOSE ABSORBED BE PREDICTED BASED ON FUNCTIONAL IMAGING?

Given that theranostics pairs are targeting the same receptors, with ^{68}Ga-labeled peptides being used most widely for the identification of patients with SSR overexpression (and therefore suitability for PRRT), it seems logical that it should be useful for predicting radiation dose absorbed when therapy such as ^{177}Lu-DOTATATE is delivered. However, the extent to which the radiopharmaceutical is retained at the cellular level, the difference in the physical half-life, and the pace at which it is cleared biologically each affect the complex relationship between activity seen on the diagnostic scan and the radiation dose absorbed with each treatment. Some correlations have been described. A study involving 11 patients receiving PRRT for meningioma[8] suggested a positive correlation between ^{68}Ga-labeled somatostatin analogue pretreatment and the estimated dose delivered following PRRT. In another study involving 21 patients with NET,[9] pretherapy ^{68}Ga-DOTATATE PET/CT may predict tumor-absorbed doses with ^{177}Lu-OCTREOTATE. However, robust correlation is currently lacking to support the use of molecular imaging to predict tumor dose absorbed in a quantitative (and spatially) useful way clinically.

THE PRINCIPLES OF INDIVIDUALIZED DOSIMETRY

The term individualized dosimetry was first popularized by Sandstrom and colleagues[10] in 2010. Many of the methods described in his publications remain the backbone for individualized dosimetry that is achievable in clinical practice. Individualized dosimetry (the process of quantifying radiation dose absorbed) typically involves serial quantitative imaging following delivery of a dose of radiopharmaceutical. Through mathematical computation, activity detected is converted into dose absorbed in organs at risk (eg, kidney and bone marrow) with the goal of modifying future dose prescriptions tailored to each patient's biology. The same mechanism can be used to quantify radiation dose absorbed by tumors. The physical and biological complexities around

individualized dosimetry mean that the degree of uncertainty around estimating dose absorbed is significant, which needs to be taken into consideration. In contrast with the processes that exist in external beam radiotherapy delivery, standardization and consensus of the methodologies is in evolution.

Guidelines published by professional organizations such as the European Association of Nuclear Medicine (EANM)[11] and Society of Nuclear Medicine and Molecular Imaging (SNMMI)[12] provide excellent state-of-the-art evidence and recommendations for clinical practice. Commentaries in recent years capture the debate of the pros and cons of including individualized dosimetry in clinical practice.[13–15] External beam radiation, another way of delivering radiation dose, has the ability to cure and palliate through disease control, and the concept of molecular radiotherapy targeting tumors with radiation through their biological characteristics is an extremely attractive tool that is expected to have a role to play in a broad spectrum of diseases in the future, including adjuvant and curative settings. A fixed-dose approach as described in the NETTER-1 randomized trial[16] is accompanied by very favorable toxicity profiles. This finding would lend support to the hypothesis that, if higher doses can be delivered safely and tailored to patient and tumor characteristics, further improvement in treatment effects can be accomplished.

Medical internal radiation dose (MIRD) formalism, originally developed for the calculation of effective dose in diagnostic procedures, is currently the basis of dosimetry evaluations in clinical practice. The traditional MIRD approach uses a so-called standard man, an anatomic model to estimate the average absorbed dose to a targeted organ from a specified source. Sandstrom and colleagues[10] provided one of the first clinical reports of this approach in the use of ^{177}Lu-DOTATATE in NETs, using single-photon emission CT (SPECT) imaging and small volume of interest (4 cm^3). Using Monte Carlo calculations as the gold standard, the methods described by Sandstrom and colleagues[10] showed SPECT and small volume of interest to be more reliable and feasible than whole-organ dosimetry. Extensive guidance on MIRD application in quantitative dosimetry has been published and is beyond the scope of this article. The recent guidance by SNMMI MIRD committee,[5] pamphlet 23,[9] provides general guidance, and pamphlet 26[17] provides specific examples from 2 institutions.

Beyond the use of MIRD, other methods, such as voxel-level dose kernel convolution and Monte Carlo simulation, provide more accurate quantification.[18] A recent report comparing these 3 methods suggests that voxel-level dose computation shows stronger agreement than MIRD,[19] although the latter is more feasible, accessible, and will likely continue to be the method of choice. In contrast with software and planning systems that are available and widely used in clinical practice for external beam radiotherapy to support dose calculations, systems in support of individualized dosimetry capable of handling three-dimensional imaging have only recently been released and are expected to have a significant impact on practice.

VARIABILITY AND STANDARDIZATION OF INDIVIDUALIZED DOSIMETRY

One of the major barrier to universal adoption of individualized dosimetry is the complexity of the process, burden on patients, and cost. The North American Neuroendocrine Tumor Society (NANETS)/SNMMI published in July 2019 consensus guidelines for the administration of ^{177}Lu-DOTATATE, guidance for dosimetry and posttreatment imaging, and a checklist of essential elements for patient-specific dosimetry. Investigators are actively exploring ways of simplifying the workflow for individualized dosimetry while preserving accuracy and reproducibility.

One important variable is the minimum number of time points that are required to construct the activity curve. Traditionally, multiple time points (eg, 3–5 evaluations over the course of 5 days) are recommended. A single-time-point imaging study after treatment has definite appeal, has been met with some success, and is gaining popularity. The method requires prior knowledge of the effective clearance rate constant (k) for a specific radiopharmaceutical in a representative population. Under conditions in which the range over which the rate constant among individuals is not too extreme, the error in estimating the total integrated activity from a single-time-point approach can be less than 10%.[13] However, the optimal time for the single measurement remains to be defined. Depending on the study population, 48 hours[20] and 96 hours[21] were suggested. The optimal choice will be a function of the tracer of interest, organs of interest, and variations within the population of interest. This approach is potentially useful for most patients with normal physiology, but less accurate for patients who potentially will benefit from it the most. Large databases of patient populations, including diverse populations such as those with borderline renal function, are needed to apply this method.

An alternative approach was reported by Del Prete and colleagues[22] comparing the single-time-point (day 3) approach with 2 time points (days 1 and 3), and a hybrid approach for different cycles using data from a sample of 79 patients. The investigators found the 2-time-point approach provided stronger correlation with the 3-time-points approach (days 0, 1, and 3) (standard in this study) for both kidney and tumor, with median relative errors of less than 2%, representing a good balance between feasibility, accuracy, and reproducibility, and was the method recommended by the investigators. The authors applied a similar approach in 81 patients who completed 3 SPECT images (days 0, 1, and 3) enrolled in our prospective clinical trial and found similar results when using the 2-time-point approach. We also explored the effect of using 2 different time points; namely, days 0 and 3 and days 1 and 3. We found days 0 and 3 to provide superior correlation to the 3-time-point approach (standard in our study). The method using days 0 and 3 seems to be particularly attractive, requiring only 1 extra visit for imaging, and may be a good strategy for widespread clinical use.[23] Further validation with different datasets is warranted.

ENSURING CONSISTENCY OF DOSE ESTIMATES ACROSS CENTERS THROUGH QUALITY ASSURANCE

Given the variations that can exist across equipment and the details in which the individualized dosimetry methodology is applied, are dose estimates equivalent and agnostic to center of acquisition? In the absence of standardized approaches at multiple levels within the individualized dosimetry workflow, the answer is almost certainly no. Arriving at a minimum standard for quantification and reporting of dose absorbed will likely be the cornerstone for universal application and future advances in treatment delivery.

Ontario, Canada, initiated a multicenter single-arm, prospective-study, individualized dosimetry ^{177}Lu-DOTATATE therapy for all patients across 4 cancer centers.[24] Each center identified its own gamma cameras that will be used for acquisition of SPECT images for the study. A study protocol with a shared image acquisition manual and a quality assurance program to support the individualized dosimetry process was designed and implemented (Table 1). In our study, the individualized dosimetry process required patients to undergo planar and SPECT images on days 0, 1, and 3 after each cycle. Treatment consisted of 4 cycles. We used a fixed dose of 7.4 GBq for cycle 1, whereas subsequent cycles were adjusted based on individualized

Table 1
Quality assurance procedures for multicenter individualized dosimetry process

Purpose	Quality Assurance Procedures
Calibration of SPECT/CT and generation of camera-specific sensitivity factor	• Study-specific laboratory manual consisting of procedures for SPECT/CT calibration was provided • A known quality of ^{177}Lu and a phantom was delivered to each center to perform the procedure • All data generated were reviewed by dosimetry working group (medical physicists) to reconcile inconsistencies before patient accrual
Verification that sensitivity factor remains valid over the duration of the study	• A known activity of ^{177}Lu (typically from the radiopharmaceutical delivered for treatment with known activity confirmed on receipt at the treatment site) was placed adjacent to the patient during each SEPCT/CT imaging session
Quality check and assurance of anonymized SPECT/CT images exported to the dosimetry center	• Quality control of all images for quality, completeness, and to ensure the sensitivity factor obtained with the standard source remained within 15% of the pretrial factor
Segmentation of liver and placement of small volume of interest (2-cm sphere) for the purpose of individualized dosimetry report	• Segmentation performed by study radiation therapist • Principal investigator checks the placement, generation of report, and clinical consistency and signs off • Study medical physicist quality checks the dosimetry report for accuracy and clinical consistency and signs off • Site investigator reviews report and clinical consistency before decision on dose prescription for next cycle

dosimetry with a kidney tolerance dose of 23 Gy. Dose escalation or deescalation was recommended based on individualized dosimetry, with a maximum of 11.1 GBq per dose.

The quality assurance program consists of the following. Before patient accrual, a phantom and calibration process was performed across the participating institutions. The procedures were adapted from published recommendations and standardized for our study. A known quality of ^{177}Lu-DOTATATE and a phantom was delivered to each center to perform the calibration procedure. All data generated were reviewed by the dosimetry working group (consisting of medical physicists and nuclear medicine physicians from each center) to reconcile inconsistences before patient accrual. Following each treatment cycle, all dosimetry images were submitted centrally (Quantitative Imaging for Personalized Cancer Medicine program) and set up to

support multicenter imaging studies. Following a quality assurance and quality control process, images were used to generate the dosimetry report by a central dosimetry team. A 2-cm spherical region of interest was placed over normal renal parenchyma, uninvolved vertebrae, and intrahepatic and extrahepatic tumors for the purpose of dosimetry calculations. MIRD-based dosimetry was applied to determine the absorbed dose to the organ based on the activity measured in the SPECT-CT images. Dosimetry reports containing estimated dose to normal and tumor regions of interest, estimated by both monoexponential and biexponential modeling, together with a recommended dose for the subsequent cycle, was issued by the principal investigator. A final quality assurance sign-off was provided by a study medical physicist for clinical use. The process established was able to identify variations in processes.

The image acquisition manual and quality assurance program were effective in standardizing our individualized dosimetry process across centers.

FROM ABSORBED DOSE TO BIOLOGICAL EFFECTIVE DOSE

Quantifying the radiation dose absorbed using the individualized dosimetry process and understanding the biological effect of radiation dose absorbed on the tumor and normal tissues require additional considerations. Radiobiological concepts are an imperfect but invaluable tool to bridge understanding. It deserves consideration if only to understand the known variables involved, to understand what is expected and what is not, from lesion-by-lesion responses to clinical outcomes such as progression-free survival, survival, and quality of life.

Biological effective dose (BED) provides a mathematical framework to understand the various biological factors at play when radiation hit cells, and quantifying, allowing BED to be refined, and validated against clinical observations. It is widely applied in external beam radiotherapy but requires additional factors when considering molecular radiotherapy.

The dose rate effect differentiates molecular radiotherapy from conventional external beam radiotherapy. With conventional external beam radiotherapy (dose rate of 1–5 Gy/min), the high dose rate and rapid treatment time mean that there is insufficient time for radiation repair to occur during treatment. In contrast, this is possible during very-low-dose-rate delivery (as in ^{177}Lu-DOTATATE therapy; $\leq$2 cGy/min), which should decrease the effect of the radiation dose absorbed and make it less efficient (**Table 2**). However, there are other mechanisms at play that are likely to more than compensate for this, accounting for the effectiveness of molecular radiotherapy. Specifically, the low-dose hyperradiosensitivity–increased radioresistance, cross-fire effect, and bystander effects deserve attention. The combined effect of μ (the effect of radiosensitivity and repair of radiation damage), λ (clearance rate constant, given by the sum of the physical decay and biological clearance), and α/β (the repair capacity of different tissues, tumor, and normal tissues) defines the relative effectiveness factor (RE) that will modulate the physical dose absorbed to estimate the BED. Expressed mathematically, BED = D × RE, where D is the dose absorbed and RE is RE per unit dose. Alternatively expressed, the radiation dose absorbed within tumor and normal tissues varies as a function of distribution of the radiopharmaceutical within tissues on delivery, physical decay, and biological clearance.[25]

One additional factor that is not represented in this equation is the effect of fractionation. Most molecular radiotherapy is fractionated (eg, 2–4) or repeated doses. From a radiobiological perspective, this has the effect of overcoming hypoxia, which may be particularly important in large tumors that are poorly vascularized. In general, preclinical models suggest that fractionated delivery reduces toxicity and improves homogeneity of dose delivery compared with single administrations.

A comprehensive approach of understanding the innate characteristics of the tumor, the physical and biological behavior of radiation dose after treatment administration, and the interplay between physical dose and radiobiological effect will likely be critical in designing novel ways of

Table 2
Comparison of radiation dose rate across radiation modalities[25,40]

Modality	Dose Rate	Notes	Dose Rate
Theranostics (molecular radiotherapy)	Very low dose rate	Eg, ^{177}Lu DOTATATE Continuous, but declining, exposure that is a function of the initial uptake and the variable half-life	$\leq$2 cGy/min
Low-dose-rate brachytherapy	Low dose rate	Eg, cervix intracavitary brachytherapy (treatment in days)	40–200 cGy/h 0.4-2 Gy/h
High-dose-rate brachytherapy	High dose rate	Eg, cervix (treatment in minutes)	1200 cGy/h
External beam radiotherapy	High dose rate	Homogeneous dose rate	100–500 cGy/min
Flash radiotherapy	Ultrahigh dose rate	Investigational	40–60 Gy/s

optimizing PRRT for NET, combined with other therapies and molecular radiotherapy at large.

IMAGING TO PREDICT OUTCOMES

PRRT is an effective mode of therapy in patients with metastatic NETs that highly overexpress SSRs.[26] Although side effects are generally mild, significant toxicities, especially hematological toxicities, can be observed in approximately 10% of patients.[27] Despite promising data, PRRT is not readily available in many cancer centers or jurisdictions and is costly. Furthermore, disease progression during or shortly after PRRT may be observed in up to 30% of patients.[28] For all these reasons, reliable selection of patients who would benefit from this therapy is paramount. Aside from baseline expression of SSRs on SSR imaging (as expressed on a 4-point scale: the Krenning score), accurate clinical and imaging biomarkers to prospectively predict therapy success and overall prognosis are lacking. There is an urgent clinical need for validated biomarkers that will help identify patients who would unlikely benefit from PRRT before initiation of therapy or shortly thereafter.

From a few prior publications, and in our experience from data in more than 90 patients treated with PRRT (unpublished data), baseline maximal SUV (SUVmax) and mean SUVmax in 5 target lesions predict response to PRRT as determined using RECIST 1.1 at 3 months after therapy.[29–31] Other investigators have tried to define an SUVmax cutoff that would help predict response, with variable results. In a study including 55 patients with metastatic NETs, baseline SUVmax less than 13 was associated with poor objective response to PRRT.[32] A different study has suggested an SUVmax cutoff of 17.9 to predict response.[33] Regardless of a specific SUV cutoff, these observations, generally generated retrospectively, would need to be confirmed prospectively in large patient cohorts. The differences observed in these 2 studies likely reflect the variability among these patient populations in terms of disease grade, site of primary tumor, and location and extent of metastatic disease, and highlight the inherent limitation of using a solitary parameter as a predictor for therapy response.

An interesting observation from a recently published study on patients with unresectable NETs treated with systemic therapies, including PRRT, is that no benefit with regard to time to progression was observed for patients that experienced objective response (defined as reduction in tumor load) compared with those who achieved stable disease[34] (**Fig. 3**). This finding suggests that early outcome data reflected in RECIST 1.1–based therapy response measures may not be accurate measures of therapy success and may not be a reliable surrogate for progression-free survival and overall survival. Others have shown that intermediate outcome data at 9 months after PRRT may correlate with overall survival. Patients with progressive disease as defined by RECIST 1.1 or Choi criteria had significantly worse overall survival compared with those with stable disease. [68]Ga DOTATATE PET/CT was able to detect new lesions earlier than CT, but no association was found between change on ^{68}Ga DOTATATE PET and overall survival.[35]

Biomarkers that accurately determine outcome to PRRT early in the course of therapy (for example, after 1 cycle of PRRT) may identify those patients who are unlikely to benefit from further therapy, and limit unnecessary toxicity. In a study including 33 patients with well-differentiated NETs treated with PRRT, change in the ratio of SUVmax in tumor to spleen after 1 cycle of PRRT compared with baseline was an independent predictor of time to progression.[36] However, the authors could not validate this observation in a local cohort of patients who underwent baseline and interim PET after 1 cycle of PRRT (unpublished data).

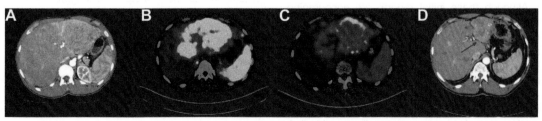

Fig. 3. A 42-year-old patient with metastatic NET, with unknown primary. Well-differentiated grade 2 NET with Ki-67 of 12%. Axial arterial phase CT image (*A*) and axial DOTATATE PET/CT (*B*) at baseline before PRRT. Large, arterially enhancing lesion with mostly homogeneous DOTATATE positivity is seen. Axial DOTATATE PET/CT(*C*) after the first cycle of PRRT shows decreasing DOTATATE positivity. The axial arterial phase CT image (*D*) shows significant reduction in size of the hepatic metastases (*red arrows*).

In recent years, there has been a heightened interest in evaluating complex quantitative metrics of tumor texture, also referred to as radiomics features, obtained from medical imaging data as predictors of treatment response and prognosis in various malignancies and clinical scenarios. A few studies have recently been published on the ability of various NET texture features to predict response to PRRT. In 1 study, investigators assessed the ability of tumor heterogeneity parameters, skewness, and kurtosis on pretherapy ^{68}Ga DOTATATE PET to predict response to PRRT. Skewness depicts the asymmetry within the gray-level distribution observed within a volume of interest and kurtosis refers to the spreading of the expected gaussian curve. The analysis was performed on a lesion level and the investigators showed that both higher skewness and kurtosis were significantly predictive of treatment failure ($P<.0001$ and $P = .004$, respectively).[37] For these parameters to be clinically useful tools to assess response to a systemic therapy, they would need to be correlated with overall patient outcome and, therefore, they may need to be acquired from all tumor sites in a patient. To perform this, segmented whole-body DT tumor volumes would need to be generated and a correlation with progression-free survival or overall survival would need to be proved. Nonetheless, these parameters are promising. A recent study showed that, in patients with G1/G2 NETs, heterogeneous expression of SSRs on ^{68}Ga DOTATATE PET, as assessed subjectively, was predictive of a shorter time to progression and inferior overall survival compared with those with tumor homogeneity ($P = .01$).[38] A further recent study including 31 patients with G1/G2 pancreatic NETs who underwent ^{68}Ga DOTATATE PET before PRRT assessed tumor texture features as predictors of therapy outcome. A median of 5 tumor lesions were segmented in each patient. The study results suggest that entropy, a measure of the inherent randomness in the gray-level intensities on a voxel-by-voxel level, was predictive of longer overall survival (AUC = 0.71; $P = .02$).[39]

Although these initial reports are encouraging, they need to be validated in larger patient cohorts, preferably from various institutions. This requirement is especially important for NETs, which are a heterogeneous group of tumors in terms of anatomic origin (eg, gastrointestinal tract, lung, pancreas), histologic differentiation, biological behavior, and outcome. To identify potent biomarkers in such a heterogeneous disease, it is likely that a large database from multiple institutions would be needed. It is also conceivable that a predictive model incorporating combinations of predictive biomarkers may result in more powerful prognostication. The reliability of these parameters, or combination of parameters, would need to be validated prospectively on an individual patient level before they could be incorporated into clinical practice.

SUMMARY

Overall, ^{68}Ga-DOTA-peptide PET imaging is a critical tool for identification, characterization of the disease sites, and therapy planning in patients with NETs. However it is important to use imaging tests that are appropriate for the stage and grading of the disease. In terms of therapy delivery, significant improvements have been seen recently for individualization of dosage. However, so far there is no robust method available to predict the absorbed dose via imaging only, and also the posttreatment time point of imaging is still a topic of debate. Imaging-based outcome prediction has been proved to be promising in several initial trials but the results found so far need to be further validated. In addition, initial evaluation of time points and imaging metrics to evaluate therapy response has shown encouraging findings, but need to be further refined as well.

DISCLOSURES

Ur Metser: no conflict of interest related to this work; Canprobe Board of Directors, member; POINT Biopharma, consultant.

Patrick Veit-Haibach: investigator-initiated studies grants from Bayer Switzerland, Roche Pharmaceuticals, Siemens Healthineers, GE Healthcare; speaker fees and travel support, Siemens Healthineers, GE Healthcare. All outside this submitted work.

Rebecca KS Wong: no conflict of interest related to this work: education grant for Clinical Research Mentorship Program, Global Access Cancer Foundation; education grant, Building Radiation Oncology Capacity Through Training; Celgene Cancer Care Links grant; Clinical trial funding provided to institution for NCT 02743741 where RW is the Principal investigator: Ontario Health, Princess Margaret Cancer Cancer Foundation; POINT Biopharma, consultant, Honoraria: Novartis, Ipsen.

CLINICS CARE POINTS

- [68]Ga PETCT has high sensitivity and specificity and is now the standard of care for staging and selection of patients for PRRT in patients with neuroendocrine tumors.

- In ^{68}Ga PETCT positive patients, additional FDG PETCT has an important complementary role in the detection of aggressive cell populations.

- A common quality assurance protocol can enable standardization of dose estimates across centers and should be implemented across theranostics centers.

- Quantifying tumor dose absorbed will likely be the cornerstone for designing novel strategies in the use of PRRT and molecular radiotherapy at large.

- On pretreatment 68Ga-DOTA-peptide PET, the tumor maximal standardized uptake value can be used for prognostication of therapy response.

REFERENCES

1. Available from: https://www.nccn.org/professionals/physician_gls/default.aspx. Accessed April 22, 2021.

2. Bauckneht M, Albano D, Annunziata S, et al. Somatostatin receptor PET/CT imaging for the detection and staging of pancreatic NET: a systematic review and meta-analysis. Diagnostics (Basel) 2020;10(8).

3. Geijer H, Breimer LH. Somatostatin receptor PET/CT in neuroendocrine tumours: update on systematic review and meta-analysis. Eur J Nucl Med Mol Imaging 2013;40(11):1770–80.

4. Liu X, Li N, Jiang T, et al. Comparison of gallium-68 somatostatin receptor and (18)F-fluorodeoxyglucose positron emission tomography in the diagnosis of neuroendocrine tumours: a systematic review and meta-analysis. Hell J Nucl Med 2020;23(2):188–200.

5. Evangelista L, Ravelli I, Bignotto A, et al. Ga-68 DOTA-peptides and F-18 FDG PET/CT in patients with neuroendocrine tumor: a review. Clin Imaging 2020;67:113–6.

6. Gaertner FC, Beer AJ, Souvatzoglou M, et al. Evaluation of feasibility and image quality of 68Ga-DOTATOC positron emission tomography/magnetic resonance in comparison with positron emission tomography/computed tomography in patients with neuroendocrine tumors. Invest Radiol 2013;48(5):263–72.

7. Beiderwellen KJ, Poeppel TD, Hartung-Knemeyer V, et al. Simultaneous 68Ga-DOTATOC PET/MRI in patients with gastroenteropancreatic neuroendocrine tumors: initial results. Invest Radiol 2013;48(5):273–9.

8. Hanscheid H, Sweeney RA, Flentje M, et al. PET SUV correlates with radionuclide uptake in peptide receptor therapy in meningioma. Eur J Nucl Med Mol Imaging 2012;39(8):1284–8.

9. Ezziddin S, Lohmar J, Yong-Hing CJ, et al. Does the pretherapeutic tumor SUV in 68Ga DOTATOC PET predict the absorbed dose of 177Lu octreotate? Clin Nucl Med 2012;37(6):e141–7.

10. Sandstrom M, Garske U, Granberg D, et al. Individualized dosimetry in patients undergoing therapy with (177)Lu-DOTA-D-Phe (1)-Tyr (3)-octreotate. Eur J Nucl Med Mol Imaging 2010;37(2):212–25.

11. European Association of Nuclear Medicine Guidelines - Dosimetry. Available at: eanm.org/publications/guidelines/dosimetry/. Accessed April 22, 2021.

12. Society of Nuclear Medicine & Molecular Imaging - clinical guidelines. Available at: snmmi.org. Accessed April 22, 2021.

13. Eberlein U, Cremonesi M, Lassmann M. Individualized dosimetry for theranostics: necessary, nice to have, or counterproductive? J Nucl Med 2017;58(Suppl 2):97S–103S.

14. Stabin MG, Madsen MT, Zaidi H. Personalized dosimetry is a must for appropriate molecular radiotherapy. Med Phys 2019;46(11):4713–6.

15. Haug AR. PRRT of neuroendocrine tumors: individualized dosimetry or fixed dose scheme? EJNMMI Res 2020;10(1):35.

16. Strosberg J, El-Haddad G, Wolin E, et al. Phase 3 trial of (177)Lu-dotatate for midgut neuroendocrine tumors. N Engl J Med 2017;376(2):125–35.

17. Ljungberg M, Celler A, Konijnenberg MW, et al. MIRD pamphlet No. 26: joint EANM/MIRD guidelines for quantitative 177Lu SPECT applied for dosimetry of radiopharmaceutical therapy. J Nucl Med 2016;57(1):151–62.

18. Argyrou M, Lyra M. Monte Carlo simulation in radionuclide therapy dosimetry. Biomed J Sci Tech Res 2019;15(1):344–52.

19. Finocchiaro D, Berenato S, Bertolini V, et al. Comparison of different calculation techniques for absorbed dose assessment in patient specific peptide receptor radionuclide therapy. PLoS One 2020;15(8):e0236466.

20. Hanscheid H, Lapa C, Buck AK, et al. Dose mapping after endoradiotherapy with (177)Lu-DOTATATE/DOTATOC by a single measurement after 4 days. J Nucl Med 2018;59(1):75–81.

21. Madsen MT, Menda Y, O'Dorisio TM, et al. Technical Note: single time point dose estimate for exponential clearance. Med Phys 2018;45(5):2318–24.

22. Del Prete M, Arsenault F, Saighi N, et al. Accuracy and reproducibility of simplified QSPECT dosimetry for personalized (177)Lu-octreotate PRRT. EJNMMI Phys 2018;5(1):25.

23. Driscoll B, Wong R, Vishway C, et al. Optimizing the SPECT imaging workflow for individualized dosimetry in Lu[177]-DOTATATE Treatment of Progressive metastatic neuroendocrine tumours. Int J Radiat Oncol Biol Phys 2020;108(3):E588–9.

24. Lu-DOTATATE treatment in patients with 68Ga-DOTATATE somatostatin receptor positive neuroendocrine

tumors (NCT02743741). Available at: clinicaltrials.gov. Accessed April 22, 2021.

25. Salvatori M, Cremonesi M, Indovina L, et al. Radiobiology and radiation dosimetry in nuclear medicine. In: al HWSe, editor. Nuclear oncology. Switzerland: Springer International; 2016. p. 305–49.

26. De Jong, Breeman WA, Kwekkeboom DJ, et al. Tumor imaging and therapy using radiolabeled somatostatin analogues. Acc Chem Res 2009;42:873–80.

27. Lin E, Chen T, Little A, et al. Safety and outcomes of (177) Lu-DOTATATE for neuroendocrine tumours: experience in New South Wales, Australia. Intern Med J 2019;49(10):1268–77.

28. Marusyk A, Polyak K. Tumor heterogeneity: causes and consequences. Biochim Biophys Acta 2010; 1805(1):105–17.

29. Miederer M, Seidl S, Buck A, et al. Correlation of immunohistopathological expression of somatostatin receptor 2 with standardised uptake values in 68Ga-DOTATOC PET/CT. Eur J Nucl Med Mol Imaging 2009;36(1):48–52.

30. Campana D, Ambrosini V, Pezzilli R, et al. Standardized uptake values of (68)Ga-DOTANOC PET: a promising prognostic tool in neuroendocrine tumors. J Nucl Med 2010;51(3):353–9.

31. Kratochwil C, Stefanova M, Mavriopoulou E, et al. SUV of [68Ga]DOTATOC-PET/CT predicts response probability of PRRT in neuroendocrine tumors. Mol Imaging Biol 2015;17(3):313–8.

32. Sharma R, Wang WM, Yusuf S, et al. (68)Ga-DOTATATE PET/CT parameters predict response to peptide receptor radionuclide therapy in neuroendocrine tumours. Radiother Oncol 2019; 141:108–15.

33. Oksuz MO, Winter L, Pfannenberg C, et al. Peptide receptor radionuclide therapy of neuroendocrine tumors with (90)Y-DOTATOC: is treatment response predictable by pre-therapeutic uptake of (68)Ga-DOTATOC? Diagn Interv Imaging 2014;95(3): 289–300.

34. Thiis-Evensen E, Poole AC, Nguyen HT, et al. Achieving objective response in treatment of non-resectable neuroendocrine tumors does not predict longer time to progression compared to achieving stable disease. BMC Cancer 2020;20(1):466.

35. Huizing DMV, Aalbersberg EA, Versleijen MWJ, et al. Early response assessment and prediction of overall survival after peptide receptor radionuclide therapy. Cancer Imaging 2020;20(1):57.

36. Haug AR, Auernhammer CJ, Wangler B, et al. 68Ga-DOTATATE PET/CT for the early prediction of response to somatostatin receptor-mediated radionuclide therapy in patients with well-differentiated neuroendocrine tumors. J Nucl Med 2010;51(9): 1349–56.

37. Onner H, Abdulrezzak U, Tutus A. Could the skewness and kurtosis texture parameters of lesions obtained from pretreatment Ga-68 DOTA-TATE PET/CT images predict receptor radionuclide therapy response in patients with gastroenteropancreatic neuroendocrine tumors? Nucl Med Commun 2020;41(10):1034–9.

38. Graf J, Pape UF, Jann H, et al. Prognostic significance of somatostatin receptor heterogeneity in progressive neuroendocrine tumor treated with Lu-177 DOTATOC or Lu-177 DOTATATE. Eur J Nucl Med Mol Imaging 2020;47(4):881–94.

39. Werner RA, Ilhan H, Lehner S, et al. Pre-therapy somatostatin receptor-based heterogeneity predicts overall survival in pancreatic neuroendocrine tumor patients undergoing peptide receptor radionuclide therapy. Mol Imaging Biol 2019;21(3):582–90.

40. Wilson JD, Hammond EM, Higgins GS, et al. Ultra-high dose rate (FLASH) radiotherapy: silver bullet or fool's gold? Front Oncol 2020;10:210.

Theragnostics in Neuroendocrine Tumors

Margarida Rodrigues, MD*, Hanna Svirydenka, MD, Irene Virgolini, MD

KEYWORDS

- Neuroendocrine tumor • Theragnostics • ^{68}Ga-DOTA-TOC • ^{18}F-FDG
- Peptide receptor radionuclide therapy • ^{177}Lu-PRRT • ^{90}Y-DOTATATE

KEY POINTS

- Somatostatin receptor (SSTR)-imaging (PET or conventional scintigraphy) is an effective tool for diagnosis, staging, planning of peptide receptor radionuclide therapy (PRRT), and evaluation of treatment response in patients with neuroendocrine tumors (NETs).
- Applying a dual-tracer approach with SSTR and PET with fludeoxyglucose F 18 imaging can help the decision-making process for therapy selection in patients with NET.
- PRRT appears to be the most effective therapeutic option in the management of patients with inoperable or metastasized NET with limited side effects if dose limits are respected.

INTRODUCTION

Neuroendocrine tumors (NET) constitute a heterogeneous group of tumors that are able to express somatostatin receptors (SSTRs) on the cell surface,[1,2] allowing the use of radiolabeled somatostatin analogs for SSTR-targeted imaging as well as peptide receptor radionuclide therapy (PRRT).

NETs are considered a relatively rare disease, although incidence rates have been rising over the past 30 years in Europe and the United States,[1,2] particularly those arising from the midgut and pancreas.[3] Located primarily with approximate 72% in the gastrointestinal tract and 25% in the bronchopulmonary system, NETs can also originate from various other sites such as the head and neck region or the prostate.[4,5] They can be asymptomatic for years and, especially those of the pancreas and intestine, they are often diagnosed at late stage when metastatic or locally advanced[6,7] and therefore inoperable, so that a systemic therapy is often required.[4,8]

The clinical course of NET can be quite heterogeneous with variable response to treatments despite possessing similar tumor characteristics and having received the same therapy. The World Health Organization (WHO) guidelines classify NET into 3 grades based on cell proliferation, the number of mitoses, and the expression of the nuclear antigen Ki-67.[4] Both proliferation index and grade strongly correlate with tumor behavior and prognosis.[9–11] High-grade, poorly differentiated NETs often have limited expression of SSTR,[9] what can lead to false negative SSTR-imaging results and makes the molecular investigation difficult.

For the choice of the most appropriate treatment for NET, information regarding anatomic location and local invasion of adjacent structures, tumor functionality, histologic tumor grading, staging, and SSTR status are required to help the decision-making process, which should be individualized for patients with NET.

CLINICAL CARE POINTS

The theragnostic principle is based on the concept of diagnostic molecular imaging, followed by an individually tailored treatment decision. Several studies have demonstrated the effectiveness of the application of SSTR-targeted imaging (PET or conventional scintigraphy) for diagnosis, staging, and planning of PRRT, as well as evaluation of response to the treatment.[4,6,7,12]

The authors have nothing to disclosure.
Department of Nuclear Medicine, Medical University of Innsbruck, Anichstrasse 35, Innsbruck 6020, Austria
* Corresponding author.
E-mail address: Margarida.Rodrigues-Radischat@i-med.ac.at

PET Clin 16 (2021) 365–373
https://doi.org/10.1016/j.cpet.2021.03.001
1556-8598/21/© 2021 Elsevier Inc. All rights reserved.

Imaging in Neuroendocrine Tumors

Assessment of liver metastases and degree of liver involvement using morphologically orientated imaging techniques, such as ultrasonography, contrast-enhanced multidetector computed tomography (CT), or MR imaging is central for accurate staging and for evaluating the response to treatment.[13] However, these methods sometimes lack specificity, as conclusions regarding malignant involvement of organ structures are based only on size criteria and the contrast enhancement pattern.[14]

SSTR expression is evaluated by SSTR-imaging with Gallium 68 (^{68}Ga)–1,4,7,10-tetraazacyclodo-decane-1,4,7,10-tetraacetic acid (DOTA)- Phe[1]-Tyr[3]-Octreotide (TOC)/ Tyr[3]-Octreotate (TATE)/ Nal[3]-Octreotide (NOC)/lanreotide PET/CT or ^{99m}Tc-hydrazinonicotinyl (HYNIC)-TOC/^{111}In-DOTA-TOC/lanreotide scintigraphy,[4,14–17] among others. The whole-body nature of the examination as well as its noninvasiveness makes SSTR-imaging (PET or scintigraphy) more appealing for imaging of NET than morphologic techniques.

Gabriel and colleagues[16] found that ^{68}Ga-DOTA-TOC PET shows a significantly higher detection rate compared with conventional SSTR scintigraphy and diagnostic CT with clinical impact in many patients. Furthermore, in terms of staging SSTR PET/CT imaging has been shown to be superior to CT and MR imaging as well.[14,17,18]

PET/computed tomography imaging with Gallium 68–labeled somatostatin analogs

The Ga-complexes of somatostatin analogs commonly show a higher binding affinity for sstr2 when compared with the corresponding complexes with indium, yttrium, or lutetium. DOTA-lanreotide when labeled with yttrium beside high affinity to sstr2 also shows high affinity to sstr5 comparable with DOTA-NOC and low affinity to sstr3 (for review see Ref.[19]).

The increased hydrophilicity of the Ga-complex results in an increased renal elimination. Together with an improved accumulation of ^{68}Ga-DOTA-TOC in the tumor lesions, these pharmacokinetic properties lead to a high lesion contrast within a short time interval post injection, which is of particular importance considering the short half-life of [68]Ga (68 minutes).[19] A detailed procedure guideline for PET-CT with ^{68}Ga-labeled somatostatin analogs peptide imaging was summarized by the Oncology Committee of the European Association of Nuclear Medicine.[20]

In the past few years, PET/CT imaging with ^{68}Ga-labeled somatostatin analogs (^{68}Ga-DOTA-TOC/TATE/NOC or ^{68}Ga-DOTA-lanreotide) has been shown to provide excellent sensitivity and specificity for diagnosing and staging NET.[16,21]

However, the very specific binding of these compounds may lead to overinterpretation of tracer accumulation. Therefore, interpretation must be done cautiously in organs showing physiologically enhanced tracer uptake, including exocrine pancreas (head/uncinate process),[22] spleen, liver, pituitary, thyroid, kidneys, adrenal glands, and salivary glands.[22] Infection/inflammation can lead to false positive results.[23]

Gabriel and colleagues[16] showed that ^{68}Ga-DOTA-TOC provided additional information that was obtained with none of the other imaging procedures in 25% (21/84) of patients with NET. Haug and colleagues[24] demonstrated the utility of ^{68}Ga-DOTA-TATE PET/CT in 104 patients with suspected NET. PET/CT showed a sensitivity of 81% and a specificity of 90% resulting in an accuracy of 87%. The Munich Group[25] also reported change in surgical management in 9 (20%) of 44 patients with NET. In a retrospective blinded review, Hofman and colleagues[26] communicated high impact on patient management including curative surgery by identifying a primary site and directing patients with multiple metastases to systemic therapy.

Our Innsbruck Group[27] reported that ^{68}Ga-DOTA-TOC showed in patients with NET a significantly higher maximum standard uptake value (SUVmax) regarding the primary tumor (n = 25) as well as liver metastases (n = 30) compared with ^{68}Ga-DOTA-LAN. Furthermore, we found that investigation only of SSTR status by ^{68}Ga-DOTA-TOC PET/CT may not reflect progression in a certain NET lesion.[28] Moreover, high-grade, poorly differentiated NET often has limited expression of SSTR,[10] what can lead to false negative SSTR-imaging results and makes the molecular investigation difficult. Therefore, applying a dual-tracer approach with SSTR and PET with fludeoxyglucose F 18 (^{18}F-FDG-PET) imaging could help the decision-making process for therapy selection in patients with NET.

PET/computed tomography imaging with fludeoxyglucose F 18

^{18}F-FDG-PET is used to assess glycolytic metabolism, and higher uptake of ^{18}F-FDG has been linked with more aggressive tumor features.[29] ^{18}F-FDG-PET is widely applied in oncology, but its use in NET has been a matter of controversy.[28]

The higher the grade of an NET, the higher is the prevalence of glucose hypermetabolic tumors.[30] A dichotomous behavior has been found between SSTR imaging and ^{18}F-FDG-PET in well-differentiated and poorly differentiated NET, where the former was more positive with SSTR imaging[30,31] and the latter with ^{18}F-FDG-PET.[32,33] ^{18}F-FDG PET/CT has thus been used increasingly in the past few years for the evaluation of high-grade NET.[29,30] The diagnostic value of ^{18}F-FDG PET in lower grade NET is limited because they are slowly proliferating tumors with lower glycolytic activity.[34] Hence, even though ^{18}F-FDG-PET has a high spatial resolution, it has not been indicated primarily for NET.

Binderup and colleagues[35] showed that although the diagnostic sensitivity of ^{18}F-FDG PET is low for NET, the prognostic value is high. This makes the low diagnostic sensitivity less important because a negative ^{18}F-FDG-PET result is predictive of low aggressiveness and a high survival rate.

Garin and colleagues[36] reported that ^{18}F-FDG-PET has a prognostic value for early tumor progression. Our Group[28] also showed that the presence of ^{18}F-FDG-positive tumors correlates strongly with a higher risk of progression. We found that initially ^{18}F-FDG-negative patients with NET may show ^{18}F-FDG-positive tumors during follow-up. Furthermore, we observed that patients with well-differentiated, G1 and G2 NET also may have ^{18}F-FDG-positive tumors initially and may develop ^{18}F-FDG-positive lesions during follow-up.

Some studies have demonstrated the association of ^{18}F-FDG PET with treatment response and progression-free survival after PRRT in NET. Zhang and colleagues[37] reported a significant benefit in overall survival and in progression-free survival for their ^{18}F-FDG-negative group. These investigators found that the presence of positive lesions on ^{18}F-FDG PET is an independent prognostic factor in patients with NET treated with PRRT. High SSTR expression combined with negative ^{18}F-FDG PET/CT imaging is associated with the most favorable long-term prognosis. However, the prognostic value of ^{68}Ga-SSTR PET imaging was found to be lower than that of the ^{18}F-FDG PET.

High ^{18}F-FDG SUV seems to strongly correlate with a short survival in patients with NET. Binderup and colleagues[35] reported that a SUVmax higher than 3 was found to be the only independent predictor of progression-free survival and that an ^{18}F-FDG SUVmax higher than 9 was strongly correlated with a greater risk of mortality in patients with NET.

Metabolic imaging with ^{18}F-FDG PET/CT complements thus the molecular imaging with ^{68}Ga-SSTR PET/CT for the prognosis of survival after PRRT.[35,37]

Peptide Receptor Radionuclide Therapy

For the choice of the most appropriate treatment for NET, information regarding anatomic location and local invasion of adjacent structures, tumor functionality, histologic tumor grading, staging, and SSTR status are required to help the decision-making process, which should be individualized for patients with NET.

Multiple treatment approaches, which are interchangeable for most patients, are now available for patients with NET presenting with metastatic disease, including surgery, locoregional therapies,[4,8,9] interferon-alpha, chemotherapy,[8,9] molecular targeted therapies,[10,38] biotherapy with somatostatin analogs,[38–40] and PRRT[4,15,21,40]; however, relapses occur after a certain time in many patients.

PRRT is a molecularly targeted radiation therapy involving the administration of a specific radiopharmaceutical composed of a β-emitting radionuclide chelated to a peptide designed to target with high affinity SSTR overexpressed on tumors. SSTR 2 is the key target molecule for both cold and radiolabeled somatostatin analogs.[4] PRRT using ^{177}Lu and/or ^{90}Y-labeled somatostatin analogs (DOTATATE, DOTATOC, or lanreotide) has been used for more than 20 years as a systemic treatment approach in metastatic and inoperable NET that expresses SSTR positivity, evaluated by SSTR-imaging (PET and/or conventional scintigraphy).[41–43]

Depending on the size of the tumor or metastasis, ^{90}Y beta rays with a range of approximately 12 mm in tissue are theoretically better suited for larger tumor lesions, whereas ^{177}Lu, with a smaller range of approximately 2 mm, is preferentially used for smaller tumors.[41] Although there is no evidence in the clinical setting, this concept has been widely applied in clinical practice for many years. In the past few years, the ^{177}Lu-labeled compound, particularly, has found its way into clinical routine in view of its more favorable properties in terms of kidney toxicity.

There are different research PRRT protocols in use with either standard dose or individualized therapy with a variable number of cycles. In most institutions, PRRT treatment scheme is individually adapted concerning the doses and time intervals, depending on tumor stage, age, tracer uptake, biochemical response, Karnofsky Index, and quality of life. The PRRT scheme that has been performed in Innsbruck for more than a decade includes a PRRT infusion administered in conjunction with an amino acid solution to protect the kidney function.[4,41]

The recommended intravenously administered activity for ^{90}Y-DOTA-TOC/TATE is 2.78 to 4.44 GBq (75–120 mCi) every 6 to 12 weeks for a total of 2 to 4 cycles, and for ^{177}Lu-DOTATATE/TOC is 5.55 to 7.4 GBq (150–200 mCi) every 6 to 12 weeks for a total of 3 to 5 cycles. Restaging with SSTR-imaging, CT, and laboratory analyses, among others, is performed after completion of the therapy cycles and in many institutions also between cycles. Combination therapies with ^{90}Y and ^{177}Lu peptides are being actively investigated.[4]

The long-acting form (cold, ie, nonradioactive) of the somatostatin analogs octreotide or lanreotide can be applied between the treatment cycles but should be at least 4 weeks apart from the radioactive cycle.[43]

In general, PRRT is used after failing first-line medical therapy. The main candidates for PRRT are those with well-differentiated and moderately differentiated NET defined as NET grade 1 or 2 according to the WHO 2010 classification.[10] Retrospective multicenter ongoing studies, such as on behalf of the World Association of Radiopharmaceutical and Molecular Therapy, are being conducted to evaluate the efficacy of PRRT also in patients with NET grade 3.

The clinical efficacy of PRRT has been demonstrated in several clinical studies[40–42] (**Fig. 1**). The documented response rate summing up complete response, partial response, minor response, and stable disease is approximately 70% to 80% for ^{90}Y-DOTATOC and for ^{177}Lu-DOTATATE.[41,42]

PRRT has been shown also effective in terms of both symptomatic control and survival.[40–42] Recently, in a 12-year follow-up after PRRT performed at our institution, Gabriel and colleagues[41] found that 32% (14 of 44 patients) of the patients with metastatic or inoperable NET disease are still alive more than 12 years after the beginning of PRRT, with a median overall survival of 79 months. Other recent study results have indicated also a benefit of PRRT concerning response rate, progression-free survival, and overall survival as compared with established therapy procedures.[40,44] In particular for metastatic midgut NETs, PRRT has been established as one major therapy strategy because only a few therapeutic alternatives are available for this tumor entity.[45]

The significant benefit of PRRT over cold somatostatin analog therapy was demonstrated by the recent randomized phase 3 clinical trial of ^{177}Lu-DOTATATE in advanced, progressive midgut NETs grade 1 or 2 (NETTER-1).[40] In this trial, PRRT resulted in a markedly longer progression-free survival and a significantly higher response rate compared with long-acting repeatable octreotide alone.

^{68}Ga-DOTA-TOC PET/CT

Initial evaluation before PRRT

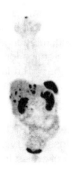

^{18}F-DG PET/CT

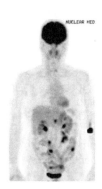

Follow-up after PRRT

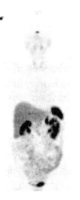

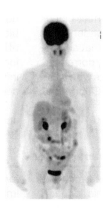

Fig. 1. A 59-year-old female patient with pancreatic NET and liver metastases before PRRT shown by ^{68}Ga-DOTA-TOC PET, whereas ^{18}F-DG PET was negative (*upper row*). Complete remission documented by ^{68}Ga-DOTA-TOC and ^{18}F-DG PET (*lower row*) after PRRT (9 cycles with ^{90}Y-DOTA-TOC, cumulative dose of 10 GBq, and 4 cycles with ^{177}Lu-DOTATATE, cumulative dose of 29 GBq).

Forrer and colleagues[46] reported that ^{177}Lu-DOTATOC therapy is feasible, safe, and efficacious in patients with relapse after ^{90}Y-DOTATOC treatment.

Health-related quality of life (HRQoL) is also significantly improved after PRRT.[40,47–49] Our group[50] examined the course of HRQoL in patients with metastatic gastroenteropancreatic NET undergoing PRRT at our institution. We found a significant improved or at least stable HRQoL on several domains from baseline to the first restaging after PRRT regarding physical, social and role functioning, fatigue, diarrhea, and appetite loss.

Several articles have been published on toxicity following PRRT proving that the treatment is safe and beneficial.[40,42,51] Dosimetry is useful to assess the radiation risk for normal and critical organs, that is, bone marrow and kidneys after PRRT. Radiolabeled SST-analogs are reabsorbed in the renal proximal tubules, hence the kidneys are exposed to a relatively high radiation dose. Renal radiation exposure can be reduced by coinfusion of amino acids during PRRT.[52] The standard activity of ^{177}Lu and ^{90}Y-labeled somatostatin analogs may be reduced in the case of pretherapeutic relevant renal impairment, or low white blood cell count.[53]

Severe toxicity (any grade greater than grade 2) according to the Common Terminology Criteria of Adverse Events (CTCAE), occur rarely.[53] Bodei and colleagues[51] reported nephrotoxicity of any CTCAE grade in 34.6% and grade 3 and 4 in 1.5% for a very inhomogeneous cohort of 807 patients studied. In our retrospective analysis[53] the vast majority of patients showed either none or only a mild to moderate decrease in kidney function as well as hematotoxicity 1 year after completion of standardized PRRT with 4 treatment cycles of either ^{90}Y-somatostatin or ^{177}Lu-somatostatin analogs. We found nephrotoxicity of any CTCAE grade in 31 (30.4%) of 102 patients and severe (CTCAE grade 3/4) in only 1 patient. In our cohort, PRRT had no statistically significant impact on leukopenia and thrombopenia. No hematotoxicity greater than grade 2 according to CTCAE was observed.

Therefore, in terms of safety, PRRT seems to have no critical impact on further oncologic treatment options in the case of disease progression.

In case of dedifferentiation, higher grade, bulky or ^{18}F-FDG-avid NET (**Fig. 2**) chemotherapy may become an option. The integration of PRRT into multimodality therapy protocols might improve response to treatment. The use of radiosensitizing

^{68}Ga-DOTA-TOC PET/CT

Initial evaluation before PRRT

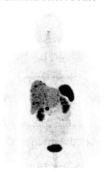

^{18}F-FDG PET/CT

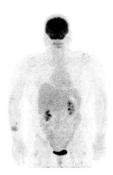

Fig. 2. A 55-year-old female patient with pancreatic NET and liver metastases before PRRT shown by ^{68}Ga-DOTA-TOC PET, whereas ^{18}F-FDG PET was negative (*upper row*). Disease progression documented by ^{68}Ga-DOTA-TOC and ^{18}F-FDG PET (*lower row*) after PRRT (5 cycles with ^{90}Y-DOTA-TOC, cumulative dose of 19.37 GBq). Biopsy of a hypermetabolic liver metastasis revealed a Ki-67 index of 40%.

Follow-up after PRRT

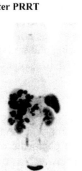

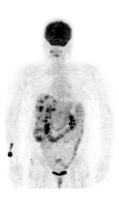

PRRT + Radiosensibilization with Low-Dose Temozolamide in G3 SSTR- and FDG-PET/CT positive NETs

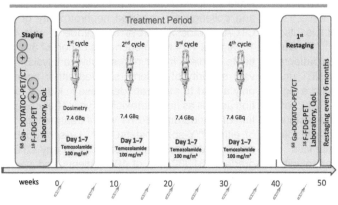

Continued Treatment with Long-Acting Somatostatin-Analogue

Fig. 3. Innsbruck scheme of PRRT in combination with radiosensibilization with low-dose temozolomide in G3 SSTR- and ^{18}F-FDG-PET/CT positive NET. QoL, evaluation of health-related quality of life.

chemotherapy in combination with ^{90}Y-somato-statin or ^{177}Lu-somatostatin analogs has shown an additive value.[54]

We investigated recently (data under publication, 2021) the efficacy of PRRT in combination with radiosensitizing chemotherapy with temozolomide (**Fig. 3**) in 20 patients with G3 NET with ^{18}F-FDG-avid lesions. At the end of the observation time, 20% of patients had complete response, 10% patients partial response, 30% patients stable disease, and 40% patients progressive disease. None of our patients showed serious adverse events after this combined treatment during follow-up.

DISCUSSION

Our group[9] showed recently that the sole investigation of SSTR status by ^{68}Ga-DOTA-TOC-PET/CT may not reflect the progression in certain NET lesions. Therefore, we recommended performing ^{18}F-FDG-PET in the initial evaluation and during follow-up of patients with NET, especially when SSTR PET/CT shows progression. ^{18}F-FDG-PET/CT along with SSTR imaging was found to help to stratify patients with G3 NET. High uptake on ^{68}Ga-SSTR PET/CT combined with negative ^{18}F-FDG PET/CT is associated with a comparatively prolonged progression-free as well overall survival.[37] ^{18}F-FDG-PET/CT is thus a complementary tool to ^{68}Ga-DOTA-TOC-PET/CT with clinical relevance for the molecular investigation of NET. These findings must be taken into account, especially for individualized and optimized therapy planning.

PRRT appears to be the most effective therapeutic option in the management of inoperable or metastasized patients with NET.[40–42] However, despite the huge potential of PRRT the nonavailability of PRRT in many countries still limits its widespread use.

The combined use of different radiolabeled somatostatin analogs, sequentially or concomitantly, may optimize the treatment outcome. Over time, several patients with differentiated NET will show progressive disease after initial response to PRRT. In these patients, re-PRRT may be a favorable option.[43]

On the other hand, PRRT also entails limited side effects that should be considered. In particular, special attention has to be paid to renal function and bone marrow reserve.[42,51] Protective measures, particularly individually adapted PRRT concerning the doses and time intervals and also concomitant application of amino acid solution to protect the kidney function should be undertaken regularly.

When NETs lose their initially high differentiation, the European Neuroendocrine Tumor Society Consensus Guidelines propose molecular targeted therapies, and in the case of higher dedifferentiation, they suggest chemotherapy.[10] Further ongoing studies are mandatory to optimize clinical protocols and assess the efficacy of PRRT in combination with radiosensitizing chemotherapy in patients with ^{18}F-FDG-avid NET lesions.

SUMMARY

Adopting a dual-tracer approach encompassing SSTR and ^{18}F-FDG-PET imaging, and assessing the SSTR expression and glycolytic metabolism, respectively, contribute toward a personalized medicine in the management of patients with NET.

PRRT with differently labeled tracers (^{90}Y or ^{177}Lu) and different somatostatin analogs is generally well tolerated, with only a few serious side effects.

Relapses occur after a certain time in many patients with NET. In these cases, the combined use of different radiolabeled somatostatin analogs, sequentially or concomitantly, as well as re-PRRT may optimize the treatment outcome.

REFERENCES

1. Reubi JC. Peptide receptors as molecular targets for cancer diagnosis and therapy. Endocr Rev 2003; 24(4):389–427.
2. Reubi JC, Schär JC, Waser B, et al. Affinity profiles for human somatostatin receptor subtypes SST1-SST5 of somatostatin radiotracers selected for scintigraphic and radiotherapeutic use. Eur J Nucl Med 2000;27(3):273–82.
3. Modlin IM, Oberg K, Chung DC, et al. Gastroenteropancreatic neuroendocrine tumours. Lancet Oncol 2008;9(1):61–72.
4. Bodei L, Mueller-Brand J, Baum RP, et al. The joint IAEA, EANM, and SNMMI practical guidance on peptide receptor radionuclide therapy (PRRNT) in neuroendocrine tumours. Eur J Nucl Med Mol Imaging 2013;40(5):800–16.
5. Quaedvlieg PF, Visser O, Lamers CB, et al. Epidemiology and survival in patients with carcinoid disease in The Netherlands. An epidemiological study with 2391 patients. Ann Oncol 2001;12(9):1295–300.
6. Hallet J, Law CH, Cukier M, et al. Exploring the rising incidence of neuroendocrine tumors: a population-based analysis of epidemiology, metastatic presentation, and outcomes. Cancer 2015;121:589–97.
7. Yao JC, Hassan M, Phan A, et al. One hundred years after "carcinoid": epidemiology of and prognostic factors for neuroendocrine tumors in 35,825 cases in the United States. J Clin Oncol 2008;26:3063–72.
8. Steinmüller T, Kianmanesh R, Falconi M, et al. Consensus guidelines for the management of patients with liver metastases from digestive (neuro) endocrine tumors: foregut, midgut, hindgut, and unknown primary. Neuroendocrinology 2008;87: 47–62.
9. Ramage JK, Goretzki PE, Manfredi R, et al. Consensus guidelines for the management of patients with digestive neuroendocrine tumors: well-differentiated colon and rectum tumor/carcinoma. Neuroendocrinology 2008;87:31–9.
10. Pavel M, Baudin E, Couvelard A, et al. ENETS consensus guidelines for the management of patients with liver and other distant metastases from neuroendocrine neoplasms of foregut, midgut, hindgut, and unknown primary. Neuroendocrinology 2012;95:157–76.
11. Rindi G. The ENETS guidelines: the new TNM classification system. Tumori 2010;96:806–9.
12. Strosberg J, Nasir A, Coppola D, et al. Correlation between grade and prognosis in metastatic gastroenteropancreatic neuroendocrine tumors. Hum Pathol 2009;40:1262–8.
13. Sundin A, Vullierme MP, Kaltsas G, et al. ENETS consensus guidelines for the standards of care in neuroendocrine tumors: radiological examinations. Neuroendocrinology 2009;90(2):167–83.
14. Gabriel M, Hausler F, Bale R, et al. Image fusion analysis of ^{99m}Tc-HYNICTyr3-octreotide SPECT and diagnostic CT using an immobilization device with external markers in patients with endocrine tumours. Eur J Nucl Med Mol Imaging 2005;32:1440–51.
15. De Jong M, Breeman WAP, Kwekkeboom DJ, et al. Tumor imaging and therapy using radiolabeled somatostatin analogues. Acc Chem Res 2009;42(7): 873–80.
16. Gabriel M, Decristoforo C, Kendler C, et al. [68]Gallium-DOTA-Tyr(3)-octreotide PET in neuroendocrine tumors: comparison with somatostatin receptor scintigraphy and computed tomography. J Nucl Med 2007;48:508–18.
17. Naswa N, Sharma P, Kumar A, et al. Gallium-68-DOTA-NOC PET/CT of patients with gastroenteropancreatic neuroendocrine tumors: a prospective single-center study. Am J Roentgenol 2011;197: 1221–8.
18. Putzer D, Gabriel M, Henninger B, et al. Bone metastases in patients with neuroendocrine tumor: ^{68}Ga-DOTA-Tyr3-octreotide PET in comparison to CT and bone scintigraphy. J Nucl Med 2009;50:1214–21.
19. Virgolini I, Gabriel M, Kroiss A, et al. Current knowledge on the sensitivity of the (68)Ga-somatostatin receptor positron emission tomography and the SUVmax reference range for management of pancreatic neuroendocrine tumours. Eur J Nucl Med Mol Imaging 2016;43(11):2072–83.
20. Virgolini I, Ambrosini V, Bomanji JB, et al. Procedure guidelines for PET/CT tumour imaging with ^{68}Ga-DOTA-conjugated peptides: ^{68}Ga-DOTA-TOC, ^{68}Ga-DOTA-NOC, ^{68}Ga-DOTA-TATE. Eur J Nucl Med Mol Imaging 2010;37:2004–10.
21. Deppen SA, Liu E, Blume JD, et al. Safety and efficacy of ^{68}Ga-DOTATATE PET/CT for diagnosis, staging, and treatment management of neuroendocrine tumors. J Nucl Med 2016;57:708–14.
22. Castellucci P, Pou Ucha J, Fuccio C, et al. Incidence of increased ^{68}Ga-DOTANOC uptake in the pancreatic head in a large series of extrapancreatic NET patients studied with sequential PET/CT. J Nucl Med 2011;52:886–90.
23. Ambrosini V, Campana D, Tomassetti P, et al. ^{68}Ga-labelled peptides for diagnosis of gastroenteropancreatic NET. Eur J Nucl Med Mol Imaging 2012;39:S52–60.
24. Haug AR, Cindea-Drimus R, Auernhammer CJ, et al. The role of ^{68}Ga-DOTATATE PET/CT in suspected

neuroendocrine tumors. J Nucl Med 2012;53: 1686–92.

25. Ilhan H, Fendler WP, Cyran CC, et al. Impact of 68Ga-DOTATATE PET/CT on the surgical management of primary neuroendocrine tumors of the pancreas or ileum. Ann Surg Oncol 2015;22:164–71.

26. Hofman MS, Kong G, Neels OC, et al. High management impact of Ga-68 DOTATATE (GaTate) PET/CT for imaging neuroendocrine and other somatostatin expressing tumours. J Med Imaging Radiat Oncol 2012;56:40–7.

27. Putzer D, Kroiss A, Waitz D, et al. Somatostatin receptor PET in neuroendocrine tumours: 68Ga-DOTA0, Tyr3-octreotide versus 68Ga-DOTA0-lanreotide. Eur J Nucl Med Mol Imaging 2013;40:364–72.

28. Nilica B, Waitz D, Stevanovic V, et al. Direct comparison of (68)Ga-DOTA-TOC and (18)F-FDG PET/CT in the follow-up of patients with neuroendocrine tumour treated with the first full peptide receptor radionuclide therapy cycle. Eur J Nucl Med Mol Imaging 2016;43(9):1585–92.

29. Kwee TC, Basu S, Saboury B, et al. A new dimension of FDG-PET interpretation: assessment of tumor biology. Eur J Nucl Med Mol Imaging 2011;38(6):1158–70.

30. Kayani I, Bomanji JB, Groves A, et al. Functional imaging of neuroendocrine tumors with combined PET/CT using 68Ga-DOTATATE (DOTA-DPhe1,Tyr3-octreotate) and 18F-FDG. Cancer 2008;112:2447–55.

31. Sharma P, Naswa N, Kc SS, et al. Comparison of the prognostic values of 68Ga-DOTANOC PET/CT and 18F-FDG PET/CT in patients with well-differentiated neuroendocrine tumor. Eur J Nucl Med Mol Imaging 2014;41:2194–21202.

32. Basu S1, Sirohi B, Shrikhande SV. Dual tracer imaging approach in assessing tumor biology and heterogeneity in neuroendocrine tumors: its correlation with tumor proliferation index and possible multifaceted implications for personalized clinical management decisions, with focus on PRRT. Eur J Nucl Med Mol Imaging 2014;41:1492–6.

33. Belhocine T, Foidart J, Rigo P, et al. Fluorodeoxyglucose positron emission tomography and somatostatin receptor scintigraphy for diagnosing and staging carcinoid tumours: correlations with the pathological indexes p53 and Ki-67. Nucl Med Commun 2002;23:727–34.

34. Adams S, Baum R, Rink T, et al. Limited value of fluorine-18 fluorodeoxyglucose positron emission tomography for the imaging of neuroendocrine tumours. Eur J Nucl Med 1998;25(1):79–83.

35. Binderup T, Knigge U, Loft A, et al. 18F-fluorodeoxyglucose positron emission tomography predicts survival of patients with neuroendocrine tumors. Clin Cancer Res 2010;16(3):978–85.

36. Garin E, Le JF, Devillers A, et al. Predictive value of 18F-FDG PET and somatostatin receptor scintigraphy in patients with metastatic endocrine tumors. J Nucl Med 2009;50:858–64.

37. Zhang J, Liu Q, Singh A, et al. Prognostic value of (18)F-FDG PET/CT in a large cohort of 495 patients with advanced metastatic neuroendocrine neoplasms (NEN) treated with peptide receptor radionuclide therapy (PRRT). J Nucl Med 2020;61(11):1560–9.

38. Pavel M, Hainsworth JD, Baudin E, et al. A randomized, double-blind, placebo-controlled, multicenter phase III trial of everolimus plus octreotide LAR vs placebo plus octreotide LAR in patients with advanced neuroendocrine tumors (NET) (RADIANT-2). Ann Oncol 2010;21(Suppl 8):viii4.

39. Rinke A, Müller HH, Schade-Brittinger C, et al. Placebo-controlled, double-blind, prospective, randomized study on the effect of octreotide LAR in the control of tumor growth in patients with metastatic neuroendocrine midgut tumors: a report from the PROMID Study Group. J Clin Oncol 2009;27:4656–63.

40. Strosberg J, El-Haddad G, Wolin E, et al. Phase 3 trial of (177)Lu-Dotatate for Midgut neuroendocrine tumors. N Engl J Med 2017;376:125–35.

41. Gabriel M, Nilica B, Kaiser B, et al. Twelve-year follow-up after peptide receptor radionuclide therapy (PRRT). J Nucl Med 2018. https://doi.org/10.2967/jnumed.118.215376.

42. Kwekkeboom DJ, de Herder WW, Kam BL, et al. Treatment with the radiolabeled somatostatin analog [177 Lu-DOTA 0,Tyr3] octreotate: toxicity, efficacy, and survival. J Clin Oncol 2008;26:2124–30.

43. Virgolini I, The Innsbruck Team. Peptide receptor radionuclide therapy (PRRT): clinical significance of re-treatment? Eur J Nucl Med Mol Imaging 2015;42:1949–54.

44. Prasad V, Horsch D, Hommann M, et al. Survival benefits and efficacy of peptide receptor radionuclide therapy (PRRT) using Y-90/Lu-177 DOTATATE in pancreatic neuroendocrine tumors (pNET) [abstract]. J Nucl Med 2009;50(suppl 2):43.

45. Strosberg JR, Halfdanarson TR, Bellizzi AM, et al. The North American Neuroendocrine Tumor Society consensus guidelines for surveillance and medical management of midgut neuroendocrine tumors. Pancreas 2017;46:707–14.

46. Forrer F, Uusijarvi H, Storch D, et al. Treatment with 177Lu-DOTATOC of patients with relapse of neuroendocrine tumors after treatment with 90Y-DOTA-TOC. J Nucl Med 2005;46:1310–6.

47. Khan S, Krenning EP, van Essen M, et al. Quality of life in 265 patients with gastroenteropancreatic or bronchial neuroendocrine tumors treated with [177Lu-DOTA0,Tyr3]octreotate. J Nucl Med 2011;52:1361–8.

48. Marinova M, Mucke M, Mahlberg L, et al. Improving quality of life in patients with pancreatic neuroendocrine tumor following peptide receptor radionuclide

therapy assessed by EORTC QLQ-C30. Eur J Nucl Med Mol Imaging 2018;45:38–46.

49. Strosberg J, Wolin E, Chasen B, et al. Health-related quality of life in patients with progressive midgut neuroendocrine tumors treated with (177)Lu-Dotatate in the phase III NETTER-1 trial. J Clin Oncol 2018;36:2578–84.

50. Martini C, Buxbaum S, Rodrigues M, et al. Quality of life in patients with metastatic gastroenteropancreatic neuroendocrine tumors receiving peptide receptor radionuclide therapy: information from a monitoring program in clinical routine. J Nucl Med 2018;59:1566–73.

51. Bodei L, Kidd M, Paganelli G, et al. Long-term tolerability of PRRT in 807 patients with neuroendocrine tumours: the value and limitations of clinical factors. Eur J Nucl Med Mol Imaging 2015;42(1):5–19.

52. Melis M, Krenning EP, Bernard BF, et al. Localisation and mechanism of renal retention of radiolabelled somatostatin analogues. Eur J Nucl Med Mol Imaging 2005;32(10):1136–43.

53. Nilica B, Svirydenka H, Fritz J, et al. Nephrotoxicity and hematotoxicity one year after four cycles of peptide receptor radionuclide therapy (PRRT). J Nucl Med 2020;61(suppl 1):307–12.

54. Kong G, Callahan J, Hofman MS, et al. High clinical and morphologic response using ^{90}Y-DOTA-octreotate sequenced with ^{177}Lu-DOTA-octreotate induction peptide receptor chemoradionuclide therapy (PRCRT) for bulky neuroendocrine tumours. Eur J Nucl Med Mol Imaging 2017;44:476–89.

Theranostics in Thyroid Cancer

Friederike Eilsberger, MD*, Andreas Pfestroff, MD

KEYWORDS

• Thyroid cancer • Radioiodine • I-131 • Sodium-iodine symporter

KEY POINTS

- Considering theranostics in thyroid cancer, the sodium-iodine symporter (NIS) is the main target structure.
- In thyroid cancer a uniquely congruent theranostics is possible by using different kinds of radioiodine.
- Besides radioiodine and the NIS, there are further possibilities for performing theranostics in thyroid cancer, as DOTA-TOC/-TATE or prostate-specific membrane antigen, particularly with regard to radioiodine refractoriness, medullary thyroid cancer, or anaplastic thyroid cancer.

INTRODUCTION

In Nuclear Medicine, radioactive isotopes of iodine have been used in clinical routine for the diagnosis and treatment of thyroid diseases, especially thyroid cancer for more than 70 years.[1,2] Even though the term was introduced much later, radioiodine therapy in thyroid cancer has been the first widely applied theranostic approach and is still the most commonly used radionuclide treatment in a malignant disease with a high response rate and the chance for a cure even in advanced disease and an excellent sensitivity and specificity for tumor lesions on posttherapeutic imaging. This article provides a brief overview of the use of different radioiodine isotopes in various clinical settings and new targets for theranostics in thyroid cancer.

SODIUM-IODINE SYMPORTER

Considering theranostics in thyroid cancer, the sodium-iodine symporter (NIS) is the main target structure. NIS, which is located in the basolateral membrane of thyrocytes, actively transports the iodine into the cell. This intracellular iodine enters the colloid on the opposite side of the cell, the apical membrane, mostly via pendrin and/or other unspecified channels. In the colloid, the iodine is

oxidized and bound to thyroglobulin (Tg) by the enzyme thyroid peroxidase and either remains in the colloid or leaves the cell incorporated into the thyroid hormones triiodothyronine or tetraiodothyronine.[3]

This specific target structure is used for therapy in differentiated thyroid cancer (DTC). DTC commonly shows a strong NIS expression, especially in a treatment-naive state and the beginning of the disease.

In 1941, Hertz and colleagues performed the first and immediately successful radioiodine therapies with iodine 130 (^{130}I) in patients with hyperthyroidism; in the same year, the first patients were also successfully treated with ^{131}I.[1,2] ^{131}I is a substrate for the NIS, and it is transported into thyroid cells instead of stable iodine during radioiodine therapy. It is incorporated into the thyroid hormones such as stable iodine and stored in the colloid bound to Tg, where it then leads to nuclear pyknosis, cell necrosis, and follicular collapse due to radioactive β-decay, which reaches an average penetration in tissue of 0.5 mm. However, there is more to ^{131}I than only the feasibility-targeted therapy mediated by the beta component. A localization of the isotope in the body is feasible, because of the gamma emissions with the help

The authors have nothing to disclose.
University Hospital Marburg, Department of Nuclear Medicine, Baldingerstrasse, 35043 Marburg, Germany
* Corresponding author.
E-mail address: friederike.mueller@staff.uni-marburg.de

PET Clin 16 (2021) 375–382
https://doi.org/10.1016/j.cpet.2021.03.007
1556-8598/21/© 2021 Elsevier Inc. All rights reserved.

pet.theclinics.com

of gamma cameras. However, the gamma component has a high energy with the main peak at 364 keV. Also because of its long half-life of 8 days and the high radiation exposure, ^{131}I is not ideal for pure imaging. As an alternative to ^{131}I, ^{123}I can also be used for diagnostic purposes. As a pure gamma emitter with lower energy gamma emission and shorter half-life, it has better properties for imaging. Its use in clinical routine is limited in many countries because of costs and supply. The usefulness of a theranostic concept in thyroid cancer has been limited so far.[4] With the increasing availability of PET, ^{124}I became of interest as a radiotracer for visualizing iodine uptake via NIS, especially due to the 2 advantages of its longer half-life of 4.2 days, which allows the collection of quantitative data for dosimetric purposes over days and the better resolution of PET compared with single-photon emission computed tomography (SPECT).

RADIOIODINE THERAPY IN DIFFERENTIATED THYROID CANCER

Most patients with differentiated thyroid carcinoma receive adjuvant radioiodine therapy (RIT) after thyroidectomy, depending on the individual risk profile. Although RIT is still being discussed controversially in low-risk and intermediate-risk patients, there is at least a consensus that all high-risk patients should routinely receive radioiodine therapy. The 3 possible aims of performing RIT are remnant ablation, adjuvant treatment, and treatment of known disease.[5] Although remnant ablation today is largely regarded as being of less importance because of improvements in ultrasound and Tg assays, the aim of adjuvant

treatment is to improve disease-specific survival, progression-free survival, and decreasing recurrence rates, by the targeted treatment of occult microscopic cancer foci such as lymph node metastases. This adjuvant treatment also destroys (not intentionally) benign remnant thyroid tissue and thereby enables iodine imaging as well as valid and reliable Tg measurements. After therapy, posttherapeutic radioiodine imaging is performed routinely. In this way, iodine avid metastases (**Fig. 1**) or persistent locoregional disease may be detected with high specificity and sensitivity, in accordance with the concept of theranostics.

RADIOIODINE IMAGING WITH ^{131}I

The supplementation of neck ultrasound, as well as Tg measurements by a diagnostic iodine-131 whole-body scintigraphy should be considered in the follow-up. Especially in cases of intense cervical uptake in the thyroid bed or iodine avid lymph nodes in posttherapy whole-body scan, the performance of a restaging including radioiodine diagnosis can be very useful, because information, for example, about the course of iodine avid metastases can be derived from the findings in combination with sonography and measurement of the stimulated Tg value.[6] In addition, if a recurrence is suspected, a previous performance of such radioiodine whole-body scan can serve as baseline imaging. It is then easy to differentiate between remaining residual thyroid as seen at baseline and new iodine avid tissue suspicious for a relapse. Diagnostic radioiodine can monitor the effect of radioiodine treatment and can be used in the assessment in the context of suspicion of relapse. Van Nostrand emphasizes this advantage

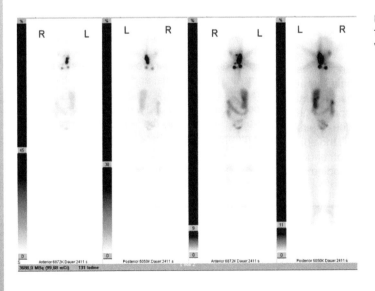

Fig. 1. Patient 1: lymph node metastases of DTC, which presented on whole-body scan after RIT.

in a paper on controversies in radioiodine imaging and therapy. He recommends that radioiodine whole-body scan should be performed 6 to 18 months after radioiodine therapy as a new baseline to be able to make a comparison between this new baseline and a new diagnostic imaging at increasing Tg.[7] The indication for radioiodine diagnostics can also be made individually and independently of the time of the first radioiodine therapy in patients without excellent response, in patients with increased anti-Tg antibody levels or impaired Tg recovery (reduced significance of the tumor marker), or in patients with persistent disease. A further useful information on a situation of recurrence is to assess the iodine avidity of the tumor manifestations in order to evaluate if another radioiodine therapy in the context of theranostics is feasible.

The use of SPECT/CT in addition to or instead of the planar whole-body scan allows an exact anatomic localization and thus better characterization of foci with increased ^{131}I uptake, both on posttherapy imaging as well as on diagnostic ^{131}I imaging.[8]

RADIOIODINE-REFRACTORY DIFFERENTIATED THYROID CANCER

The final definition of iodine-refractory differentiated thyroid cancer is still subject of brisk scientific discussions. Tuttle and colleagues[5] emphasize that there is currently no definition or fixed criteria by which patients can be safely classified as radioiodine negative, rather an individual assessment should be made about many factors to evaluate the probability of iodine refraction.

Until a commonly accepted and well-founded definition of radioiodine refractoriness is available, the criteria remain vague, but generally speaking, radioiodine-refractory disease means that treatment with ^{131}I is no longer effective and the discontinuation of this therapeutically concept must be considered. Based on this, patients with one or more vital tumor lesions without iodine uptake are currently considered ^{131}I refractory (**Figs. 2 and 3**). An additional point is tumor progression within a short period of time (6 or 12 months) after radioiodine therapy, regardless of the radioiodine avidity of these lesions. Also, patients showing tumor manifestations with high metabolism in PET with fludeoxyglucose 18F or patients with disease progression after radioiodine treatment with a cumulative activity of 22.2 GBq are sometimes considered to be ^{131}I refractory.[9]

In theranostics thyroid cancer radioiodine refractoriness implies a limitation of the usability of the main target structure, namely the NIS. The loss of the expression of this leads to a loss of the therapeutic option of radioiodine therapy, as well as the detectability and visualization of the metastases. The experimental approach for restoring the expression of the NIS and thus the radioiodine avidity has been able to achieve good preclinical results in recent years.[10,11]

REDIFFERENTIATION THERAPY

The mechanism responsible for developing radioiodine refractoriness lies with genetic alterations in the MAPK signaling pathway. The activation of the MAPK pathway in thyroid carcinoma leads, among other effects, to the downregulation of the expression of genes responsible for the NIS and Tg

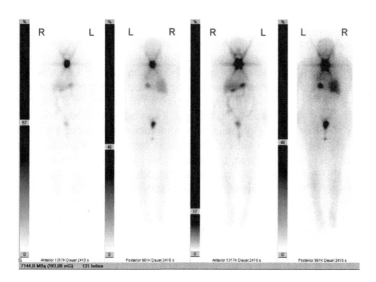

Fig. 2. Patient 2: radioiodine refractory lung metastases on whole-body scan after RIT.

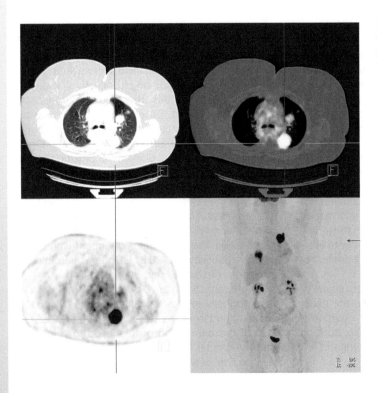

Fig. 3. Patient 2: radioiodine refractory lung metastases on whole-body scan after RIT, which show high uptake in FDG-PET/CT (compare **Fig. 2**).

synthesis.[12] The *BRAF*[V600E] mutation is the most common genetic alteration in papillary thyroid cancer (PTC); in addition, RAS mutations are found in 10% to 20% of PTCs and 40% to 50% of patients with follicular thyroid cancer (FTC).

By inhibiting the MAPK signaling pathway through the inhibition of BRAF, preclinical studies in radioiodine-refractory thyroid cancer have demonstrated a reexpression of the NIS. Nagarajah and colleagues[11] were able to show that this upregulation caused the tumors to become radioiodine sensitive again in vitro and in vivo.

Preclinical experience with MAPK inhibition suggests an increase in radioiodine uptake, but no prolongation in retention time, which seem to be confirmed in first patient data.[13]

The active transport of iodine via NIS into the cell correlates with the expression level of the symporter and can be quantified in vivo by [124]I PET imaging. The effective half-life, in other words the fate of the absorbed iodine in various organs or tumor manifestations, can be determined by performing multiple time-point PET imaging over several days. The advantages of [124]I PET dosimetry become particularly clear when it comes to quantifying the changes in iodine uptake or iodine kinetics after manipulation of NIS. It is also possible to differentiate whether the manipulation affects the uptake or the kinetics or both.

The [124]I PET results in the previous first patients showed an approximately 14-fold increase in radioiodine uptake, whereas the effective half-life remained unchanged; this is probably because in these tumors the MAPK inhibitor alone is not sufficient to restore cell polarity and thus form a functional colloidal structure, which is crucial for the binding of the radioiodine to the Tg, leading to an increased effective half-life.[13] Redifferentiation therapy with the MAPK inhibitors selumetinib and dabrafenib in BRAF- and NRAS-positive tumors is currently still an experimental therapeutic approach. However, due to the limited number of well-tolerated alternatives, especially for progressive diseases, redifferentiation offers a new therapeutic option. PET imaging with [124]I is able to perform an evaluation in this setting of redifferentiation therapy. According to the results of the corresponding therapy, it can be determined whether the iodine uptake could possibly be used for therapy with radioiodine in terms of theranostics. In addition, the activity that can or should be applied can be calculated via dosimetry. Pretherapeutic dosimetry is particularly important in patients who have received redifferentiation therapy, as the planned radioiodine therapy in many cases will be the last and in many cases advanced disease is present. Pretherapeutic dosimetry is possible according to 2 forms. On the one hand according to the method developed by Benua and colleagues,[14] the "As High As Safely Administrable", which is based on the calculation of an activity that, with maximum ^{131}I administration, seeks to avoid toxicities such as bone marrow depression, pulmonary fibrosis, or pneumonitis, and the "As Low As Reasonably Achievable" (ALARA) approach, which is based on the calculation of the lowest possible activity to reach the desired dose in tumor lesions.[14,15] The response of metastases to radioiodine therapy is closely related to the effective dose achieved and the radiation sensitivity of the tumor cells. Maxon defined a threshold value of 80 Gy as the dose to be achieved for successful treatment of metastases.[15] In patients with known multiple metastases, the "maximum activity to be tolerated" is determined in each individual case. As risk organs, the doses of blood as surrogate parameters for the bone marrow, the lung dose, and the whole-body activity are determined at different points in time within the framework of pretherapeutic dosimetry after oral application of approximately 10 MBq [131]I. The maximum activity to be applied should not exceed a maximum dose in the blood (bone marrow) of 2 Gy, a maximum whole-body activity of 4.4 GBq after 48 hours, and a maximum activity in the lung of 3 GBq after 24 hours. These limits represent thresholds to avoid damage to the bone marrow or healthy lung parenchyma.

FURTHER POSSIBILITIES OF THERANOSTICS IN THYROID CANCER

Besides the traditional theranostics that uses NIS as its target, there are further possibilities, for example, the expression of somatostatin receptors (SSTR) or the expression of the prostate specific membrane antigen (PSMA), that could provide alternative diagnostic possibilities und therapy options.

Somatostatin Receptor Targeting

The expression of somatostatin receptors is generally known as a characteristic of endocrine, especially neuroendocrine tumors. In order to target somatostatin receptors, somatostatin analogues and also antagonists have been developed. Initially, indium 111(111I)- and technetium 99m-radiolabeled peptides were used for diagnostic purposes, along with beta-emitters for therapeutic approaches. The first reported somatostatin receptor–targeted treatments of patients with thyroid cancer were published by Krenning and colleagues[16] in 1999. Initially, the group performed imaging with ^{111}In-DTPA-octreotide. If the tumor masses were well visualized, which means a good somatostatin receptor expression, the

patients received peptide receptor radionuclide therapy (PRRT) with repetitive administrations of high activities of this compound. The publication of a pilot study followed in 2005, presenting the result of PRRT with 22.4 to 30.1 GBq of lutetium 177 (^{177}Lu)-DOTATATE in 5 patients with radioiodine-refractory differentiated thyroid cancer (DTC). Before therapy an ^{111}In-octreotide scintigraphy was performed for visualizing the expression of SSRT. After therapy one patient with Hürthle cell thyroid carcinoma had stable disease, one showed minor remission, and one had partial remission. The patient with PTC had stable disease and the response of the one patient with FTC was progressive disease.[17] Although there were also a few newer studies, the results of this therapeutically approach are not consistently convincing,[18,19] just like studies regarding the SSTR expression in radioiodine-refractory DTC.[20] At this point, it is worth mentioning a work by Binse and colleagues,[21] in which the investigators described the uptake of gallium 68 (^{68}Ga)-DOTATOC in ^{18}F-FDG negative lesions.

Besides theranostics in differentiated thyroid cancer, SSTR targeting can be used in medullary thyroid cancer (MTC), which inherently has no NIS expression, as a possible option, although there is only limited experience on its efficacy. Iten and colleagues[22] published a clinical phase II trial with 31 patients with metastasized MTC who received a median cumulative activity of 12.6 GBq yttrium 90-DOTATOC. Nine patients showed a response, which was associated with longer survival from the time of diagnosis and from the time of first PRRT. Besides, the treatment response and survival were not associated with the grade of visual scintigraphic tumor uptake.[22]

Beukhof and colleagues[23] came to a different conclusion in their evaluation. In a retrospective evaluation of treatment effects of PRRT in 10 patients with MTC, 4 had stable disease at first follow-up, and all of them exhibited a positive SSTR type 2a expression of the tumor by immunohistochemistry and a high uptake on ^{111}In-octreotide scintigraphy, so it was concluded by the investigators that these characteristics must be present for a reasonable and successful therapy.[23]

Prostate-Specific Membrane Antigen Targeting

Originally the prostate-specific membrane antigen targeting (PSMA) is established in diagnostic purposes and treatment in prostate cancer. PSMA is a membrane-bound glycoprotein with the function of a glutamic acid–releasing carboxypeptidase enzyme, which is biologically expressed by the

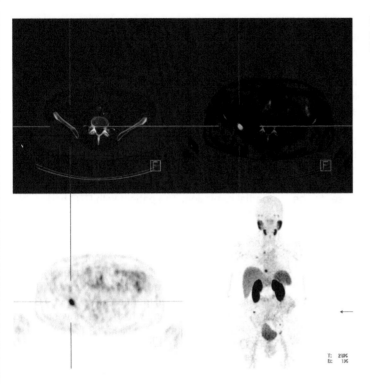

Fig. 4. Patient 3: ^{68}Ga-PSMA-PET/CT in radioiodine-refractory DTC showing high uptake in bone metastases.

prostate and among others, proximal renal tubule cells, small intestine, central and peripheral nervous system, but expression was likewise shown in the neovasculature of various malignancies, for example, in DTC[24–26] (**Figs. 4** and **5**).

There are very few cases in the literature of patients with iodine-refractory DTC initially receiving a ^{68}Ga-PSMA PET/CT and afterward, if a good PSMA expression was demonstrated, receiving ^{177}Lu-PSMA therapy, in some of these rare patients partial, temporary response was reachable.[27] But to be truly able to evaluate the

diagnostic and therapeutic potential of this approach, further research is needed.

In addition to the iodine-refractory DTC, PSMA expression is a very interesting point in poorly differentiated and dedifferentiated (anaplastic) thyroid cancer. Heitkötter and colleagues[28] were able to show a strong expression in the neovasculature in these tumor entities. In the clinical practical implementation, there are case reports of high uptake in ^{68}Ga-PSMA PET/CT in the primary tumor, cervical, and mediastinal lymph nodes.[29] With regard to theranostics, the consolidation of

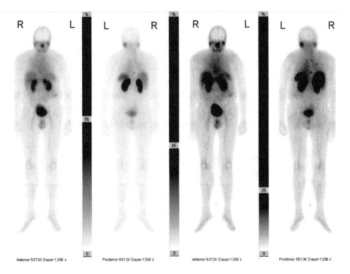

Fig. 5. Patient 3: whole-body scintigraphy after ^{177}Lu-PSMA radioligand therapy showing uptake in bone metastases.

knowledge concerning PSMA expression and the opportunity to make use of it may lead to new therapeutically options in patients with anaplastic thyroid cancer.

SUMMARY

With regard to theranostics in thyroid carcinoma, there are very elegant possibilities, especially for the differentiated variants. Because the diagnostic nuclides ^{123}I and [124]I have the same kinetics to the therapeutic nuclide ^{131}I, a uniquely congruent theranostics is possible, which is in contrast to the use of carrier molecules that have different kinetics when bound to ^{68}Ga or [177]Lu.[30,31] Furthermore, radioiodine therapy is the only theranostic approach that achieves a cure in nearly most cases. Compared, for example, with theranostics in prostate carcinoma, complete remission can rarely be achieved. The rates of a complete remission here are around 10% for the application of actinium 225–PSMA and around 2.5% for a biochemical complete remission for the therapy with ^{177}Lu-PSMA.[32–34]

The visualization of metastases is better in scans after ^{131}I therapy than in iodine diagnostics; when using ^{123}I or ^{131}I in low activity, the whole-body scan after therapy shows a better sensitivity and specificity.[35] In this respect ^{131}I theranostics is superior to theranostics with DOTA-TOC/-TATE or PSMA. In PET/CT imaging with ^{68}Ga more lesions can be seen than in the posttherapeutic ^{177}Lu scan, among other things due to the better resolution.[36] Sainz-Esteban and colleagues[37] were able to show that the sensitivity, positive predictive value, and accuracy for ^{177}Lu whole-body scan in comparison with ^{68}Ga-DOTA-TATE-PET/CT were 91%, 97%, and 88%; 9% of the lesions seen on PET/CT were not imaged on ^{177}Lu whole-body scan after therapy.

In summary, the unique status of iodine in theranostics (for thyroid cancer) has to be emphasized.

CLINICS CARE POINTS

- In patients with differentiated thyroid cancer a uniquely congruent theranostic is possible by using different kinds of iodine nuclides, which provide the same kinetics.
- There are further targeting structures such as somatostatin receptors or the expression of the prostate specific membrane antigen.
- These further structures may represent an even more important diagnostic and therapeutic tool in the future for patients with radioiodine-refractory DTC, medullary thyroid cancer, or anaplastic thyroid cancer.

REFERENCES

1. Becker DV, Sawin CT. Radioiodine and thyroid disease: the beginning. Semin Nucl Med 1996;26(3): 155–64.
2. Sawin CT, Becker DV. Radioiodine and the treatment of hyperthyreodism: the early history. Thyroid 1997; 7(2):163–76.
3. Brent GA. Mechanisms of thyroid hormone action. J Clin Invest 2012;122(9):3035–43.
4. Luster M, Clarke SE, Dietlein M, et al. Guidelines for radioiodine therapy of differentiated thyroid cancer. Eur J Nucl Med Mol Imaging 2008;35:1941–59.
5. Tuttle RM, Ahuja S, Avram AM, et al. Controversies, consensus, and collaboration in the use of 131I therapy in differentiated thyroid cancer: a joint statement from the American thyroid association, the European association of nuclear medicine, the society of nuclear medicine and molecular imaging, and the European thyroid association. Thyroid 2019;29(4): 461–70.
6. Verburg FA, Schmidt M, Kreissl MC, et al. Iod-131-Ganzkörperszintigraphie beim differenzierten Schilddrüsenkarzinom. Stand 1/2019, AWMF-Registrierungsnummer: 031-013
7. Van Nostrand D. Selected controversies of radioiodine imaging and therapy in differentiated thyroid cancer. Endocrinol Metab Clin North Am 2017;46: 783–93.
8. Ahmed N, Niyaz K, Borakati A, et al. Hybrid SPECT/CT imaging in the management of differentiated thyroid carcinoma. Asian Pan J Canver Prev 2018; 19(2):303–8.
9. Cabanillas ME, McFadden DG, Durante C. Thyroid cancer. Lancet 2016;388:2783–95.
10. Chakravarty D, Santos E, Ryder M, et al. Small-molecule MAPK inhibitors restore radioiodine incorporation in mouse thyroid cancers with conditional BRAF activation. J Clin Invest 2011;121:4700–11.
11. Nagarajah J, Le M, Knauf JA, et al. Sustained ERK inhibition maximizes responses of BrafV600E thyroid cancers to radioiodine. J Clin Invest 2016;126: 4119–24.
12. Knauf JA, Kuroda H, Basu S, et al. RET/PTC-induced dedifferentiation of thyroid cells is mediated through Y1062 signaling through SHC-RAS-MAP kinase. Oncogene 2003;22(28):4406–12.
13. Kreißl MC, Jentzen W, Janssen M, et al. 124I/131I-Theranostics of sodium-iodine-symporter in thyroid cancer. Der Nuklearmediziner 2019;42:15–20.
14. Benua RS, Cicale NR, Sonenberg M, et al. The relation of radioiodine dosimetry to results and complications in the treatment of metastatic thyroid cancer. Am J Roentgenol Radium Ther Nucl Med 1962;87:171e82.
15. Maxon HR, Thomas SR, Hertzberg VS, et al. Relation between effective radiation dose and outcome of

radioiodine therapy for thyroid cancer. N Engl J Med 1983;309:937e41.

16. Krenning EP, De Jong E, Kooij PPM, et al. Radiolabelled somatostatin analogue(s) for peptide receptor scintigraphy and radionuclide therapy. ANN Oncol 1999;10:23–9.

17. Teunissen JJM, Kwekkeboom DJ, Kooil PPM, et al. Peptide receptor radionuclide therapy for non–radioiodine-avid differentiated thyroid carcinoma. J Nucl Med 2005;46:107–14.

18. Budiawan H, Salavati A, Kulkarni HR, et al. Peptide receptor radionuclide therapy of treatment-refractory metastatic thyroid cancer using 90-Yttrium and 177-Lutetium labeled somatostatin analogs: toxicity, response and survival analysis. Am J Nucl Med Mol Imaging 2014;4:39–52.

19. Versari A, Sollini M, Frasoldati A, et al. Differentiated thyroid cancer: a new perspective with radiolabeled somatostatin analogues for imaging and treatment of patients. Thyroid 2014;24:715–26.

20. Jois B, Asopa R, Basu S. Somatostatin receptor imaging in non-(131)I-avid metastatic differentiated thyroid carcinoma for determining the feasibility of peptide receptor radionuclide therapy with (177) Lu-DOTATATE: low fraction of patients suitable for peptide receptor radionuclide therapy and evidence of chromogranin A level-positive neuroendocrine differentiation. Clin Nucl Med 2014;39:505–10.

21. Binse I, Poeppel TD, Ruhlmann M, et al. 68Ga-DOTATOC PET/CT in patients with iodine- and 18F-FDG-Negative differentiated thyroid carcinoma and elevated serum thyroglobulin. J Nucl Med 2016;57:1512–7.

22. Itel F, Müller B, Schindler C, et al. Response to [90Yttrium-DOTA]-TOC treatment is associated with long-term survival benefit in metastasized medullary thyroid cancer: a phase II clinical trial. Clin Cancer Res 2007;13:6696–702.

23. Beukhof CM, Brabander T, Van Nederveen FH, et al. Peptide receptor radionuclide therapy in patients with medullary thyroid carcinoma: predictors and pitfalls. BMC Cancer 2019;19(1):325.

24. Barinka C, Sacha P, Sklenar J, et al. Identification of the N-glycosylation sites on glutamate carboxypeptidase II Necessary for proteolytic activity. Protein Sci 2004;13(6):1627–35.

25. Kinoshita Y, Kuratsukuri K, Landas S, et al. Expression of prostate-specific membrane antigen in normal and malignant human tissues. World J Surg 2006;30:628–36.

26. Taywade SK, Damle NA, Bal CS. PSMA expression in papillary thyroid carcinoma opening a new horizon in management of thyroid cancer? Clin Nucl Med 2016;41:263–5.

27. De Vries LH, Lodewijk L, Braat AJA, et al. 68 Ga-PSMA PET/CT in radioactive iodine-refractory differentiated thyroid cancer and first treatment results with 177 Lu-PSMA-617. EJNMMI Res 2020;10:18.

28. Heitkötter B, Steinestel K, Trautmann M, et al. Neovascular PSMA expression is a common feature in malignant neoplasms of the thyroid. Oncotarget 2018;9:9867–74.

29. Damle NA, Bal CB, Singh TP, et al. Anaplastic thyroid carcinoma on 68 Ga-PSMA PET/CT: opening new frontiers. Eur J Nucl Med Mol Imaging 2018;45:667–8.

30. Weineisen M, Schottelius M, Simecek J, et al. 68Ga- and 177Lu-labeled PSMA I%T: Optimization of a PSMA-targeted theranostic concept and first proof-of-concept human studies. J Nucl Med 2015;56(8):1169–76.

31. Umbrich CA, Benesova M, Schmid RM, et al. 44Sc-PSMA-617 for radiotheranostics in tandem with 177Lu-PSMA-617 – preclinical investigation in comparison with 68Ga-PSMA-11 and 68Ga-PSMA-617. EJNMMI Res 2017;7:9.

32. Yadav MP, Ballal S, Sahoo RK, et al. Efficacy and safety of 255-Ac-PSMA-617 targeted alpha therapy in metastatic castration-resistant Prostate Cancer patients. Theranostics 2020;10(20):9264–377.

33. Kratochwil C, Bruchertseifer F, Rathke H, et al. α-Therapy of metastatic castration-resistant prostate cancer with 225 Ac-PSMA-617: swimmer-plot analysis suggests efficacy regarding duration of tumor control. J Nucl Med 2018;59(5):795–802.

34. Kulkarni HR, Singh A, Schuchardt C, et al. PSMA-based radioligand therapy for metastatic castration-resistant prostate cancer: the bad berka experience since 2013. J Nucl Med 2016;57(3):97–104.

35. Robertson M, Voss S, Grant F, et al. I-123 and I-131 scintigraphy discordance in pediatric thyroid cancer; effect of previous I-131 therapy. J Nucl Med 2015;56(3):423.

36. Maffey-Steffan J, Scarpa L, Svirydenka A, et al. The 68 Ga/177 Lu-theragnostic concept in PSMA-targeting of metastatic castration-resistant prostate cancer: impact of post-therapeutic whole-body scintigraphy in the follow-up. Eur J Nucl Med Mol Imaging 2020;47(3):695–712.

37. Sainz-Esteban A, Prasas V, Schuchardt C, et al. Comparison of sequential planar 177Lu-DOTA-TATE dosimetry scans with 68Ga-DOTA-TATE PET/CT images in patients with metastasized neuroendocrine tumours undergoing peptide receptor radionuclide therapy. Eur J Nucl Med Mol Imaging 2012;39(3):501–11.

Prostate Cancer Theranostics
From Target Description to Imaging

Ian L. Alberts, MD, MA[a,*], Robert Seifert, MD[b,c,d,e], Kambiz Rahbar, MD[b,d],
Ali Afshar-Oromieh, MD[a]

KEYWORDS

- Prostate cancer • Biochemical recurrence • Prostate-specific membrane antigen • PSMA
- PSMA-PET/CT

KEY POINTS

- Prostate-specific membrane antigen–PET/computed tomography (PSMA-PET/CT) is an established modality in the staging of recurrent prostate cancer, demonstrating superior diagnostic performance compared with conventional imaging modalities, such as CT or MR imaging, and previous-generation nuclear medicine modalities, such as scintigraphy and choline-based radiotracers.
- There is increasing evidence, including clinical trial data, that PSMA-PET/CT has a role in the staging of high-risk prostate cancer.
- PSMA is highly expressed on prostate cancer cells, but is not specific, potentially causing pitfalls. Some prostate cancers express no, or low levels of PSMA, and various factors including the use of hormone deprivation therapy can influence PSMA expression.
- Although a large body of robust evidence shows the superiority of PSMA-PET/CT compared with the present alternatives, further work is needed to elucidate potential differences between PSMA-based radiotracers and to establish the influence of PSMA-PET/CT on clinical outcomes for patients.
- PSMA-PET/CT has an important role for identifying patients suitable for PSMA therapy.

INTRODUCTION

Prostate cancer (PC) is the most common malignancy in men, and the second leading cause of cancer-related death in men.[1] Despite initial therapy at early-stage disease, biochemical recurrence remains a commonly encountered entity and presents a challenge for conventional imaging modalities given their limited abilities to detect disease at early stages of recurrence. Although the exact timing of salvage radiotherapy (SRT) remains a topic of debate, early SRT may be beneficial for some patients,[2] and imaging has a demonstrable impact on therapeutic strategy and decision-making.[3]

Although PC screening with prostate-specific antigen (PSA) is a topic of some controversy, since the advent of PSA testing the proportion of patients presenting with advanced disease has fallen. Nevertheless, a small number of patients continue to suffer from disease at an incurable stage at presentation.[4] Furthermore, despite significant advances in therapeutics in recent decades, a number of patients develop advanced disease (where the disease has spread beyond the prostate bed). Compared with

[a] Department of Nuclear Medicine, Inselspital, Bern University Hospital, University of Bern, Bern, Switzerland;
[b] Department of Nuclear Medicine, University Hospital Münster, Münster, Germany; [c] Department of Nuclear Medicine, University Hospital Essen, Essen, Germany; [d] West German Cancer Centre, Universitätsklinikum Essen, Hufelandstr. 55, 45147 Essen, Germany; [e] German Cancer Consortium (DKTK), German Cancer Research Center, Im Neuenheimer Feld 280, D-69120 Heidelberg, Germany
* Corresponding author.
E-mail address: Ian.alberts@insel.ch

PET Clin 16 (2021) 383–390
https://doi.org/10.1016/j.cpet.2021.03.003
1556-8598/21/© 2021 The Author(s). Published by Elsevier Inc. This is an open access article under the CC BY-NC-ND license (http://creativecommons.org/licenses/by-nc-nd/4.0/).

almost 100% 5-year survival for local or regional disease, the 5-year survival rate for advanced disease is 31%,[5] where therapeutic options remain of limited efficacy. For example, palliative radium-223 dichloride (Xofigo) therapy is associated with a modest medial overall survival of 14.9 versus 11.3 months when compared with placebo.[6] Nuclear medicine therefore was faced with two concomitant challenges: first, to identify correctly and accurately individuals at early-stage disease, where the likelihood of a definitive cure is greatest, as well as to offer solutions to individuals who have progressed to, or present with, advanced disease. The discovery of ligands for the prostate-specific membrane antigen (PSMA) has allowed nuclear medicine and molecular imaging to rise to both of these challenges in a manner that combines both therapy and diagnostics: theranostics.

PROSTATE-SPECIFIC MEMBRANE ANTIGEN

Before embarking on a description of PSMA in the imaging and therapy of PC, it is worth pausing to consider the broader function of this key molecular target. PSMA, also known as glutamate carboxypeptidase II (GCPII) or N-acetyl-L-aspartyl-L-glutamate peptidase I (NAALADase I), is a 750 amino-acid type II transmembrane glycoprotein, weighing approximately 100 kDa.[7] First described in studies of monoclonal antibodies to a novel antigenic marker in PC in the late 1980s,[8–10] it has rapidly become clear that despite its name, the expression of this transmembrane protein is not restricted to PC. It also can be found in normal prostatic tissue and the vascular endothelium in a wide variety of solid tumors,[11,12] but not in blood vessels of normal tissues. Physiologic PSMA expression is reported in the lacrimal and salivary glands, the liver, the spleen, the kidneys, and the intestines.[13] PSMA-ligand uptake has also been observed in benign inflammatory lymph nodes,[14] and numerous publications have demonstrated PSMA-avid peripheral nerve ganglia and in central nervous tissue.[15–20] The role of PSMA in the prostate and its exact role in PC remains elusive. PSMA appears to have NAALDase activity and folate hydrolase activity, and therefore has many potentially interesting roles in both glutamate and folate metabolism, with implications for the diagnosis and treatment of various cancers as well as neurologic disorders.

PROSTATE-SPECIFIC MEMBRANE ANTIGEN-BASED IMAGING AND THERANOSTICS

The discovery that PSMA is exquisitely overexpressed on PC cells[9] led to it becoming the focus of great attention as a potential target for treatment and therapy. Conventional imaging methods such as CT and MR imaging have limited performance in PC,[21] and traditional nuclear medicine techniques such as bone scintigraphy have a limited role in the exclusion of advanced disease. Instead, various alternatives have been advanced in recent decades: PET imaging with radiolabeled choline tracers have been used,[22] capitalizing on the overexpression of choline kinase in PC.[23] In tandem, PSMA-based imaging probes were developed, first with the introduction of In-111 capromab-pendetide (ProstaScint), a radiolabeled anti-PSMA antibody.[24] However, it was the introduction of PSMA-PET ligands that revolutionized the molecular imaging of PC.[25] ^{68}Ga-PSMA-11 (also known has PSMA-HBED, HBED-CC or PSMA-DFKZ), following its first clinical introduction in 2011,[13] has rapidly established itself as the examination of choice in recurrent PC and increasing data are accumulating about its important role in the staging of high-risk primary PC.[26]

FACTORS INFLUENCING PROSTATE-SPECIFIC MEMBRANE ANTIGEN EXPRESSION

As described previously, PSMA is not prostate specific. A number of publications also report the phenomenon of PSMA-negative PC. Although an additional PSMA-PET/CT in the context of a negative choline-PET/CT has been described as a potential imaging sequence in jurisdictions in which PSMA-PET might not be universally available, the reverse scenario has received relatively little attention, although there is a role for an additional choline-PET/CT in PSMA-nonexpressing PC.[27] Some investigators suggest PET with fludeoxyglucose ^{18}F-FDG as an adjunct to PSMA imaging before PSMA-based radioligand therapy to identify de-dedifferentiated tumor sites lacking PSMA expression (differentiated PC is normally not FDG avid).[28]

In addition to variation in tumor biology, PSMA expression can also be modulated by the patient's hormone status. Androgen deprivation therapy (ADT) is an established modality in the treatment of castration-sensitive PC (CSPC), and as such it is estimated that up to a third of all patients referred for PSMA-PET/CT imaging are receiving ADT.[29] However, the influence of ADT on PSMA-PET/CT is unclear. Preclinical data indicate upregulated PSMA expression following short-term ADT,[30–32] making it a potential pre-imaging or therapeutic maneuver to increase lesion uptake. However, there is a paucity of clinical information regarding the effect of long-term ADT on PSMA-PET/CT. A variegated PSMA-imaging response was observed following short-term ADT in CSPC patients in case reports,[31,33] in cohorts with small patient numbers[34–36] and in studies of retrospective design.[37–39]

The exact relationship between androgen receptor activity and PSMA expression remains elusive. The PSMA receptor is encoded in the folate hydrolase 1 (FOLH1) gene, the expression of which is downregulated by androgens.[40] As a consequence, ADT leads to an upregulation of FOLH1 expression, potentially explaining a relationship between androgen deprivation and heightened PSMA expression.[36] This mechanism may also explain the clinical finding of association between ADT and increased probability of a pathologic PSMA-PET/CT,[38,41] although this may well be a result of selection bias with patients at more advanced clinical stage being more likely to have ADT prescribed. However, it needs to be emphasized, that only a short duration of treatment for ADT (defined in various publications as 2 days-4 weeks) has been observed to lead to PSMA overexpression[32,42] or increased uptake of PSMA-ligands.[31] Following long-duration ADT, the opposite response is seen,[38] possibly due to a shrinking of the tumor in CSPC. PSMA expression is likely mediated by a more complex series of cellular signaling pathways. For example, the phosphatidylinositol 3-kinase (PI3K)–AKT pathway is also implicated in PC progression, with downstream implications for cell survival, metabolism, anti-apoptosis, and differentiation.[43] Cross-talk between the PI3K-AKT pathway and androgen receptor pathways has been reported.[44] When coupled with the finding that PSMA initiates upstream signaling of the PI3K-AKT pathway, a more complex picture emerges, which requires further studies to fully explain.[45]

The current iteration of guidelines makes no clear suggestion on the conduct of PSMA-PET/CT with ADT.[46] Although it is generally recommended to conduct imaging before commencing ADT therapy, the utility of pausing treatment or the length of pause required to return to baseline PSMA expression remains unclear, and requires further investigation.

THE PROSTATE-SPECIFIC MEMBRANE ANTIGEN RADIOLIGANDS

There are now a number of PSMA-based radiotracers described in the literature with various properties, advantages, and disadvantages that may be bewildering to the nonexpert. The first PSMA-based radiotracer introduced into clinical routine was ^{68}Ga-PSMA-11. In almost a decade of world-wide use, a large body of experience

and evidence has been gathered for this tracer, largely replacing previous-generation scintigraphy agents and PET agents, such as ^{18}F-Choline and Fluciclovine. Other PSMA radiotracers for PET imaging have also been introduced with important differences. Use of ^{68}Ga-PSMA-11 is currently still hampered by the radiotracer's short half-life (68 minutes).[47] In contrast, ^{18}F is readily available through cyclotron production, potentially increasing accessibility of PSMA radiotracers to centers with existing radio-pharmacy facilities, although this advantage must be considered alongside the possibility for cyclotron production of [68]Ga[48] and the increasing sensitivity of latest-generation digital PET/CT scanners, which may afford lower applied activities[49] The lower positron energy of ^{18}F may theoretically improve imaging resolution. The longer half-life makes its logistics and handling easier, and may enable acquisition of later images in which lesion uptake and contrast are higher, improving lesion detection and in the discrimination between specific and nonspecific causes of radiotracer uptake.[20,50,51] Although ^{18}F-labeled PSMA-11 has been described in the literature, it has not been widely implemented.[52] ^{18}F-PSMA-1007, ^{18}F-rhPSMA-7, or ^{18}F-DCFPyL are promising alternatives. One advantage of the first two mentioned radiotracers is the very low level of excretion of the radiotracer via the urinary bladder in the first two to three hours. This may aid in the detection of local recurrences. However, whereas a matched-pair retrospective cohort for ^{68}Ga-PSMA-11 and ^{18}F-PSMA-1007 revealed no increased detection rate for the latter, noteworthy was the fivefold increased rate of nonspecific PSMA-avid lesions detected by ^{18}F-PSMA-1007,[53] which can represent a diagnostic conundrum.[54] Such indeterminate lesions can result in unnecessary investigations, treatments, and interventions,[55,56] representing a potential important pitfall with this tracer. ^{18}F-DCFPyl is another important PSMA radioligand, which undergoes renal excretion and is a promising candidate for routine PSMA imaging, with some preliminary data suggesting improved tumor-to-background ratio and potentially greater detection of pathologic lesions, although adequately powered studies with predefined endpoints are required to confirm this.[57]

THERANOSTIC IMAGING

In advanced or end-stage disease, in which existing conventional therapeutic options have been exhausted or declined by the patient, PSMA-endoradioligand therapy is a promising alternative and may offer a life-prolonging treatment for men with metastatic castration-resistant PC (mCRPC), which the ongoing TheraP trial seeks to confirm.[58]

When selecting candidates for PSMA therapy, an adequate PSMA expression on most PC lesions must be demonstrated to spare the patient any potentially futile therapy with significant side effects. A second consideration is prediction of therapy response, in which pretherapy dosimetry may be of additional utility.[59] One important consideration here is the pharmacokinetics and behavior of the radiotracer; for the purposes of therapy planning these are assumed to be identical, or that differences, for example, in the radioligand's internalization are negligible. Whereas the limited intraindividual comparative data for PSMA radioligands appear to suggest a difference in lesion radiotracer uptake (SUVmax[57]), Ferdinandus and colleagues[60] report a univariate analysis of individuals undergoing PSMA therapy, with no relationship between therapy response and PSMA uptake. Although the commonly used therapeutic tracers are ^{177}Lu-PSMA-617 or ^{177}Lu-PSMA-I&T, these radioligands are infrequently used (but available) as ^{68}Ga-labeled diagnostic tracers. Further studies into the differences between radiotracers for therapy planning and prediction of response is required, as well as in therapy monitoring.

CONTROVERSIES IN PSMA IMAGING

Given the rapid pace of development, a number of controversies and unresolved issues remain to be addressed in the molecular imaging of PC with PSMA probes. Ideally, the best-available evidence would inform the choice of radiotracer for a specific patient at a specific time. In the hierarchy of evidence-based medicine, these would be systematic analyses of multiple, blinded and randomized trials designed to meet specific endpoints with minimization of bias. For a number of valid logistical and regulatory reasons, such data have been difficult to obtain for nuclear medicine studies. A large body of retrospective cohort studies and meta-analyses thereof demonstrate high detection rates for PSMA radioligands, for example, for ^{68}Ga-PSMA-11[41,61] and more recently, for ^{18}F-based radiotracers.[62,63] However, there are only limited confirmatory prospective data, which are restricted to a small selection of the available radiotracers. Such data are often of crucial importance for the approval, licensing and remuneration of nuclear medicine studies in various jurisdictions and world-wide implantation of PSMA-imaging services has not been ubiquitous.[64] Fendler and colleagues[65] report trial data confirming the diagnostic accuracy of ^{68}Ga-PSMA-11, and Morris

and colleagues[66] report details of an ongoing trial for ^{18}F-DCDPyl, for example. In the comparison of radiotracers, mostly noncontrolled, nonrandomized cohort studies with small patient numbers are available.[57] Only Calais and colleagues[67] have hitherto reported data for a prospective comparative imaging trial in ^{18}F-Fluciclovine and ^{68}Ga-PSMA-11 PET/CT and further trial data are now needed for the comparison of the PSMA radioligands. Few studies report any data for patient outcomes. Although the impact of PSMA-PET on radiation therapy planning has long been known,[68] no data exist to suggest that individuals undergoing PSMA-guided PET/CT have better outcomes, and trials are under way to resolve this important question.[69] Indeed, although the detection of advanced metastatic disease may divert the patient from futile local therapy, this commonly occurs in more advanced disease, where the magnitude of the difference between PSMA and previous-generation radiotracers is small.[70] Whereas the combination of new radiotracers,[62] optimum imaging protocols,[71,72] and advanced digital scanners[73] act in concert to increase the detection rate at earlier stages of recurrence, the clinical rationale behind this approach remains unclear and there is uncertainty in the oncological literature about the best management approach for these patients. Although the ORIOLE Phase II trial suggests a role for stereotactic ablative radiotherapy in men with oligometastatic PC[74] this approach lacks a firm solid-evidence base at present and is a topic of debate in the urologic literature.[75]

Finally, there is increasing evidence for the superiority of PSMA-PET/CT in high-risk primary PC compared with conventional imaging modalities. The prospective ProPSMA study recently reported higher accuracy, high clinical impact with 31% of patients undergoing a change in management plan following PET/CT and with good cost efficacy, replacing a battery of studies with a single diagnostic test.[21]

SUMMARY

Since its introduction, PSMA-PET/CT has rapidly established itself as the investigation of choice for imaging PC, largely replacing previous-generation imaging modalities, such as choline-PET/CT, and conventional imaging modalities, such as CT or MR imaging. Demonstrating high diagnostic accuracy, PSMA-PET/CT is able to detect disease at very early stages of recurrence, where the chances of a definitive cure may be at their greatest. It also has an increasingly recognized role in the staging of men with high-risk primary PC. A number of PSMA radioligands are in established clinical routine, and there is currently only limited data and no single tracer can clearly be advocated over the others at present. Further clinical trial data, comparing and contrasting radiotracers and reporting outcome-based data are necessary to further increase the implementation of this very promising imaging modality.

CLINICS CARE POINTS

- PSMA PET/CT is well-established imaging tool for recurrent prostate cancer.
- There is increasing recognition of the utility of PSMA PET/CT in high risk primary prostate cancer.
- Despite the increasing emphasis on early detection of disease in recurrence, studies are required to show improvement in patient-level outcomes when using PSMA PET/CT.
- A number of PSMA-radioligands are available for use, with limited evidence to guide their choice.
- PSMA PET/CT has a clear role in theragnostics, where PSMA radioligands can identify patients suitable for PSMA-therapy.

DISCLOSURE

K. Rahbar has received consultant fees from Bayer and ABX, lectureship fees from Janssen Cilag, Amgen, AAA, Siemens, and SIRTEX, and has received travel expenses from Endocyte as an unpaid member of the steering committee of the VISION phase III trial.

REFERENCES

1. Siegel RL, Miller KD, Jemal A. Cancer statistics, 2019. CA Cancer J Clin 2019;69:7–34.
2. Fossati N, Karnes RJ, Colicchia M, et al. Impact of early salvage radiation therapy in patients with persistently elevated or rising prostate-specific antigen after radical prostatectomy. Eur Urol 2017. https://doi.org/10.1016/j.eururo.2017.07.026.
3. Hope TA, Aggarwal R, Chee B, et al. Impact of (68) Ga-PSMA-11 PET on management in patients with biochemically recurrent prostate cancer. J Nucl Med 2017;58:1956–61.
4. Catalona WJ. Prostate cancer screening. Med Clin North Am 2018;102:199–214.
5. Available at: https://www.cancer.net/cancer-types/prostate-cancer/statistics.
6. Parker C, Nilsson S, Heinrich D, et al. Alpha Emitter radium-223 and survival in metastatic prostate cancer. New Engl J Med 2013;369:213–23.
7. Shimkets WJLRA. The oncogenomics handbook. Totowa (NJ): Humana Press; 2005.
8. Horoszewicz JS, Kawinski E, Fau - Murphy GP, et al. Monoclonal antibodies to a new antigenic marker in epithelial prostatic cells and serum of prostatic cancer patients. Anticancer Res 1987;7(5B):927–35.
9. Israeli RS, Powell CT, Corr JG, et al. Expression of the prostate-specific membrane antigen. Cancer Res 1994;54:1807.
10. Israeli RS, Powell CT, Fair WR, et al. Molecular cloning of a complementary DNA encoding A prostate-specific membrane antigen. Cancer Res 1993;53:227.
11. Malik D, Kumar R, Mittal BR, et al. 68Ga-Labeled PSMA uptake in nonprostatic malignancies: has the time come to remove "PS" from PSMA? Clin Nucl Med 2018;43:529–32.
12. Chang SS. Overview of prostate-specific membrane antigen. Rev Urol 2004;6:S13–8.
13. Afshar-Oromieh A, Malcher A, Eder M, et al. PET imaging with a [68Ga]gallium-labelled PSMA ligand for the diagnosis of prostate cancer: biodistribution in humans and first evaluation of tumour lesions. Eur J Nucl Med Mol Imaging 2013;40:486–95.
14. Afshar-Oromieh A, Sattler LP, Steiger K, et al. Tracer uptake in mediastinal and paraaortal thoracic lymph nodes as a potential pitfall in image interpretation of PSMA ligand PET/CT. Eur J Nucl Med Mol Imaging 2018;45:1179–87.
15. Krohn T, Verburg FA, Pufe T, et al. [(68)Ga]PSMA-HBED uptake mimicking lymph node metastasis in coeliac ganglia: an important pitfall in clinical practice. Eur J Nucl Med Mol Imaging 2015;42:210–4.
16. Werner RA, Sheikhbahaei S, Jones KM, et al. Patterns of uptake of prostate-specific membrane antigen (PSMA)-targeted (18)F-DCFPyL in peripheral ganglia. Ann Nucl Med 2017;31:696–702.
17. Kanthan GL, Hsiao E, Vu D, et al. Uptake in sympathetic ganglia on 68Ga-PSMA-HBED PET/CT: a potential pitfall in scan interpretation. J Med Imaging Radiat Oncol 2017;61:732–8.
18. Hubble D, Robins PRE. Uptake in sympathetic ganglia on 68Ga-PSMA-HBED PET/CT: a potential pitfall in scan interpretation. J Med Imaging Radiat Oncol 2018;62:377–8.
19. Rischpler C, Beck TI, Okamoto S, et al. 68)Ga-PSMA-HBED-CC uptake in cervical, coeliac and sacral ganglia as an important pitfall in prostate cancer PET imaging. J Nucl Med 2018. https://doi.org/10.2967/jnumed.117.204677.
20. Alberts I, Sachpekidis C, Dijkstra L, et al. The role of additional late PSMA-ligand PET/CT in the differentiation between lymph node metastases and ganglia. Eur J Nucl Med Mol Imaging 2020;47:642–51.

21. Hofman MS, Lawrentschuk N, Francis RJ, et al. Prostate-specific membrane antigen PET-CT in patients with high-risk prostate cancer before curative-intent surgery or radiotherapy (proPSMA): a prospective, randomised, multicentre study. Lancet 2020;395:1208–16.

22. Hara T, Kosaka N, Fau - Kishi H, et al. PET imaging of prostate cancer using carbon-11-choline. J Nucl Med 1998;39(6):990–5.

23. Samper Ots P, Luis Cardo A, Vallejo Ocana C, et al. Diagnostic performance of (18)F-choline PET-CT in prostate cancer. Clin translational Oncol 2019;21: 766–73.

24. Rahbar KA-O, Afshar-Oromieh A, Jadvar H, et al. PSMA theranostics: current status and future directions. Mol Imaging 2018;17. 1536012118776068.

25. Eder M, Schäfer M, Bauder-Wüst U, et al. 68Ga-Complex lipophilicity and the targeting property of a urea-based PSMA inhibitor for PET imaging. Bioconjug Chem 2012;23:688–97.

26. Hofman MS, Lawrentschuk N, Francis RJ, et al. Prostate-specific membrane antigen PET-CT in patients with high-risk prostate cancer before curative-intent surgery or radiotherapy (proPSMA): a prospective, randomised, multicentre study. Lancet. 2020 Apr 11;395(10231):1208–16. https://doi.org/10.1016/S0140-6736(20)30314-7.

27. Alberts I, Sachpekidis C, Fech V, et al. PSMA-negative prostate cancer and the continued value of choline-PET/CT. Nuklearmedizin Nucl Med 2020;59:1.

28. Hofman MS, Violet J, Hicks RJ, et al. [177Lu]-PSMA-617 radionuclide treatment in patients with metastatic castration-resistant prostate cancer (LuPSMA trial): a single-centre, single-arm, phase 2 study. Lancet Oncol 2018;19:825–33.

29. Vaz S, Hadaschik B, Gabriel M, et al. Influence of androgen deprivation therapy on PSMA expression and PSMA-ligand PET imaging of prostate cancer patients. Eur J Nucl Med Mol Imaging 2020;47:9–15.

30. Kranzbuhler B, Salemi S, Umbricht CA, et al. Pharmacological upregulation of prostate-specific membrane antigen (PSMA) expression in prostate cancer cells. Prostate 2018;78:758–65.

31. Hope TA, Truillet C, Ehman EC, et al. 68Ga-PSMA-11 PET imaging of response to androgen receptor inhibition: first human experience. J Nucl Med 2017;58:81–4.

32. Evans MJ, Smith-Jones PM, Wongvipat J, et al. Noninvasive measurement of androgen receptor signaling with a positron-emitting radiopharmaceutical that targets prostate-specific membrane antigen. Proc Natl Acad Sci U S A 2011;108:9578–82.

33. Zacho HD, Petersen LJ. Bone flare to androgen deprivation therapy in metastatic, hormone-sensitive prostate cancer on 68Ga-Prostate-specific membrane antigen PET/CT. Clin Nucl Med 2018;43: e404–6.

34. Aggarwal R, Wei X, Kim W, et al. Heterogeneous flare in prostate-specific membrane antigen positron emission tomography tracer uptake with initiation of androgen pathway blockade in metastatic prostate cancer. Eur Urol Oncol 2018;1:78–82.

35. Emmett L, Yin C, Crumbaker M, et al. Rapid modulation of PSMA expression by androgen deprivation: serial (68)Ga-PSMA-11 PET in men with hormone-sensitive and castrate-resistant prostate cancer commencing androgen blockade. J Nucl Med 2019;60:950–4.

36. Ettala O, Malaspina S, Tuokkola T, et al. Prospective study on the effect of short-term androgen deprivation therapy on PSMA uptake evaluated with (68) Ga-PSMA-11 PET/MRI in men with treatment-naive prostate cancer. Eur J Nucl Med Mol Imaging 2019. https://doi.org/10.1007/s00259-019-04635-7.

37. Onal C, Guler OC, Torun N, et al. The effect of androgen deprivation therapy on (68)Ga-PSMA tracer uptake in non-metastatic prostate cancer patients. Eur J Nucl Med Mol Imaging 2020;47:632–41.

38. Afshar-Oromieh A, Debus N, Uhrig M, et al. Impact of long-term androgen deprivation therapy on PSMA ligand PET/CT in patients with castration-sensitive prostate cancer. Eur J Nucl Med Mol Imaging 2018;45:2045–54.

39. Gupta P, Murthy V, Agarwal A, et al. 68Ga-prostate-specific membrane antigen PETCT-based response to androgen deprivation therapy in patients with prostate cancer. Nucl Med Commun 2019;40:1283–8.

40. Setti L, Kirienko M, Dalto SC, et al. FDG-PET/CT findings highly suspicious for COVID-19 in an Italian case series of asymptomatic patients. Eur J Nucl Med Mol Imaging 2020. https://doi.org/10.1007/s00259-020-04819-6.

41. Afshar-Oromieh A, Holland-Letz T, Giesel FL, et al. Diagnostic performance of (68)Ga-PSMA-11 (HBED-CC) PET/CT in patients with recurrent prostate cancer: evaluation in 1007 patients. Eur J Nucl Med Mol Imaging 2017;44:1258–68.

42. Meller B, Bremmer F, Sahlmann CO, et al. Alterations in androgen deprivation enhanced prostate-specific membrane antigen (PSMA) expression in prostate cancer cells as a target for diagnostics and therapy. EJNMMI Res 2015;5:66.

43. Caromile LA, Dortche K, Rahman MM, et al. PSMA redirects cell survival signaling from the MAPK to the PI3K-AKT pathways to promote the progression of prostate cancer. Sci Signaling 2017;10:eaag3326.

44. Lee SH, Johnson D, Luong R, et al. Crosstalking between androgen and PI3K/AKT signaling pathways in prostate cancer cells. J Biol Chem 2015;290:2759–68.

45. Kaittanis C, Andreou C, Hieronymus H, et al. Prostate-specific membrane antigen cleavage of vitamin B9 stimulates oncogenic signaling through metabotropic glutamate receptors. J Exp Med 2017;215: 159–75.

46. Fendler WP, Eiber M, Beheshti M, et al. 68)Ga-PSMA PET/CT: joint EANM and SNMMI procedure guideline for prostate cancer imaging: version 1.0. Eur J Nucl Med Mol Imaging 2017;44:1014–24.

47. Rösch F. 68Ge/68Ga generators: past, present, and future. In: Baum RP, Rösch F, editors. Theranostics, Gallium-68, and other Radionuclides. Berlin, Heidelberg: Springer Berlin Heidelberg; 2013. p. 3–16.

48. Nelson BJB, Wilson J, Richter S, et al. Taking cyclotron 68Ga production to the next level: Expeditious solid target production of 68Ga for preparation of radiotracers. Nucl Med Biol 2020;80-81:24–31.

49. Surti S, Viswanath V, Daube-Witherspoom ME, et al. Benefit of improved performance with state-of-the art digital PET/CT for lesion detection in oncology. J Nucl Med 2020. https://doi.org/10.2967/jnumed.120.242305.

50. Alberts IA-O, Sachpekidis C, Gourni E, et al. Dynamic patterns of [(68)Ga]Ga-PSMA-11 uptake in recurrent prostate cancer lesions. Eur J Nucl Med Mol Imaging 2020;47(1):160–7.

51. Werner RA, Derlin T, Lapa C, et al. 18F-Labeled, PSMA-targeted radiotracers: leveraging the advantages of radiofluorination for prostate cancer molecular imaging. Theranostics 2020;10:1–16.

52. Piron S, De Man K, Schelfhout V, et al. Optimization of PET protocol and interrater reliability of (18)F-PSMA-11 imaging of prostate cancer. EJNMMI Res 2020;10:14.

53. Rauscher I, Kronke M, Konig M, et al. Matched-pair comparison of (68)Ga-PSMA-11 PET/CT and (18)F-PSMA-1007 PET/CT: frequency of pitfalls and detection efficacy in biochemical recurrence after radical prostatectomy. J Nucl Med Med 2020;61:51–7.

54. Afaq A, Wan MYS, Priftakis D, et al. Assessment of benign bone marrow uptake with 18F-PSMA-1007 in prostate cancer using PET/MRI. J Nucl Med 2020;61:1255.

55. Yin Y, Werner RA, Higuchi T, et al. Follow-up of lesions with equivocal radiotracer uptake on PSMA-targeted PET in patients with prostate cancer: predictive values of the PSMA-RADS-3A and PSMA-RADS-3B categories. J Nucl Med 2019;60:511–6.

56. De Coster L, Sciot R, Everaerts W, et al. Fibrous dysplasia mimicking bone metastasis on (68)GA-PSMA PET/MRI. Eur J Nucl Med Mol Imaging 2017;44:1607–8.

57. Dietlein M, Kobe C, Kuhnert G, et al. Comparison of [(18)F]DCFPyL and [(68)Ga]Ga-PSMA-HBED-CC for PSMA-PET imaging in patients with relapsed prostate cancer. Mol Imaging Biol 2015;17:575–84.

58. Hofman MS, Emmett L, Violet J, et al. TheraP: a randomized phase 2 trial of (177) Lu-PSMA-617 theranostic treatment vs cabazitaxel in progressive metastatic castration-resistant prostate cancer (Clinical Trial Protocol ANZUP 1603). BJU Int 2019;124(Suppl 1):5–13.

59. Seifert R, Seitzer K, Herrmann K, et al. Analysis of PSMA expression and outcome in patients with advanced Prostate Cancer receiving (177)Lu-PSMA-617 Radioligand Therapy. Theranostics 2020;10:7812–20.

60. Ferdinandus J, Eppard E, Gaertner FC, et al. Predictors of response to radioligand therapy of metastatic castrate-resistant prostate cancer with 177Lu-PSMA-617. J Nucl Med 2017;58:312–9.

61. Tan N, Bavadian N, Calais J, et al. Imaging of prostate specific membrane antigen targeted radiotracers for the detection of prostate cancer biochemical recurrence after definitive therapy: a systematic review and meta-analysis. J Urol 2019;202:231–40.

62. Rahbar K, Afshar-Oromieh A, Seifert R, et al. Diagnostic performance of (18)F-PSMA-1007 PET/CT in patients with biochemical recurrent prostate cancer. Eur J Nucl Med Mol Imaging 2018;45:2055–61.

63. Giesel FL, Knorr K, Spohn F, et al. Detection efficacy of (18)F-PSMA-1007 PET/CT in 251 patients with biochemical recurrence of prostate cancer after radical prostatectomy. J Nucl Med 2019;60:362–8.

64. Afaq A, Ell PJ, Bomanji JB. Is it time to fund routine NHS usage of PSMA PET-CT? Nucl Med Commun 2019;40:975–9.

65. Fendler WP, Calais J, Eiber M, et al. Assessment of 68Ga-PSMA-11 PET accuracy in localizing recurrent prostate cancer: a prospective single-arm clinical trial. JAMA Oncol 2019;5:856–63.

66. Morris MJ, Pouliot F, Saperstein L, et al. A phase III, multicenter study to assess the diagnostic performance and clinical impact of 18F-DCFPyL PET/CT in men with suspected recurrence of prostate cancer (CONDOR). J Clin Oncol 2019;37:TPS5093.

67. Calais J, Ceci F, Eiber M, et al. 18F-fluciclovine PET-CT and 68Ga-PSMA-11 PET-CT in patients with early biochemical recurrence after prostatectomy: a prospective, single-centre, single-arm, comparative imaging trial. Lancet Oncol 2019;20:1286–94.

68. Grubmuller B, Baltzer P, D'Andrea D, et al. 68)Ga-PSMA 11 ligand PET imaging in patients with biochemical recurrence after radical prostatectomy - diagnostic performance and impact on therapeutic decision-making. Eur J Nucl Med Mol Imaging 2018;45:235–42.

69. Calais J, Czernin J, Fendler WP, et al. Randomized prospective phase III trial of (68)Ga-PSMA-11 PET/CT molecular imaging for prostate cancer salvage radiotherapy planning [PSMA-SRT]. BMC cancer 2019;19:18.

70. Pernthaler B, Kulnik R, Gstettner C, et al. A prospective head-to-head comparison of 18F-fluciclovine with 68Ga-PSMA-11 in biochemical recurrence of prostate cancer in PET/CT. Clin Nucl Med 2019;44:e566–73.

71. Uprimny C, Bayerschmidt S, Kroiss AS, et al. Impact of forced diuresis with furosemide and hydration on

the halo artefact and intensity of tracer accumulation in the urinary bladder and kidneys on [68Ga]Ga-PSMA-11-PET/CT in the evaluation of prostate cancer patients. Eur J Nucl Med Mol Imaging 2020. https://doi.org/10.1007/s00259-020-04846-3.

72. Haupt F, Dijkstra L, Alberts I, et al. 68Ga-PSMA-11 PET/CT in patients with recurrent prostate cancer—a modified protocol compared with the common protocol. Eur J Nucl Med Mol Imaging 2020;47:624–31.

73. Alberts I, Prenosil G, Sachpekidis C, et al. Digital versus analogue PET in [(68)Ga]Ga-PSMA-11 PET/CT for recurrent prostate cancer: a matched-pair comparison. Eur J Nucl Med Mol Imaging 2020;47:614–23.

74. Phillips R, Shi WY, Deek M, et al. Outcomes of observation vs stereotactic ablative radiation for oligometastatic prostate cancer: the ORIOLE phase 2 randomized clinical trial. JAMA Oncol 2020;6: 650–9.

75. Briganti A, Gandaglia G, Montorsi F. Metastasis-directed therapy for oligorecurrent prostate cancer—not all that glitters is gold. JAMA Oncol 2020;6:1638–9.

Prostate Cancer Theranostics
PSMA Targeted Therapy

Robert Seifert, MD[a,b,c,d], Ian L. Alberts, MD, MA[e], Ali Afshar-Oromieh, MD[e],
Kambiz Rahbar, MD[a,c],*

KEYWORDS

- Prostate cancer • Theranostics • Prostate-specific membrane antigen • PSMA

KEY POINTS

- Prostate cancer theranostics has significantly changed the management of patients with prostate cancer.
- Prostate-specific membrane antigen–targeted radioligand therapy has shown promising results in patients with advanced metastasized castration-resistant prostate cancer.
- Clinical phase II and III trials are currently running globally to bring this new therapeutic to approval.

INTRODUCTION

Prostate cancer is one of the leading causes of cancer-related death in men.[1] After radical prostatectomy or external beam radiation therapy as the main primary therapies, the blood tumor marker prostate-specific antigen (PSA) level shall drop below detectability or to low levels, respectively. Both local and systemic therapeutic options are present in case of increasing PSA levels (which is termed biochemical recurrence). Systemic therapy options include androgen deprivation therapy (ADT), which was first proposed by Huggins who received the Nobel Prize in medicine in 1966 for this discovery. However, conventional ADT generally does not remain effective forever, and after a while, the prostate cancer ultimately becomes resistant to this type of treatment. This status is called castration resistance. Metastasized castration-resistant prostate cancer (mCRPC) is a challenging social and economic burden with the need for effective therapeutic options and individualized therapy sequences.

Since 2004, various agents have been approved for the treatment of mCRPC that prolonged overall survival and progression-free survival (PFS).[2–9] The treatment of patients with those agents depends on the metastatic tumor burden, prior performed therapies and the expected toxicity profile.[10]

Abiraterone or enzalutamide represent second-generation ADT substances that are used to treat patients who became resistant to first-generation ADT. In case of treatment failure of abiraterone or enzalutamide, the change to the other therapeutic agent is associated with a significantly lower response rate compared with the initial usage of the agent (only 8% and 18% response rate after conversion).[11,12] After resistance to abiraterone or enzalutamide, chemotherapy with docetaxel is recommended, if the performance status of the patient is sufficient.[13] Cabazitaxel is used as second-line chemotherapy. In case of symptomatic bone metastases without visceral metastases, radium-223 has been approved since 2013.[6] However, higher mortality and bone fracture rates have been reported in therapy regimes combining radium-223 with abiraterone.[14]

[a] Department of Nuclear Medicine, University Hospital Münster, Münster, Germany; [b] Department of Nuclear Medicine, University Hospital Essen, Essen, Germany; [c] West German Cancer Center (WTZ); [d] German Cancer Consortium (DKTK); [e] Department of Nuclear Medicine, University Hospital, Inselspital Bern, Bern, Switzerland
* Corresponding author. Department of Nuclear Medicine, University Hospital Muenster, Albert-Schweitzer-Campus, 48149 Münster, Germany.
E-mail address: rahbar@uni-muenster.de

PET Clin 16 (2021) 391–396
https://doi.org/10.1016/j.cpet.2021.03.004

Overview of Prostate-Specific Membrane Antigen–Targeted Therapy

Recently, prostate-specific membrane antigen (PSMA) targeting small molecule ligands have shown promising results in imaging and as a therapeutic option in patients with prostate cancer.[15–24] Both the lutetium-177–labeled PSMA-617 as well as PSMA-I&T (Lu-PSMA) has shown promising results in patients with mCRPC. The largest patient cohort reported in a German multicenter study using PSMA-617 comprised 145 patients and showed a biochemical response rate in 45% of patients (PSA decline of 50% and more according to prostate cancer work group III criteria).[25] Grade 3 and 4 anemia, thrombocytopenia, and leukopenia were reported in 10%, 4%, and 3%, respectively. A dry mouth was reported in 8% of the patients. Only grade 1/2 nephrotoxicity was reported (in 12% of patients). Grade 3/4 liver toxicity or nausea were not observed.

Biochemical response was associated with longer overall survival in a group of 104 patients with end-stage mCRPC receiving 177Lu-PSMA-617 radioligand therapy. This study revealed that a PSA decline of 20.87% and more was associated with a significantly longer overall survival of 16 versus 11 months ($P < .001$), which remained an independent prognosticator in a multivariate analysis.[24]

An Australian phase II study reported a biochemical response in 57% of the patients, which was higher than those previously observed in retrospective studies.[26] This increase might be because the patients were selected based on PSMA positivity assessed not only by PSMA PET but also by F-18 fluorodeoxyglucose (18F-FDG) PET computed tomography (CT). Patients with mismatch findings (positive in 18F-FDG PET but negative in PSMA PET), which might be caused by tumor dedifferentiation, were not included in the study.

The ligand PSMA I&T can be used both for imaging and therapy for patients with prostate cancer. When used as 177Lu-PSMA-I&T, it shows biochemical response in 38% of patients.[27] Grade 3/4 anemia was observed in 10%, thrombocytopenia in 4%, and neutropenia in 6%.

Besides from the beta radiation emitting lutetium-177, alpha radiation emitting actinium-225 has also been used for PSMA-targeted therapy. Actinium-225–labeled PSMA-617 showed a biochemical response in 63% of patients with a tumor control duration of 9 months in median.[28] Tumor control was denoted the time from the start of PSMA therapy till changed treatment regime. Actinium-225 as an alpha emitter might be more effective than lutetium-177 but has a poorer toxicity profile and comparative data confirming its purported efficacy is lacking. In particular, permanent xerostomia was a main cause for therapy termination.[29] Xerostomia might have a higher frequency in actinium-225 ligands due to alpha radiation. Therefore, future developments of PSMA ligands should therefore focus on reducing the affinity to salivary glands to facilitate a low toxicity profile.

Overview of Recent and Ongoing Prospective Prostate-Specific Membrane Antigen Trials

An overview of the current running studies using radiolabeled PSMA-617 is given in **Table 1**.

The entire prostate cancer therapy community is eagerly awaiting the results of the phase III VISION trial.[30] In this open-label prospective study patients are randomized on a 2:1 basis to receive Lu-PSMA plus standard of care (SOC) therapy or SOC alone with overall survival and radiological PFS as endpoints. Patients must have received at least one line of chemotherapy, but no more than 2, and must have had received at least one of the second-generation ADT abiraterone or enzalutamide. The results of this study will hopefully lead to the approval of Lu-PSMA and thereby make it available for larger group of patients.

Initial results of TheraP, a randomized phase II trial of Lu-PSMA radioligand therapy versus cabazitaxel in mCRPC progressing after docetaxel, were presented at annual meeting of the society of clinical oncology in 2020.[31] In the presented analysis, 98 patients had received Lu-PSMA and 85 patients were treated with cabazitaxel. Lu-PSMA-treated patients showed a higher rate of biochemical response than those treated with cabazitaxel (67% vs 33%). In addition, total rates of grade 3/4 hematoxicity were lower in patients treated with Lu-PSMA compared with cabazitaxel (35 % vs 54%). A phase III trial implementing this protocol is needed to confirm these results.[31]

IMAGING AND THERAPY

With the rise of advanced image analysis techniques, semiautomated approaches for the delineation of all metastases in PSMA PET/CT have been proposed.[32,33] It was shown that the comprehensive analysis of PSMA expression in all metastases could identify patients with favorable, intermediate, and poor outcome.[34] Interestingly, patients with best outcome had exclusively metastases with strong PSMA expression, whereas patients with side by side presence of strong and weak PSMA expression had intermediate outcome. Patients with a generally low PSMA expression had poor outcome. This might be

Table 1
Overview of the current running prospective studies using ^{177}Lu-PSMA-617

Study (NCT) n (Number of Patients)	Phase	Study Description	End Points
LuPARP NCT03874884 n = 52	I	^{177}Lu-PSMA-617 therapy and olaparib in patients with metastatic castration-resistant prostate cancer	Dose-limiting toxicities
NCT03042468 n = 48	I	Phase I dose-escalation study of fractionated 177Lu-PSMA-617 for progressive metastatic CRPC	Dose-limiting toxicities
PRINCE NCT03658447 n = 37	Ib/II	Phase Ib/II study of radionuclide [177]lutetium-PSMA-617 therapy in combination with pembrolizumab for treatment of metastatic castration-resistant prostate cancer (mCRPC)	Safety PSA response
NCT0354165 n = 48	Ib/II	^{177}Lu-J591 and 177Lu-PSMA-617 combination for mCRPC	Dose-limiting toxicities PSA response
TheraP NCT03392428 n = 200	II	A randomized phase II trial of ^{177}Lu-PSMA-617 (Lu-PSMA) theranostic vs cabazitaxel in metastatic castration resistant prostate cancer (mCRPC) progressing after docetaxel	PSA response rate Safety
VISION NCT03511664 n = 750	III	An international, prospective, open-label, multicenter, randomized phase III study of ^{177}Lu-PSMA-617 in the treatment of patients with progressive PSMA-positive metastatic castration-resistant prostate cancer	Overall survival

explained by tumor dedifferentiation: in the course of the disease, the expression of the PSMA molecule is lost, whereas neuroendocrine cell markers are gained.[35,36] Thereby, the appearance of metastases with low PSMA expression might resemble the presence of dedifferentiated prostate cancer cells. However, an alternative explanation might be that Lu-PSMA might deliver more dosage to metastases with strong PSMA expression, which in turn results in favorable outcome. Future studies are needed to elucidate these initial findings.

There are divergent reports on the prognostic value of the baseline total tumor volume. Ferdinandus and colleagues[37] have stated that the PSMA PET–derived tumor volume is not a significant predictor of overall survival time. In contrast, Seifert and colleagues[38,39] could show that the total tumor volume is a significant predictor of overall survival in a single center analysis, which was corroborated in a bicentric analysis. Currently used dose regimes are not tumor volume specific. The concentration of the administered therapeutic ligand is therefore dependent on the total tumor volume, which is sometimes denoted as tumor sink-in effect. Therefore, it seems plausible that the total tumor volume is a negative prognosticator of overall survival, as the maximal dose delivered through Lu-PSMA should depend on the ratio of applied dose per tumor volume. This thought is underlined by the fact that the metric total lesion quotient (denoted in analogy to the FDG PET metric total lesion glycolysis), which is obtained by dividing the tumor volume by the medium PSMA uptake, is an even better prognosticator of overall survival time.[39] Therefore, future studies should evaluate this novel parameter further.

FUTURE DIRECTIONS

Future directions of PSMA-targeted therapy will likely focus on combinational therapies, dose escalation, personalized doses, and on optimized patient selection.

A combination of PSMA-targeted radioligand therapy and second-generation ADT combined with inhibitors of double-strand DNA break repair mechanisms (poly(ADP)-ribose polymerase inhibitors) may improve therapeutic efficacy at low toxicity and should be investigated in future studies.[40]

Only a small number of studies have evaluated the relevance of the applied radiation dosage in Lu-PSMA therapy regimes. Seifert and colleagues[41] have retrospectively evaluated the response of patients treated with 7.5 GBq every 6 weeks compared with those treated with 6 GBq every 8 weeks. The median number of cycles was 4 in the 7.5 GBq group versus 3 in the 6.0 GBq group. As expected, the 7.5 GBq group showed better response to therapy, which was however not statistically significant. Rathke and colleagues[42] have applied single doses of up to 9.3 GBq. However, to date there is no systematic analysis whether higher doses result in better outcome.

All retrospective and prospective studies have one thing in common: it is still not known why some patients respond and some patients do not respond to PSMA-targeted therapy. This might be partly explained by the heterogeneity of prostate cancer, especially in later stages: it is a rather complex disease with various classification and gradings systems already at the beginning of the disease, for example, Gleason score, initial PSA, and others. Moreover, prostate cancer lesions are heterogeneous within the same patient, which becomes visible by PSMA-targeted imaging showing different PSMA expression in different metastatic lesions. This heterogeneity of PSMA expression might be a predictor for efficacy of PSMA-targeted therapy. The tumor and its metastases undergo an evolutionary process within the course of disease, which is also influenced by the therapies performed. Although the topic of different tumor types and clones is complex, currently only the presence of liver metastases is known to be a negative predictor for outcome of patients treated with Lu-PSMA therapy.[43] Therefore, precision medicine might be needed to predict the response of a patient with prostate cancer to Lu-PSMA by analyzing patient-specific tumor characteristics. To give an example, several studies could show that androgen receptor splice variant 7 in circulating tumor cells is a negative predictor of response to abiraterone and enzalutamide because of the lack of the ligand-binding domain on tumor cells.[44] To unleash the full potential of radionuclide therapy in prostate cancer, those kinds of studies are needed for patients receiving Lu-PSMA as well.

DISCLOSURES

KR has received consultant fees from Bayer and ABX; lectureship fees from Janssen Cilag, Amgen, AAA, and SIRTEX; and has received travel expenses from Endocyte as an unpaid member of the steering committee of the VISION phase III trial.

REFERENCES

1. Siegel RL, Miller KD, Jemal A. Cancer statistics, 2017. CA Cancer J Clin 2017;67(1):7–30.
2. Beer TM, Armstrong AJ, Rathkopf DE, et al. Enzalutamide in metastatic prostate cancer before chemotherapy. N Engl J Med 2014;371(5):424–33.
3. de Bono JS, Oudard S, Ozguroglu M, et al. Prednisone plus cabazitaxel or mitoxantrone for metastatic castration-resistant prostate cancer progressing after docetaxel treatment: a randomised open-label trial. Lancet 2010;376(9747):1147–54.
4. Kantoff PW, Higano CS, Shore ND, et al. Sipuleucel-T immunotherapy for castration-resistant prostate cancer. N Engl J Med 2010;363(5):411–22.
5. Parker C, Nilsson S, Heinrich D, et al. Alpha emitter radium-223 and survival in metastatic prostate cancer. N Engl J Med 2013;369(3):213–23.
6. Petrylak DP, Tangen CM, Hussain MHA, et al. Docetaxel and estramustine compared with mitoxantrone and prednisone for advanced refractory prostate cancer. N Engl J Med 2004;351(15):1513–20.
7. Ryan CJ, Smith MR, de Bono JS, et al. Abiraterone in metastatic prostate cancer without previous chemotherapy. N Engl J Med 2013;368(2):138–48.
8. Scher HI, Fizazi K, Saad F, et al. Increased survival with enzalutamide in prostate cancer after chemotherapy. N Engl J Med 2012;367(13):1187–97.
9. Tannock IF, de Wit R, Berry WR, et al. Docetaxel plus prednisone or mitoxantrone plus prednisone for advanced prostate cancer. N Engl J Med 2004; 351(15):1502–12.
10. Cornford P, Bellmunt J, Bolla M, et al. EAU-ESTRO-SIOG guidelines on prostate cancer. Part II: treatment of relapsing, metastatic, and castration-resistant prostate cancer. Eur Urol 2017;71(4): 630–42.
11. Noonan KL, North S, Bitting RL, et al. Clinical activity of abiraterone acetate in patients with metastatic castration-resistant prostate cancer progressing after enzalutamide. Ann Oncol 2013;24(7):1802–7.
12. Brasso K, Thomsen FB, Schrader AJ, et al. Enzalutamide antitumour activity against metastatic castration-resistant prostate cancer previously treated with docetaxel and abiraterone: a multicentre analysis. Eur Urol 2015;68(2):317–24.
13. Heidenreich A, Bastian PJ, Bellmunt J, et al. EAU guidelines on prostate cancer. Part II: treatment of advanced, relapsing, and castration-resistant prostate cancer. Eur Urol 2014;65(2):467–79.
14. Smith M, Parker C, Saad F, et al. Addition of radium-223 to abiraterone acetate and prednisone or prednisolone in patients with castration-resistant prostate cancer and bone metastases (ERA 223): a

randomised, double-blind, placebo-controlled, phase 3 trial. Lancet Oncol 2019;20(3):408–19.

15. Afshar-Oromieh A, Zechmann CM, Malcher A, et al. Comparison of PET imaging with a 68Ga-labelled PSMA ligand and 18F-choline-based PET/CT for the diagnosis of recurrent prostate cancer. Eur J Nucl Med Mol Imaging 2013;41(1):11–20.

16. Afshar-Oromieh A, Avtzi E, Giesel FL, et al. The diagnostic value of PET/CT imaging with the 68Ga-labelled PSMA ligand HBED-CC in the diagnosis of recurrent prostate cancer. Eur J Nucl Med Mol Imaging 2015;42(2):197–209.

17. Sheikhbahaei S, Afshar-Oromieh A, Eiber M, et al. Pearls and pitfalls in clinical interpretation of prostate-specific membrane antigen (PSMA)-targeted PET imaging. Eur J Nucl Med Mol Imaging 2017;44(12):2117–36.

18. Rahbar K, Weckesser M, Huss S, et al. Correlation of intraprostatic tumor extent with ^{68}Ga-PSMA Distribution in patients with prostate cancer. J Nucl Med 2016;57(4):563–7.

19. Brauer A, Grubert LS, Roll W, et al. (177)Lu-PSMA-617 radioligand therapy and outcome in patients with metastasized castration-resistant prostate cancer. Eur J Nucl Med Mol Imaging 2017;44(10):1663–70.

20. Rahbar K, Bode A, Weckesser M, et al. Radioligand therapy with 177Lu-PSMA-617 as A novel therapeutic option in patients with metastatic castration resistant prostate cancer. Clin Nucl Med 2016;41(7):522–8.

21. Rahbar K, Afshar-Oromieh A, Seifert R, et al. Diagnostic performance of 18F-PSMA-1007 PET/CT in patients with biochemical recurrent prostate cancer. Eur J Nucl Med Mol Imaging 2018;45(12):2055–61.

22. Rahbar K, Afshar-Oromieh A, Bögemann M, et al. 18F-PSMA-1007 PET/CT at 60 and 120 minutes in patients with prostate cancer: biodistribution, tumour detection and activity kinetics. Eur J Nucl Med Mol Imaging 2018;65(1):5–6.

23. Seifert R, Schafigh D, Bogemann M, et al. Detection of local relapse of prostate cancer with 18F-PSMA-1007. Clin Nucl Med 2019;44(6):e394–5. https://doi.org/10.1097/RLU.0000000000002543.

24. Rahbar K, Boegemann M, Yordanova A, et al. PSMA targeted radioligandtherapy in metastatic castration resistant prostate cancer after chemotherapy, abiraterone and/or enzalutamide. A retrospective analysis of overall survival. Eur J Nucl Med Mol Imaging 2018;45(1):12–9.

25. Rahbar K, Ahmadzadehfar H, Kratochwil C, et al. German multicenter study investigating ^{177}Lu-PSMA-617 radioligand therapy in advanced prostate cancer patients. J Nucl Med 2017;58(1):85–90.

26. Hofman MS, Violet J, Hicks RJ, et al. [177 Lu]-PSMA-617 radionuclide treatment in patients with metastatic castration-resistant prostate cancer (LuPSMA trial): a single-centre, single-arm, phase 2 study.

Lancet Oncol 2018;19(6):825–33. https://doi.org/10.1016/S1470-2045(18)30198-0.

27. Heck MM, Tauber R, Schwaiger S, et al. Treatment outcome, toxicity, and predictive factors for radioligand therapy with 177Lu-PSMA-I&T in metastatic castration-resistant prostate cancer. Eur Urol 2019;75(6):920–6.

28. Kratochwil C, Bruchertseifer F, Rathke H, et al. Targeted α-therapy of metastatic castration-resistant prostate cancer with 225 Ac-PSMA-617: swimmerplot analysis suggests efficacy regarding duration of tumor control. J Nucl Med 2018;59(5):795–802.

29. Kratochwil C, Bruchertseifer F, Rathke H, et al. Targeted Alpha Therapy of mCRPC with ^{225} Actinium-PSMA-617: swimmer-Plot analysis suggests efficacy regarding duration of tumor-control. J Nucl Med 2018. https://doi.org/10.2967/jnumed.117.203539.

30. Rahbar K, Bodei L, Morris MJ. Is the "VISION" of radioligand therapy for prostate cancer becoming reality? An overview of the phase III trial and the importance for the future of theranostics. J Nucl Med 2019;60(11):1504–6. https://doi.org/10.2967/jnumed.119.234054.

31. Hofman MS, Emmett L, Sandhu SK, et al. TheraP: a randomised phase II trial of 177 Lu-PSMA-617 (LuPSMA) theranostic versus cabazitaxel in metastatic castration resistant prostate cancer (mCRPC) progressing after docetaxel: initial results (ANZUP protocol 1603). J Clin Oncol 2020;38(15_suppl):5500.

32. Seifert R, Weber M, Kocakavuk E, et al. AI and machine learning in nuclear medicine: future perspectives. Semin Nucl Med 2020. https://doi.org/10.1053/j.semnuclmed.2020.08.003.

33. Strack C, Seifert R, Kleesiek J. Artificial intelligence in hybrid imaging. Radiologe 2020;Volume 60:405–12. https://doi.org/10.1007/s00117-020-00646-w.

34. Seifert R, Seitzer K, Herrmann K, et al. Analysis of PSMA expression and outcome in patients with advanced Prostate Cancer receiving 177 Lu-PSMA-617 Radioligand Therapy. Theranostics 2020;10(17):7812–20.

35. Bakht MK, Derecichei I, Li Y, et al. Neuroendocrine differentiation of prostate cancer leads to PSMA suppression. Endocr Relat Cancer 2019;26(2):131–46.

36. Derlin T, Werner RA, Lafos M, et al. Neuroendocrine differentiation and response to PSMA-targeted radioligand therapy in advanced metastatic castration-resistant prostate cancer: a single-center retrospective study. J Nucl Med 2020;61(11):1602–6.

37. Ferdinandus J, Violet J, Sandhu S, et al. Prognostic biomarkers in men with metastatic castration-resistant prostate cancer receiving [177Lu]-PSMA-617. Eur J Nucl Med Mol Imaging 2020;47(10):2322–7.

38. Seifert R, Herrmann K, Kleesiek J, et al. Semi-automatically quantified tumor volume using Ga-68-

PSMA-11-PET as biomarker for survival in patients with advanced prostate cancer. J Nucl Med 2020. https://doi.org/10.2967/jnumed.120.242057.

39. Seifert R, Kessel K, Schlack K, et al. PSMA PET total tumor volume predicts outcome of patients with advanced prostate cancer receiving [177Lu]Lu-PSMA-617 radioligand therapy in a bicentric analysis. Eur J Nucl Med Mol Imaging 2020. https://doi.org/10.1007/s00259-020-05040-1.

40. Fendler WP, Cutler C. More A than B for prostate cancer? J Nucl Med 2017;58(11):1709–10.

41. Seifert R, Kessel K, Schlack K, et al. Radioligand therapy using [177Lu]Lu-PSMA-617 in mCRPC: a pre-VISION single-center analysis. Eur J Nucl Med

Mol Imaging 2020;47:2106–12. https://doi.org/10.1007/s00259-020-04703-3.

42. Rathke H, Giesel FL, Flechsig P, et al. Repeated 177 Lu-labeled PSMA-617 radioligand therapy using treatment activities of up to 9.3 GBq. J Nucl Med 2018;59(3):459–65.

43. Kessel K, Seifert R, Schäfers M, et al. Second line chemotherapy and visceral metastases are associated with poor survival in patients with mCRPC receiving 177 Lu-PSMA-617. Theranostics 2019; 9(17):4841–8.

44. Antonarakis ES, Lu C, Wang H, et al. AR-V7 and resistance to enzalutamide and abiraterone in prostate cancer. N Engl J Med 2014;371(11):1028–38.

Theranostics in Brain Tumors

Hossein Shooli, MD[a], Reza Nemati, MD[b], Hojjat Ahmadzadehfar, MD, MSc[c],
Mariam Aboian, MD, PhD[d], Esmail Jafari, MSc[a], Narges Jokar, MSc[a], Iraj Nabipour, MD[e],
Habibollah Dadgar, MSc[f], Ali Gholamrezanezhad, MD, FEBNM, DABR[g], Mykol Larvie, MD, PhD[h],
Majid Assadi, MD, FASNC[a],*

KEYWORDS

- Theranostics • Brain tumor • PET/CT • PET/MR imaging • Neuro-oncology • Neurotheranostics
- Radioneurotheranostics

KEY POINTS

- Theranostic nuclear oncology, mainly in neuro-oncology (neurotheranostics), aims to combine cancer imaging and therapy using the same molecular targeting platform.
- The ability of radioneurotheranostic agents to interact with cancer cells at the molecular level with high specificity can significantly improve the effectiveness of cancer therapy and helps to identify patients who are most likely to benefit from tumor molecular radionuclide therapy.
- A variety of biologic targets are under investigation for treating brain tumors.
- PET-based precision imaging can substantially improve the therapeutic efficacy of radiotheranostic approach in brain tumors.

INTRODUCTION

Brain tumors are divided into primary brain tumors, which originate from the brain itself, and metastatic brain tumors, which originate from the tumors of other body parts. According to the World Health Organization (WHO) grading system, primary brain tumors are classified as low-grade tumors (grade I–II) and high-grade tumors (grade III–IV). Furthermore, the most common metastatic brain tumors originate from the breast, lung, and skin (melanoma).[1] Among the high grade gliomas, there is differentiation based on origin of the tumor, such as secondary high grade gliomas are transformed from lower grade gliomas. On the other hand, primary glioblastomas commonly do not have a precursor lesion.[2] Among primary brain gliomas, glioblastoma (GBM) is the most frequent and most lethal primary brain tumor.

Conflicts of interest: The authors declare that they have no commercial or financial conflict of interest.
Financial disclosures: National Center for Advancing Translational Science (NCATS), CTSA grant KL2 TR001862 to Mariam Aboian. Other authors have nothing to disclose.
[a] Department of Molecular Imaging and Radionuclide Therapy (MIRT), The Persian Gulf Nuclear Medicine Research Center, Bushehr Medical University Hospital, School of Medicine, Bushehr University of Medical Sciences, Moallem St, Bushehr, Iran; [b] Department of Neurology, Bushehr Medical University Hospital, Bushehr University of Medical Sciences, School of Medicine, Bushehr, Iran; [c] Department of Nuclear Medicine, Klinikum Westfalen, Dortmund, Germany; [d] Department of Radiology, Yale University School of Medicine, New Haven, CT, USA; [e] Department of Internal Medicine (Division of Endocrinology), Bushehr Medical University Hospital, The Persian Gulf Tropical Medicine Research Center, The Persian Gulf Biomedical Sciences Research Institute, Bushehr University of Medical Sciences, Bushehr, Iran; [f] Cancer Research Center, RAZAVI Hospital, Imam Reza International University, Mashhad, Iran; [g] Department of Diagnostic Radiology, Keck School of Medicine, University of Southern California (USC), 1520 San Pablo Street, Suite L1600, Los Angeles, CA 90033, USA; [h] Department of Radiology, Cleveland Clinic, Cleveland, OH, USA
* Corresponding author. Department of Molecular Imaging and Radionuclide Therapy, The Persian Gulf Nuclear Medicine Research Center, Bushehr Medical University Hospital, School of Medicine, Bushehr University of Medical Sciences, Moallem St, Bushehr, Iran 7514633341.
E-mail addresses: assadipoya@yahoo.com; asadi@bpums.ac.ir

PET Clin 16 (2021) 397–418
https://doi.org/10.1016/j.cpet.2021.03.005

Current standard of care includes debulking surgery, radiotherapy, and chemotherapy (temozolomide).[3] However, the prognosis is still poor despite the available multimodal treatments. Moreover, extensive tumor heterogeneity is one of the greatest challenges that might explain lack of progress in identifying effective treatments.[3] Tumor heterogeneity includes intratumoral heterogeneity and significant heterogeneity in tumor characteristics among patients, there is also heterogeneity in temporal evolution of tumor biology over the course of disease (temporal heterogeneity). Furthermore, the infiltrative nature of brain tumor cells into the adjacent healthy tissue leads to tumor recurrence and worsens the prognosis.[4] Thus, these underlying mechanisms enable tumor cells to resist an across-the-board therapeutic strategy.[3]

To deal with these highly heterogeneous tumors, it is necessary to provide a tailored therapy by giving the right drug to the most appropriate patient according to individual molecular and genetic profile, which is known as precision medicine. The National Institutes of Health (NIH) describes precision medicine as "an emerging approach for disease treatment and prevention that takes into account individual variability in genes, environment, and lifestyle for each person."[5] This definition requires clinicians and investigators to provide an individually tailored treatment for every patient with cancer that targets cancer cells with the least damage to healthy tissues.[5,6] In the context of neuro-oncologic cancer care, the concept of precision medicine is epitomized by a radiotheranostic approach.

In theranostic nuclear oncology, the diagnostic radionuclide and the therapeutic radionuclide are integrated within an identical pharmaceutical molecular targeting platform (targeting molecule), which is referred to as a theranostic pair.[7] At the first step, a diagnostic radiotracer is coupled with a tumor-specific biomarker that not only visualizes the target expression on the tumor, but also reflects the unique molecular pathology of the tumor cells noninvasively. Once a sufficient level of target expression is identified on the tumor, the therapeutic radionuclide is coupled with the same tumor-specific biomarker and is administered in order to deliver an ablative radiation dose enough to achieve a therapeutic response.[8] Thus, given the extensive tumor heterogeneity and lack of an effective and tailored treatment strategy, theranostic-based precision oncology can offer an unrivalled patient-oriented therapeutic strategy, aiming at delivering the right radiotheranostic drug to the right patient.

This review article discusses the currently available biological targets in theranostic research for brain tumors as well as other targets with theranostic potentials that are not used in a theranostic setting yet. Moreover, it reviews clinical theranostic investigations that have been conducted from the first application of theranostics in brain tumors to date. In addition, it highlights the exclusive potentials of PET imaging in addressing current challenges of theranostic applications in brain tumor treatment.

BIOLOGICAL TARGETS FOR TARGETED THERAPY
Clinical Phase Targets

Tenascin-C
Tenascin-C (TN-C) is a glycoprotein of extracellular matrix (ECM) that is expressed in a few physiologic and some important pathologic conditions. It is physiologically expressed in the fetus during embryogenesis and organogenesis for a transient period of time.[9] Moreover, it is highly expressed in some pathologic conditions, including inflammation, wound healing, and tumor pathogenesis.[9] In tumor pathogenesis, TN-C has an important role in the migration of tumor cells within the ECM and to other body parts.[10] Many glioma tumors, such as GBM overexpress TN-C, whereas other healthy tissues express it to a lesser extent.[9,11,12] Furthermore, overexpression of TN-C is associated with a high proliferation rate, tumoral angiogenesis, and progressive pattern of tumor growth.[13]

TN-C is a potential molecular target because it is highly exressed in gliomas, it has crucial role in biology of gliomas, and it has negligible expression in normal healthy tissues. Up to this point, some monoclonal antibodies (mAbs) have been developed to target TN-C, which can be categorized as murine mAbs and chimeric antibodies. Murine anti–TN-C mAbs include ST2146, F16, P12, ST2485, 81C6, BC-2, and BC-4, while ch81C6 is a chimeric antibody.[14]

Targeted therapy using radiolabeled anti–TN-C mAbs is done in a molecular radioimmunotherapy setting in which radiolabeled mAbs are administered locoregionally or injected into systemic circulation. A phase II clinical trial showed encouraging outcomes, indicating that a phase III clinical trial is needed.[15] Nonetheless, these anti–TN-C radiopharmaceuticals have not been used in a radiotheranostic setting for treating brain tumors yet. Radiotheranostic approach can improve therapeutic efficacy of anti-TN-C by adding a patient selection step before the therapy. This step allows to identify patients with adequate target expression[16] (**Fig. 1**).

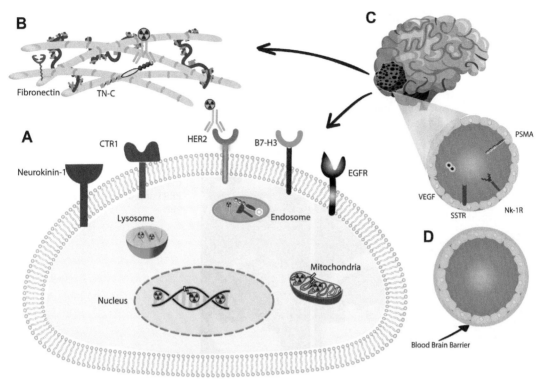

Fig. 1. Potential biological targets for a radiotheranostic approach in brain tumor treatment. (*A*) Brain tumor cell, (*B*) extracellular matrix of brain tumors, (*C*) neovasculature of brain tumors (*D*) normal vasculature of brain. CTR1, copper transporter 1; EGFR, epidermal growth factor receptor; HER2, human epidermal growth factor 2; Nk-1R, neurokinin type 1 receptor; PSMA, prostate-specific membrane antigen; SSTR, somatostatin receptor; VEGF, vascular endothelial growth factor.

Epidermal growth factor receptor

Epidermal growth factor receptor (EGFR) is a transmembrane cell receptor that is a biological receptor for protein ligands that belong to the epidermal growth factor family.[17] Once the specific ligand binds to EGFR, the receptor is phosphorylated and activates intracellular signaling pathways, which regulate cellular proliferation, cell differentiation, and survival.[17] Many cancers overexpress EGFR, including brain tumors; for example, GBM overexpresses it in more than 57% of cases.[16] Given that EGFR has a significant role in tumor cell proliferation and survival, it is considered as an attractive biological target for targeted therapy.

This target has been used in radioimmunotherapy clinical trials in which radiolabeled anti-EGFR mAbs were administered to brain tumors with immunohistochemically confirmed overexpression of EGFR. However, this target has not been studied in a radiotheranostic setting yet.

Application of radiolabeled anti-EGFR mAbs in a radiotheranostic setting can be of great potential because this approach is capable of identifying patients with tumor molecular signature that is most likely to benefit from anti-EGFR targeted therapy. Therefore, while tissue biopsy cannot completely reflect the molecular and genetic profile of these heterogeneous tumors, radiotheranostics are able to provide this critical information.

Somatostatin receptor

Somatostatin receptor (SSTR) belongs to a family of G protein–coupled 7-transmembrane receptors. Five SSTR subtypes ($SSTR_{1-5}$) have been identified.[18] Somatostatin (SST), the ligand for SSTR, is a neuropeptide that is produced by immune, inflammatory, and neuroendocrine cells and is involved in neuromodulation (sensory, motor, and cognition) and inhibition of cell growth via autocrine and paracrine pathways.[19,20] Many brain tumors overexpress SSTR, such as, gliomas and meningiomas, medulloblastomas, pituitary adenomas, and primitive neuroendocrine tumors.[20,21] Dutour and colleagues[22] showed that glioma and meningioma tumors, which are the most frequent primary brain tumors, overexpressed different subtypes of SSTRs. They also found that, although different brain tumors had different profiles of SSTR overexpression, they expressed at least 1

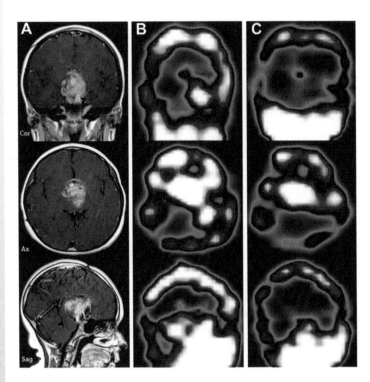

Fig. 2. A 7-year-old girl with a lesion measuring 48 × 40 × 32 mm in suprasellar cistern according to the brain MR imaging (*A*), and pathology confirmed astrocytoma that underwent 2 cycles of peptide receptor radionuclide therapy (PRRT) with ^{177}Lu-DOTATATE. Posttherapy scintigraphy after the first cycle (*B*) revealed intensive uptake of radiotracer in the lesion that decreased significantly in posttherapy scintigraphy of the second cycle (*C*). The patient showed marked clinical improvement after PRRT and does not have any symptom yet.

type of SSTR.[22] Moreover, they documented different profiles of SSTR expression between low-grade and high-grade gliomas. Up to now, 4 types of 1,4,7,10-tetraazacyclododecane-1,4,7,10-tetraacetic acid (DOTA)-peptides have been developed for clinical imaging, including 1,4,7,10-tetraazacyclododecane-N,N',N'',N'''-tetraacetic acid]-d-Phe1, Tyr3-octreotate (DOTATATE), 1,4,7,10-tetraazacyclododecane-1,4,7,10-tetraacetic acid-1-Nal3-octreotide (68Ga-DOTANOC), 1,4,7,10-tetraazacyclododececane-1-(glutaric acid)-4,7,10-triacetic acid (DOTAGA), and 1,4,7,10-tetraazacyclododecane-N,N',N'',N'''-tetraacetic acid-d-Phe1-Tyr3-octreotide (DOTATOC) (**Figs. 2–4**). These peptides have been labeled with beta-emitter and alpha emitter radionuclides and are currently applied in an increasing number of studies.[14,20,23]

Neurokinin type 1 receptor

Neurokinin type 1 receptor (NK-1R) is a G protein–coupled 7-transmembrane receptor that belongs to the mammalian tachykinin receptor family. It exerts its biological effect by activating phospholipase C enzyme, which produces inositol triphosphate.[24] The biological ligand of NK-1R is substance P.[23] Brain tumors (any WHO grade) overexpress NK-1R on the cell surface and within the neovasculature. Therefore, substance P and NK-1R have gained increasing attraction as a biological target for targeted therapies in brain

tumors. Radiolabeled substance P is administered locally for targeting NK-1R in glioma tumors as an adjuvant or primary treatment when patients are not amenable to other treatments (**Table 1**).[25]

Prostate-specific membrane antigen

Prostate-specific membrane antigen (PSMA) is a type II transmembrane glycoprotein that is located in the cytosol of normal prostate cells; however, it attaches to the cancer cell membrane in prostate carcinoma, forming a membrane-bound protein.[26] Furthermore, PSMA expression is not limited to the prostate, because it has been detected in the brain, kidneys, salivary glands, and intestine. In addition, PSMA is overexpressed by the endothelium of the neovasculature of many types of solid tumors, including brain tumors, whereas it is absent on the normal endothelium.[26,53]

In the context of targeted therapies, vasculature-targeted therapy is of great potential in brain tumors considering their extensive neovascularization. In 2019, Verma and colleagues[27] studied the level of PSMA expression in high-grade gliomas compared with low-grade gliomas using ^{68}Ga-PSMA 11 PET/computed tomography (CT) and histopathologic examination. They found that the PSMA 11 uptake on PET/CT was significantly higher in high-grade gliomas compared with low-grade gliomas and correlated well with the histologic proliferation index in both tumor types.

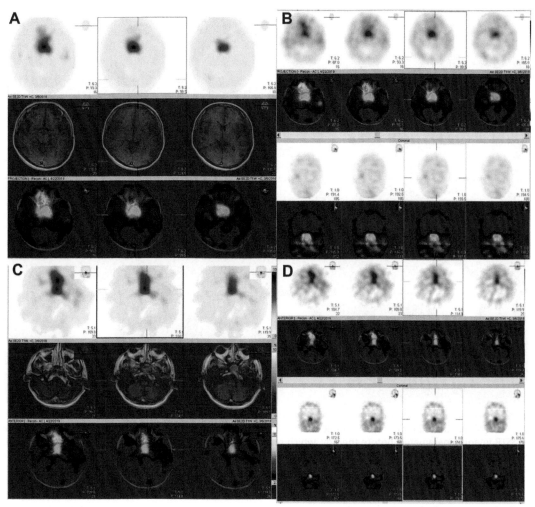

Fig. 3. Posttreatment brain single-photon emission computed tomography (SPECT)/MR imaging after the initial PRRT (*A*, *B*) compared with the third PRRT course (*C*, *D*) in a patient with a functioning pituitary adenoma showing remarkable response.

Taken together, the noninvasive PSMA-based theranostic platform may open a new horizon in the management of these highly heterogeneous and aggressive tumors of the brain (**Fig. 5**).

Human epidermal growth factor 2

Human epidermal growth factor 2 (HER2) is a member of the human growth factor receptor family that is overexpressed in about 30% of breast cancers.[28] It is involved in tumor cell proliferation, cell survival, and angiogenesis; moreover, it is considered an independent factor for metastatic disease.[29] HER2-positive breast cancers are more likely to metastasize to the brain in up to 37% of cases.[30] Targeted therapy for breast cancer using trastuzumab, a monoclonal antibody targeting HER2 receptors, is a well-stablished treatment strategy.[29] However, breast cancer metastasis to the brain significantly accelerates

progression to death for patients who have otherwise treatable primary tumors.[31] Therefore, there is still a need for effective treatment strategies to treat brain metastasis of HER2-positive breast cancer (**Fig. 6**). Puttemans and colleagues[31] studied the therapeutic efficacy of 2Rs15d, a novel anti-HER2 Camelid single-domain antibody fragment, for treating intracranial metastases of breast cancer in a theranostic setting in mice. The results were promising and radiolabeled 2Rs15d was able to increase the survival in trastuzumab-resistant tumors (see **Table 1**). These results warrant future translational studies to assess the therapeutic effect of 2Rs15d in vivo.

Copper transporter 1

Copper is a key nutrient in mammals and works as a cofactor in various principal biological processes. Furthermore, copper metabolism is

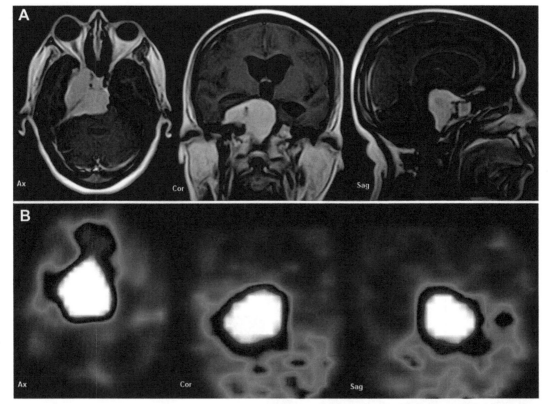

Fig. 4. A 41-year-old woman presented with a history of right cerebellopontine angle meningioma measuring 50 × 48 × 40 mm according to the brain MR imaging (A). The patient underwent PRRT with ^{177}Lu-DOTATATE using SSTR imaging parameters before therapy, which revealed intensive uptake of the radiotracer in the involved region according to the posttherapy scintigraphy (B). She had a stable disease with some improvement in the clinical status.

precisely regulated via several cell transporters and copper-binding proteins. Among these copper transporters, copper transporter 1 (CTR1) is the main transporter because it transfers a large amount of copper into the cell.[32,33] Nonetheless, in various cancer types, patients have an altered copper metabolism, and an increased level of copper has been detected both in serum samples and in tumor tissues.[34]

Radioactive copper has been used for many years to study copper metabolism in patients with Wilson disease.[35] PET-based radioactive copper is used for cancer imaging to evaluate copper metabolism in cancer lesions.[36,37] Moreover, copper-based PET imaging has shown a high tumor uptake in GBM lesions in animal models.[38]

In the context of theranostic nuclear oncology, only 1 preclinical study used ^{64}Cu-CuCl$_2$ as a theranostic agent to treat GBM in an animal model. However, clinical data are still lacking. In a preclinical study, Ferrari and collegues[39] evaluated the theranostic potential of ^{64}Cu-CuCl$_2$ for the treatment of a xenografted GBM mouse model. The

results were promising and the uptake of the radiotheranostic agent by xenografted GBM was significant. At the tissue level, ^{64}Cu-CuCl$_2$ prevented GBM cells from neurosphere formation, a globular structure of tumor cells and a prerequisite for the formation of tumor mass. ^{64}Cu-CuCl$_2$ positively affected survival, with a survival rate of 73.3% and 0% at 20 weeks of follow-up in the treatment and control group, respectively (see **Fig. 1**).

ROUTES OF DRUG DELIVERY TO BRAIN TUMORS
Systemic Drug Delivery

Systemic drug delivery involves the administration of a therapeutic into the systemic circulation, either intravenously or intra-arterially. Although systemic administration is the principal route of drug delivery in many solid tumors, there is an exception for intra-axial brain tumors because of the barricading function of the blood-brain barrier (BBB). An intact BBB is a biologically active and highly selective semipermeable structure that

Table 1
Clinical and preclinical studies of radiotheranostic approach in the treatment of brain tumors

Brain Tumor Type	Target	Diagnostic Radiotracer	Therapeutic Radiopharmaceuticals (Route of Delivery)	Results/Comments
Clinical Studies				
GBM[48] (2002) (MAURITIUS trial)	SSTR	^{111}In-DOTA–lanreotide	^{90}Y-DOTA–lanreotide (IV administration)	• n = 43 • One to 4 treatment cycles were administered at a dose of 11–100 mCi • Regressive disease (n = 5), stable disease (n = 14), and progressive disease (n = 24) were observed
Glioma tumors (grade II–IV)[23] (2006)	NK-1R	^{125}I-Bolton-Hunter-SP	^{177}Lu-DOTAGA-SP ^{90}Y-DOTAGA-SP ^{213}Bi-DOTAGA-SP (locoregional administration)	• n = 20 • Diagnostic radiotracer assessed the expression level of NK-1R in tissue samples • 13 patients achieved disease stabilization and/or improvement in neurologic status • A transient toxicity profile was documented
Recurrent meningiomas[55] (2009)	SSTR	^{99m}Tc-octreotide	^{90}Y-DOTATOC (IV administration)	• n = 29 (grade I = 14, grade II = 9, and grade III = 6) • 2–6 cycles of treatment were administered at a cumulative dose of 5–15 GBq • 19 patients (66%) showed stable disease; however, 10 patients (33%) developed progressive disease
Recurrent high-grade gliomas[56] (2010)	SSTR	^{68}Ga-DOTATOC	^{90}Y-DOTATOC (locoregional administration)	• n = 3 • All patients responded to the therapy, 1 patient showed complete remission, and 2 patients showed PR • Only minor toxicities were reported
Primary glioma tumors (grade II–IV)[49] (2010)	NK-1R	^{111}I-DOTA–substance P	^{213}Bi-DOTA–substance P (locoregional administration)	• n = 5 • Targeted alpha-emitter radionuclide therapy was studied in critically located gliomas • mOS: 19 mo • mPFS: 17 mo • No local or systemic toxicity was reported

(continued on next page)

Table 1
(continued)

Brain Tumor Type	Target	Diagnostic Radiotracer	Therapeutic Radiopharmaceuticals (Route of Delivery)	Results/Comments
Primary GBM[57] (2010)	NK-1R	[111]I-DOTAGA-SP	^{90}Y-DOTAGA-SP (locoregional administration)	• n = 17 • 15 patients experienced stable disease or clinical improvement • A low toxicity profile was reported
Progressive meningiomas[58] (2016)	SSTR	^{68}Ga-DOTATOC/-TATE	^{90}Y-DOTATOC ^{177}Lu-DOTATATE (IV administration)	• n = 20 • Median treatment cycle was 3 with a median administered dose per cycle of 7400 MBq • mPFS: 32.2 mo (grade I), 7.2 mo (grade II), and 2.1 mo (grade III) • Uptake on ^{68}Ga-DOTA-TOC/-TATE was positively correlated with PFS
Metastatic brain lesions[51] (2017)	PSMA	^{99m}Tc-MIP1427 PSMA	[225]Ac-PSMA-617 (locoregional administration)	• n = 3, with cerebral metastasis from castration-resistant prostate cancer • One patient achieved PR • For castration-resistant prostate cancers with advanced-stage metastasis, the investigators suggested a treatment activity of 100 kBq/kg of 225Ac-PSMA-617 per cycle repeated every 8 wk
Metastatic brain lesions[52] (2017)	PSMA	^{68}Ga-PSMA-11	^{177}Lu-PSMA-617	• n = 2, with cerebral metastasis from castration-resistant prostate cancer • Along with radionuclide targeted therapy, local external beam radio-therapy was also applied • Significant tumor regression was achieved in both patients
Secondary GBM[2] (2018)	NK-1R	^{68}Ga-DOTA–substance P	[213]Bi-DOTA–substance P (locoregional administration)	• n = 9 • Secondary GBM evolving from low-grade gliomas (I–II) • mPFS: 5.8 mo • mOS: 16.4 mo • Only mild and transient toxicities were reported
Recurrent GBM[50] (2019)	NK-1R	^{68}Ga-DOTA–substance P	[213]Bi-DOTA–substance P (locoregional administration)	• n = 20 • mPFS: 2.7 mo • mOS: 23.6 mo • Median survival time from first treatment cycle was 7.5 mo

(continued on next page)

Table 1
(continued)

Brain Tumor Type	Target	Diagnostic Radiotracer	Therapeutic Radiopharmaceuticals (Route of Delivery)	Results/Comments
High-grade gliomas (primary and recurrent tumors)[41] (2019)	SSTR	^{68}Ga-DOTATATE	^{177}Lu-DOTATATE (IV administration)	• n = 10 • Response to the therapy was observed as complete remission (n = 1), partial remission(n = 3), stable disease (n = 2), progressive disease (n = 4) • Treatment was well tolerated in old patients with/without severe disabilities • No treatment-related toxicity was reported
Meningioma[59] (2019)	SSTR	^{68}Ga-DOTATATE	^{177}Lu-DOTATATE (IV administration)	• n = 5 • A total of 2–6 (mean, 4) cycles of treatment were administered with a mean administered dose of 19.86 GBq • Two complete remission (40%), 1 PR (20%), and 2 progressive disease (40%) were achieved • Mean PFS: 26.2 mo • No major toxicity was reported
Preclinical Studies				
GBM[39] (2015)	CTR1	^{64}Cu-CuCl$_2$	^{64}Cu-CuCl$_2$	• Significant uptake was observed in xenografted GBM, whereas the brain uptake was not significant • At tissue level, copper irradiation inhibited tumor cells' capacity of neurosphere formation • ^{64}Cu-CuCl$_2$ significantly increased survival rate at 20 wk (70%–73.3% vs 0%)
HER2-positive metastatic brain lesions[31] (2020)	HER2	[111]In-2Rs15d	[131]I-2Rs15d [225]Ac-2Rs15d	• [111]In-2Rs15d, compared with ^{111}In-trastuzumab, showed a superior affinity profile for binding to HER2-positive brain lesion • [131]I-2Rs15d and [225]Ac-2Rs15d increased the survival time in trastuzumab-resistant tumor models

Abbreviations: CTR1, copper transporter 1; HER2, human epidermal growth factor receptor 2; mOS, median of overall survival; mPFS, median of progression-free survival; PSMA, prostate-specific membrane antigen; SP, substance P.

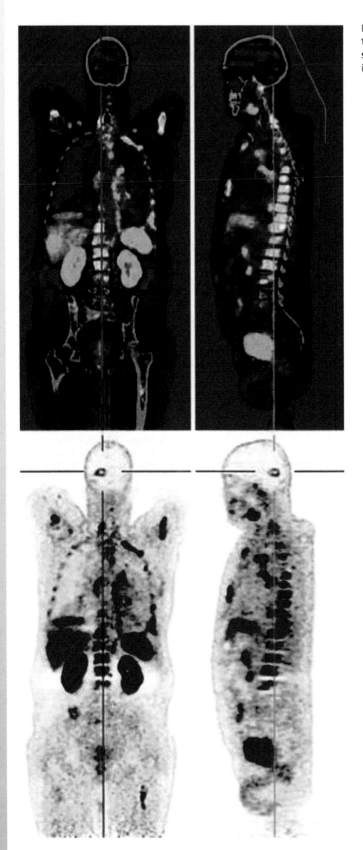

Fig. 5. 68Ga-PSMA PET/CT scan of a patient with prostate cancer and widespread metastases. There is focal uptake in the posterior brain.

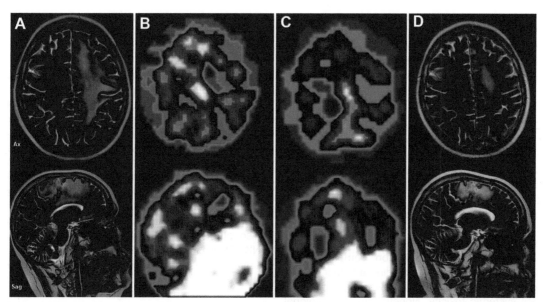

Fig. 6. A 46-year-old woman with HER2-expressing breast cancer and brain metastases according to the MR imaging (*A*). She was refractory to chemotherapy and radiotherapy and underwent 2 cycles of ^{177}Lu trastuzumab (Herceptin). Pretherapy MR imaging (*A*) showed peritumoral edema and a large area of peripheral gadolinium enhancement (T1 post-gadolinium imaging not included). Posttherapy scintigraphy after the first cycle (*B*) revealed intensive radiotracer uptake in the lesion and its peripheral region, which decreased significantly in posttherapy scintigraphy of the second cycle (*C*). Brain MR imaging performed 2 weeks after the second cycle of therapy showed a significant decrease in edema and the peripheral GAD enhancement (not shown) (*D*).

prevents many solutes of the systemic circulation from passing across the BBB and entering the extracellular fluid of the central nervous system (CNS). Nonetheless, small molecule and molecules that are the substrate for transporters on luminal side of the BBB can pass through it.[40]

Brain tumors have variable degree of blood brain barrier permeability. The degree of BBB interruption increases with an increase in the WHO tumor grade. However, even high-grade brain tumors with extensive BBB disruption have some areas with intact BBB, making systemic drug delivery challenging.[20] In contrast to intra-axial tumors, extra-axial tumors, such as meningiomas, are not covered by the BBB; therefore, there is no interference for systemic drug delivery to extra-axial tumors.

In principle, systemic administration of radiopharmaceuticals for treating brain tumors is possible and their therapeutic efficiency has been documented.[41] In the radioimmunotherapy setting, Emrich and colleagues[42] reported a therapeutic response following intravenous (IV) injection of ^{125}I-labeled EGFR-mAb 425 in patients with high-grade gliomas. Moreover, Zalutsky and colleagues[43] found that, after IV administration of [131]I-81C6 (anti-TN-C mAb), the tumor uptake was 25 times higher compared with the adjacent

healthy tissue, which was supported by histopathologic examinations. In the radiotheranostic setting, the authors administered IV ^{177}Lu-DOTA-TATE to patients with high-grade gliomas, which resulted in a promising therapeutic response.[41]

It is controversial whether intra-arterial administration is an advantage for drug delivery to CNS tumors. Several studies found no significant difference between IV and intra-arterial administration of radiopharmaceuticals for treating intra-axial tumors.[43,44] In contrast, some studies reported a significant advantage for intra-arterial administration of radiopharmaceuticals compared with IV administration.[45,46] Given the available documents, it can be suggested that a precise patient selection is needed to determine the route of drug delivery, and the method of molecular imaging including PET, CT, and MRI.

According to current evidence, a PET-based theranostic platform is capable of offering better diagnosis and pre-treatment patient selection than immunohistochemistry. One reason is that PET-based molecular imaging can noninvasively evaluate the whole body in 1 scan, which is a significant advantage compared with single-tissue sampling. Moreover, static and dynamic PET molecular imaging using different radiotracers enables clinicians to comprehensively visualize cancer biology before and after treatment at different time points. Taken together, a radiotheranostic molecular platform can select patients who are most likely to benefit from the treatment more accurately using a diagnostic/therapeutic molecular pair.

Local Drug Delivery

Locoregional drug delivery is defined as the direct injection of the radiopharmaceutical into the tumor tissue, tumor cyst, or a surgically created resection cavity. For brain tumors, this method is preferred to systemic administration mainly because it allows to bypass the BBB as the most important physical barrier to systemic drug delivery to brain tumors. There are other advantages for locoregional administration compared with systemic drug delivery, including a higher tumor-to-normal ratio for radiation absorbed dose and less systemic toxicity. Nonetheless, locoregional drug delivery is an advanced procedure that needs specialty trained physicians and personnel and requires hospitalization. Other potential risks include intraventricular leak of radiopharmaceuticals, intracerebral hemorrhage, local phlebitis, catheter infection, subdural hygromas, subgaleal collections, catheter dysfunction, iatrogenic damage to critical structures of the brain, local inflammation, and local pain.[3,14]

Clinical Radiotheranostic Studies

Although the first-in-human application of radiotheranostics for cancer therapy was 75 years ago, it was not translated into clinical investigations to treat brain tumors until the last decade.[47] However, the first attempt for treating brain tumors was made in 1999 when Merlo and colleagues[44] evaluated the therapeutic efficacy of locoregional administration of ^{90}Y-DOTATOC into brain tumors. They treated 7 patients with low-grade gliomas and 4 patients with anaplastic gliomas using ^{90}Y-DOTATOC, which resulted in 1 complete remission (CR) and 4 cases of stable disease (SD) in the low-grade cohort and 2 SD in anaplastic gliomas. Eventually, they concluded that intratumoral injection of radiolabeled analogues of SSTR could successfully target SSTR-positive glioma tumors in vivo. In 2019, the authors reported the initial results of an ongoing study in which we evaluated the therapeutic efficacy of the IV administration of ^{177}Lu-DOTATATE in high-grade gliomas.[41] Ten patients were included that received 1 to 4 cycles of treatment at 1-month intervals, which resulted in 1 case of CR, 3 cases of partial remission (PR), 2 cases of SD, and 4 cases of progressive disease (PD). The treatment was

tolerated well and no local or systemic toxicity was reported.

With recent discoveries in cancer biology, novel targeted agents (such as peptide ligands and mAbs), and the production of efficient radionuclides, radiolabeled targeted therapeutics are increasingly used for treatment of brain tumors. Three years after the first application of radiopharmaceuticals for the treatment of brain tumors, the first report on the implementation of radiotheranostics in brain tumor treatment was published in 2002 as part of the Multicenter Analysis of a Universal Receptor Imaging and Treatment Initiative, a European Study (MAURITIUS trial).[48] Furthermore, biological targets other than SSTR were also studied in a theranostic setting, including NK-1R and PSMA (see **Table 1**).

NK-1R was the second target used after SSTR in a radiotheranostic setting for treating brain tumors. Cordier and colleagues[49] treated 20 patients with critically located glioma tumors using locoregional administration of an alpha-emitter radionuclide labeled with an NK-1r analogue, ^{213}Bi-DOTA–substance P. The median progression-free survival (mPFS) and the median overall survival (mOS) were 17 and 19 months, respectively. Moreover, no local or systemic toxicity was reported. More recently, in 2019, Królicki and colleagues[50] administered ^{213}Bi-DOTA–substance P to patients with recurrent GBM locoregionally. The patients received 1 to 7 doses of intracavitary or intratumoral injection at 2-month intervals. The treatment was tolerated well with only mild and transient side effects. mPFS and mOS were 2.7 and 23.6 months, respectively.

PSMA is another biological target used for radiotheranostic-based treatment of brain tumors. Only 2 studies used a theranostic setup for these tumors, and both of them investigated metastatic brain lesions originating from castration-resistant prostate cancer.[51,52] As mentioned in **Table 2**, ^{18}F-DCFPyL, ^{89}Zr-Df-IAB2M, and ^{68}Ga-PSMA11 were studied as PET-based diagnostics with promising results. The results showed that PSMA uptake on PET scan not only showed a high tumor-to-background ratio, but also it was in good agreement with the PSMA expression level in histopathologic examinations.[27,53,54] However, it is yet to be determined whether PSMA-targeted therapies can be used for treating primary brain tumors. **Table 1** summarizes a list of theranostic investigations for the treatment of brain tumors.

Although the biological targets discussed earlier have shown an added value for CNS tumor therapeutics, only a few targets have been used in neuroradiotheranostic setting. After more than a decade of theranostic practice in neuro-

Table 2
Clinical and preclinical studies investigating potential biological targets, radiotracers, and radiopharmaceuticals that can be used in a radiotheranostic approach in brain tumors

Brain Tumor Type	Target	Diagnostic Radiotracer	Therapeutic Radio-pharmaceuticals	Results/Comments
Clinical Studies				
Metastatic brain lesions[60] (2013)	Fibronectin	^{124}I-L19SIP	Not used in this study (it is available as ^{131}I-1s9SIP)	• N = 6, metastatic lesions originated from breast cancer (n = 3) and non–small cell lung cancer (n = 3) • High TBR on PET imaging • There was a considerable difference in lesion's uptake within individual patients and between different patients, highlighting intralesional and interlesional heterogeneity • Immuno-PET seems to be a promising noninvasive modality for personalized decision making
Diffuse intrinsic pontine gliomas[61] (2017)	VEGFR	^{89}Zr-Bevacizumab	NA	• n = 7 • There was a considerable intratumoral and intertumoral heterogeneity in radiopharmaceutical uptake on PET scan
Secondary high-grade gliomas[54] (2017)	PSMA	^{18}F-DCFPyL	NA	• n = 3 • Secondary high-grade glioma tumors evolve from low-grade gliomas (I–II) • Histopathologic examination revealed that PSMA was overexpressed by the tumor's neovasculature endothelium
Primary glioma tumors (grade II–IV)[62] (2018)	VEGFR	^{123}I-VEGF	NA	• n = 23 • Grade IV gliomas showed a significant uptake but grade II–III showed negative results on PET scan
Recurrent high-grade gliomas[53] (2018)	PSMA	^{89}Zr-Df-IAB2M	NA	• n = 3 • Excellent TBR • Expressed on tumor neovasculature endothelium • May be of great potential for antivasculature targeted therapy

(continued on next page)

Table 2
(continued)

Brain Tumor Type	Target	Diagnostic Radiotracer	Therapeutic Radio-pharmaceuticals	Results/Comments
Diffuse pontine glioma[63] (2018) (clinical trial phase 1)	B7-H3 antigen	NA	[124]I-8H9	• n = 28, divided into 7 dose-escalation cohorts • Although it was used for posttherapy imaging, it was not applied for pretreatment assessment of target expression and patient qualification • Radiopharmaceuticals were administered using a convection-enhanced delivery system • mOS: 15.3 mo • No dose-limiting toxicities were reported • The promising results warrant further investigation • This target is also overexpressed by adult GBMs[64]
Gliomas (low-grade and high-grade tumors)[27] (2019)	—	^{68}Ga-PSMA-11	Not in this study (it is available as ^{177}Lu-PSMA-617)	• n = 10 • PSMA uptake was significantly higher in high-grade gliomas compared with low-grade tumors • PSMA uptake on PET scan was in a good agreement with histologic proliferative indices • High TBR on PET imaging
High-grade gliomas (grade III–IV)[65] (2020)	CXCR-4	^{99m}Tc-CXCR4-L	NA	• n = 9 • Tracer uptake had a high TBR in high-grade gliomas
Glioma tumors[66] (2020)	TSPO	^{18}F-GE-180	NA	• n = 58 • Primary and recurrent gliomas were studied • Correlation between genetic profile and imaging biomarkers was assessed • Uptake on ^{18}F-GE-180 PET scan increased in higher tumor grades • Radiotracer was capable of reaching out to nonenhancing areas on MR imaging

(continued on next page)

Table 2
(continued)

Brain Tumor Type	Target	Diagnostic Radiotracer	Therapeutic Radio-pharmaceuticals	Results/Comments
Preclinical Studies				
High-grade gliomas (grade III–IV)[67] (2019)	FAP	^{68}Ga-FAPI-02 ^{68}Ga-FAPI-04	Not used in this study (it is available as ^{90}Y-FAPI-04)	• n = 18 • FAPI-02 showed higher binding specificity to FAP compared with FAPI-04 • Normal brain showed a negligible uptake
Metastatic brain lesions of breast cancer[68] (2020)	VCAM-1	NA	^{212}Pb-αVCAM-1[a]	• ^{212}Pb-αVCAM-1 was taken up by metastatic lesion with a TBR of 6 • ^{212}Pb-αVCAM-1 significantly reduced metastatic burden compared with EBRT • ^{212}Pb-αVCAM-1 increased OS

This table summarizes a list of preclinical and clinical evaluation of biological targets that are of theranostic potential in the treatment of brain tumors. Moreover, it lists clinical studies investigating biological targets of brain tumors that have been conducted in a diagnostic or therapeutic setting and can be used in a personalized theranostic setting.

Abbreviations: CXCR-4, chemokine-4 receptor; FAP, fibroblast activation protein; FAPI, fibroblast activation protein inhibitor; NA, not available; ; TBR, tumor-background ratio; TSPO, 18-kDa translocator protein; VCAM-1, vascular cell adhesion molecule-1; VEGFR, vascular endothelial growth factor receptor.

[a] An anti–VCAM-1 antibody radiolabeled with ^{212}Pb (^{212}Pb-αVCAM-1).

oncologic diseases, there is still an urgent need for identification of novel biological targets to pave the ground for more inclusive and tailored therapeutic opportunities. It is imperative to develop radionuclides with different characteristics covering every aspect of cancer imaging and therapy that will, eventually improve cancer care. The multiplicity of radionuclide agents will allow to examine cocktails of various therapeutic isotopes in the same patient and will pave the way for precision therapy.

In order to meet these objectives, many efforts have been made in the context of radiotheranostics in brain tumors. These studies, which are done in preclinical or clinical settings, have contributed to significant progress by identification of novel targets, new radionuclides, and efficient radiotheranostic molecular platforms. **Table 2** presents a selection of biological targets, radiotracers, and radiotherapeutics that are of theranostic potential.

PET-BASED PRECISION IMAGING AND CURRENT CHALLENGES OF THERANOSTICS IN NEURO-ONCOLOGY

Although many efforts have been made to develop an efficient treatment strategy for brain

tumors, a successful strategy is still lacking because of several challenging issues resulting in treatment failure. Therefore, the prognosis remains poor and an efficient therapeutic strategy is yet to be developed. Challenging problems that might explain treatment failure in brain tumors include the barricading function of the BBB, pharmacokinetic failure (insufficient dose delivery to the tumor), pharmacodynamic failure (lack of therapeutic response despite adequate drug activity to the targeted site), activation or development of escape/resistance pathways, intratumoral heterogeneity, patient to patient tumor heterogeneity, temporal biological evolution of tumor in the disease course (temporal heterogeneity), brain tumor stem cells, and infiltrative nature of brain tumor cells. Thus, these underlying mechanisms enable tumor cells to resist an across-the-board therapeutic strategy.[3]

Recent advances and initiatives in molecular imaging, characterized many PET-based approaches that can overcome most of the current shortcomings related to treatment failure in neuro-oncology (**Fig. 7**).[46]

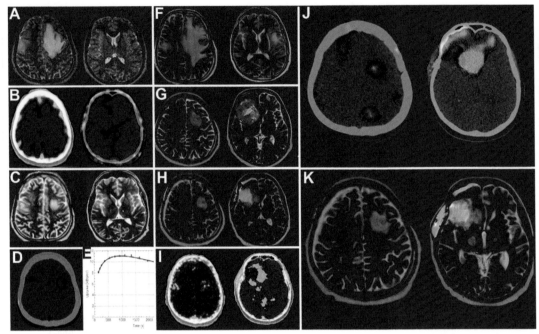

Fig. 7. A 41-year-old patient with a high-grade glioma tumor in the left frontal lobe (*A*). The patient underwent surgery in combination with chemoradiation immediately. Follow-up MR imaging and ^{68}Ga-DOTATATE PET/CT within 1 month postsurgery were normal (*B*). Three months later, although the patient was clinically stable and his scheduled MR imaging (*C*) was unremarkable, his monitoring static and dynamic ^{18}F-fluoroethyl-ʟ-tyrosine (FET) PET (*D, E*) showed multiple uptake foci in addition to the uptake within the tumor bed. The patient was under observation for up to 4 months. MR imaging was performed 4 months later because of worsening of the patient's condition, which showed recurrence in the left frontal lobe (*F*). Debulking surgery was performed for the second time. Follow-up MR imaging performed 3 months after the second surgery revealed a reduction in the left frontal tumor but multiple metastatic lesions were found in the right frontal lobe and the brain stem (*G*). Therefore, the patient was discussed in a multidisciplinary tumor board and was potentially considered for ^{177}Lu-DOTATATE therapy because of his clinical and imaging characteristics (*H*), especially high somatostatin receptor expression in lesions according to the ^{68}Ga-DOTATATE PET/CT (*I*). The patient received 2 cycles of ^{177}Lu-DOTATATE therapy (11.5 GBq) (*J*) that resulted in a short-term SD according to the follow-up MR imaging (*K*) and clinical status.

TARGET EXPRESSION ASSESSMENT AND TUMOR HETEROGENEITY

In the context of radiotheranostics, the first prerequisite is sufficient overexpression of a tumor-specific target throughout the tumor, for which histopathologic confirmation is the method of choice. Although histologic examination is the gold standard for tumor diagnosis, grading, and genetic profiling, it is subject to sampling error, false-positive, and false-negative results. Brain tumors are not only highly heterogeneous between patients (intertumoral heterogeneity), they also have spatial and temporal heterogeneity within each patient, making single-tissue sampling inaccurate to truly determine target expression in a cancer lesion.[46] Furthermore, tissue sampling in brain tumors is challenging because of its invasive nature and associated risk of iatrogenic injury. Therefore, single-tissue biopsy is insufficient to reflect the whole genomic profile of brain tumors. There are many unanswered questions regarding how to determine target expression accurately and overcome tumor heterogeneity.

Molecular imaging is of particular interest because it may help to achieve these objectives and overcome brain tumor heterogeneity. PET-based molecular imaging has enabled clinicians to visualize and quantify gene expression, cancer cell receptors, and biological processes throughout the body at same time noninvasively. Moreover, the combination of molecular imaging and anatomic imaging in a hybrid imaging system such as PET/CT or PET/MR can offer precise biological data with detailed anatomic localization. Recent developments in immuno-PET and tyrosine kinase inhibitor (TKI) PET modalities have significantly contributed to quantitative evaluation of immunotherapy targets and have opened new

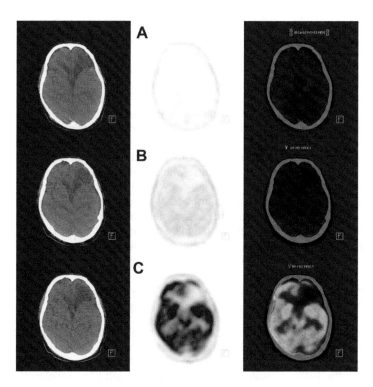

Fig. 8. ^{68}Ga-DOTATATE PET/CT (*A*), FET-PET/CT (*B*), and FDG-PET/CT (*C*) of a patient with a history of left frontal tumor that underwent surgery and chemoradiotherapy and was referred for evaluation of recurrence. No evidence of local tumor recurrence was noted in the left frontal lobe in 3 scan studies. The hypometabolic region in the left frontal lobe is consistent with previous resection.

horizons in theranostic applications of radiolabeled immunetherapeutics.[46]

Furthermore, PET imaging can overcome tumoral heterogeneity in a personalized manner. PET imaging can evaluate the whole brain to identify receptor-positive and receptor-negative segments of a brain tumor. At the next step, it can use different radiotracers to evaluate other targets with therapeutic potentials in receptor-negative segments in order to overcome intratumoral heterogeneity.

In a theranostic setting, PET-based target expression is a milestone because it confirms a sufficient level of target expression in a tumor; a

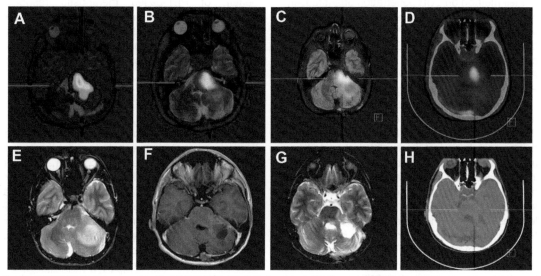

Fig. 9. FET-PET/MR imaging (*A–C*), FET-PET/CT (*D*), MR imaging (*E–G*), and CT (*H*) of a patient with a history of high-grade glioma that underwent surgery and chemoradiotherapy and was referred for assessment of tumoral recurrence. The study showed recurrence on the left side of the pons and the left cerebellar hemisphere.

therapeutic radionuclide can then be used on the same molecular platform (see **Table 1**) (**Figs. 8 and 9**).

PHARMACOKINETIC ASSESSMENT AND BIODISTRIBUTION

Pharmacokinetic failure is one of the main challenges interfering with drug delivery to brain tumors. The barricading function of the BBB is the leading cause of pharmacokinetic failure. Nonetheless, endeavors to address the BBB challenge have a long history and many investigators tried to establish an efficient solution using different methods or manipulations. As the first method, chemical disruption of the BBB using hyperosmotic agents was studied to enhance intracranial drug delivery.[69] Another method is mechanical disruption, in which radiotherapy, microwave, or high-intensity focused ultrasonography is used to interrupt the BBB and increase the tumor absorbed dose. Furthermore, vector-mediated drug delivery is another approach in which the BBB is bypassed by coupling a drug to molecules that are biologically transported across the BBB (eg, nanoparticles, viral vectors, liposomes, and exosomes). The aforementioned locoregional administration is another novel technical initiative that is capable of bypassing the BBB and delivering the drug with a high tumor ratio relative to healthy organs. Although these endeavors slightly improved the situation, an efficient strategy is yet to be developed.

One reason for the failure could be that nearly none of the studies assessed the effectiveness of their method on BBB penetration quantitatively. Interestingly, an increasing body of evidence shows the added value of PET imaging in studying drug delivery across the BBB.[46,70–72] Lesniak and colleagues[73] were the first researchers who used PET imaging to accurately quantify the effect of BBB manipulation on drug delivery to the brain in mice in 2019. They studied intra-arterial injection of ^{89}Zr-bevacizumab compared with IV injection in combination with BBB opening via mannitol to compare brain uptake in different conditions. Intra-arterial injection combined with BBB opening increased the brain uptake of ^{89}Zr-bevacizumab by more than 10 times. Moreover, another study was conducted in 2019 by Varrone and colleagues[74] in which the investigators used TKI-PET for quantitative assessment of the pharmacokinetics and biodistribution of osimertinib in the healthy brain with an intact BBB in vivo. They injected ^{11}C-osimertinib TKI-PET tracer into 8 healthy patients and found a rapid and high uptake of ^{11}C-osimertinib in the healthy brain,

indicating the theranostic potential of this TKI and justifying further well-designed studies in a theranostic setting.

Taken together, unique PET imaging is of significant value for a whole-body, noninvasive, and quantitative assessment of the pharmacokinetics of radiotheranostics in a patient-oriented model. PET-based assessment of pharmacokinetics evaluates the BBB passage of radiotheranostics as well as their binding affinity and stability, dose retention, and whole-body biodistribution for each drug in every patient. Accordingly, this PET-based molecular diagnosis can pave the way toward personalized decision making in which the right drug can be delivered to the most appropriate patient based on both the tumor biology profile and the patient's physiologic status.

EVALUATION OF PHARMACODYNAMICS AND CANCER BIOLOGY MONITORING

After an accurate biological profiling of the tumor and selecting the predominant target for a radiotheranostic approach, the next step is PET-based evaluation of the diagnostic and pharmacokinetic properties of a specific theranostic molecular platform in every patient in a personalized model. The next crucial step is to assess the pharmacodynamics of the radiopharmaceutical. This step relies on a series of posttreatment PET scans with the same radiotracer used in the diagnostic stage, aiming at early assessment of molecular treatment response. This posttreatment approach can detect early therapeutic response or resistance much earlier than anatomic changes. Another clinical benefit of PET-based theranostic response assessment is to monitor tumor biology that is subject to evolution during the course of the disease. PET imaging allows precision patient-centered model of posttreatment evaluation in neuro-oncology.

FUTURE DIRECTIONS

The unique characteristics of molecular theranostic nuclear oncology may help to meet the essentials of the precision medicine concept. Precision medicine is a concept that tries to integrate interaction, translation, and transduction of biological information between genetic profile, cells, microenvironment, or macroenvironment at intracellular, cell, tissue, and organ levels. The ultimate goal is to incorporate all factors in a disease-specific and patient-oriented model for disease management. Major breakthroughs have been made in innovative radiopharmaceuticals, radionuclide generators, novel radioisotopes, and advanced molecular imaging techniques, especially hybrid imaging using PET/CT and PET/MR, which facilitate a theranostic approach.

In the foreseeable future, receptor-ligand constellations can be radiolabeled with a vast range of theranostic radionuclides other than 68-gallium and 177-lutetium. Novel alpha, beta, gamma, and Auger electron-emitting radiometals have been produced such as 67-gallium, 161-terbium, 225-actinium, 166-holmium, 47-scandium, 212-lead/212 bismuth, 213-bismuth, and 149-terbium. These radionuclides are in different stages of investigations, including preclinical or clinical research; however, the current supply is still inadequate. Although, drug regulatory and reimbursement processes are very slow, the number of radiotheranostic agents is increasing very rapidly. In our department, several radiotheranostic agents (eg, 177Lu-pentixather, targeting CXCR4 [chemokine-4 receptor]; 177Lu-rituximab [anti-CD20 antibody], and 177Lu-trastuzumab, targeting HER2) are currently under investigation in a clinical setting.

Furthermore, cancers can be characterized according to radiomics, an emerging translational field of research aiming to analyze a large number of medical images especially hybrid PET/CT and PET/MR imaging. Radiomic approaches extract quantitative features from images and can be used to identify disease-specific patterns using artificial intelligence.

Eventually, mathematical modeling makes a connection between system biology and precision medicine through integration of -omics profile and molecular imaging data. This mathematical model considers spatial, temporal, intertumoral, and intratumoral heterogeneity and quantitatively monitors the damage acquired by the tumor and healthy tissues. Theranostic molecular nuclear oncology offers a noninvasive quantifiable PET-based evaluation that can take into account many aspects of tumor heterogeneity and monitor the cancer biology and physiologic processes of the healthy tissues in a personalized manner.

However, radiotheranostics suffer from several challenges that prevent them from being translated into routine clinical oncology practice. Individual dosimetry is a time-consuming process and is not universally available in all clinical centers. Incorporation of single-photon emission CT (SPECT)–based and PET-based dosimetry into clinical setting has contributed to theranostic practice, taking a step forward as a realistic model for the precision medicine concept.

Another challenge for theranostic practice is to find a comprehensive strategy to organize multidisciplinary teams for a patient-oriented interdisciplinary collaboration to treat cancers. Nuclear medicine specialists need to gain a comprehensive understanding of cancer biology and need to be fluent in the new language of genomics and proteomics.

Personalized care covers patient surveillance and disease monitoring after a targeted radiotheranostic therapy. Minimal residual disease may remain untreated after therapy completion, representing an unsolved challenge leading to disease recurrence. There are several novel methods to identify minimal residual disease in a cancer patient, including the detection of circulating tumor cells, tumor cell-free DNA, tumor nucleic acids, or tumor exosomes in the blood sample. Moreover, a theranostic molecular platform is of particular potential to detect, quantify, localize, treat, and eventually confirm tumor eradication noninvasively in a personalized manner. A combination of novel blood-based approaches and radiotheranostic agents can improve the diagnostic accuracy and treatment precision.

The ultimate goal should not be to rely on isolated parameters in separated disease-based, drug-based, and patient-based models. For comprehensive predictive, preventive, personalized, and participatory management, it is required to integrate the individual biology profile (genomics, proteomics, and metabolomics) into tumor characteristics and theranostic molecular platform properties, considering all patient variations and tumor heterogeneities in a universal model.

SUMMARY

Theranostics has been implemented successfully and is used for personalized cancer management and precision medicine. However, there are still several unmet essentials in neurotheranostics that require extensive multidisciplinary collaboration in which basic and clinical teams of different disciplines should work together to address current challenges and offer more tailored therapeutics in neuro-oncology.

Molecular imaging has a matchless capacity to diagnose the disease precisely and can offer patient-centered management in combination with a tailored therapy on the same molecular platform selected based on the individual's biology-driven data. It also allows clinicians to visualize cancer biology noninvasively and has provided a biological basis for predicting disease progression and disease prognostication. In this regard, radiotheranostics are capable of designing a road map to realize the concept of precision medicine in neuro-oncologic care. The ultimate goal is to assimilate each isolated factor into a comprehensive and personalized approach, which accounts for all these issues in an integrated model.

CONFLICT OF INTEREST

The authors declare that they have no commercial or financial conflict of interest.

FINANCIAL DISCLOSURES

National Center for Advancing Translational Science (NCATS), CTSA grant KL2 TR001862 to Mariam Aboian. Other authors have nothing to disclose.

CLINICS CARE POINTS

Nuclear oncology theranostics allows to noninvasively identify the most appropriate patients for a specific radiopharmaceutical.

Given extensive tumor heterogeneity, the most appropriate target should be selected in a personalized manner.

PET-based precision imaging can be used for assessment of target expression, distribution of radiopharmaceuticals, and disease monitoring after the therapy.

REFERENCES

1. Soffietti R, Ducati A, Rudà R. Brain metastases. Handbook of clinical neurology, vol. 105. Netherlands: Elsevier; 2012. p. 747–55.
2. Krolicki L, Bruchertseifer F, Kunikowska J, et al. Prolonged survival in secondary glioblastoma following local injection of targeted alpha therapy with (213) Bi-substance P analogue. Eur J Nucl Med Mol Imaging 2018;45(9):1636–44.
3. Gan HK, van den Bent M, Lassman AB, et al. Antibody–drug conjugates in glioblastoma therapy: the right drugs to the right cells. Nat Rev Clin Oncol 2017;14(11):695.
4. Dijkers EC, Oude Munnink TH, Kosterink JG, et al. Biodistribution of 89Zr-trastuzumab and PET imaging of HER2-positive lesions in patients with metastatic breast cancer. Clin Pharmacol Ther 2010; 87(5):586–92.
5. Collins FS, Varmus H. A new initiative on precision medicine. N Engl J Med 2015;372(9):793–5.
6. Ghasemi M, Nabipour I, Omrani A, et al. Precision medicine and molecular imaging: new targeted approaches toward cancer therapeutic and diagnosis. Am J Nucl Med Mol Imaging 2016;6(6):310–27.
7. Turner JH. Recent advances in theranostics and challenges for the future. Br J Radiol 2018; 91(1091):20170893.
8. Herrmann K, Schwaiger M, Lewis JS, et al. Radiotheranostics: a roadmap for future development. Lancet Oncol 2020;21(3):e146–56.
9. Herold-Mende C, Mueller MM, Bonsanto MM, et al. Clinical impact and functional aspects of tenascin-C expression during glioma progression. Int J Cancer 2002;98(3):362–9.
10. Martin D, Brown-Luedi M, Chiquet-Ehrismann R. Tenascin-C signaling through induction of 14-3-3 tau. J Cell Biol 2003;160(2):171–5.
11. Leins A, Riva P, Lindstedt R, et al. Expression of tenascin-C in various human brain tumors and its relevance for survival in patients with astrocytoma. Cancer 2003;98(11):2430–9.
12. Ventimiglia JB, Wikstrand CJ, Ostrowski LE, et al. Tenascin expression in human glioma cell lines and normal tissues. J Neuroimmunol 1992;36(1): 41–55.
13. Kim CH, Bak KH, Kim YS, et al. Expression of tenascin-C in astrocytic tumors: its relevance to proliferation and angiogenesis. Surg Neurol 2000;54(3): 235–40.
14. Gholamrezanezhad A, Shooli H, Jokar N, et al. Radioimmunotherapy (RIT) in brain tumors. Nucl Med Mol Imaging 2019;53(6):374–81.
15. Reardon DA, Akabani G, Edward Coleman R, et al. Phase II trial of murine 131I-labeled antitenascin monoclonal antibody 81C6 administered into surgically created resection cavities of patients with newly diagnosed malignant gliomas. J Clin Oncol 2002;20(5):1389–97.
16. Brennan CW, Verhaak RG, McKenna A, et al. The somatic genomic landscape of glioblastoma. Cell 2013;155(2):462–77.
17. Herbst RS. Review of epidermal growth factor receptor biology. Int J Radiat Oncol Biol Phys 2004; 59(2):S21–6.
18. Patel YC. Molecular pharmacology of somatostatin receptor subtypes. J Endocrinol Invest 1997;20(6): 348–67.
19. Reichlin S. Somatostatin. N Engl J Med 1983; 309(24):1495–501.
20. Shooli H, Dadgar H, Wáng YJ, et al. An update on PET-based molecular imaging in neuro-oncology: challenges and implementation for a precision medicine approach in cancer care. Quant Imaging Med Surg 2019;9(9):1597–610.
21. Assadi M, Nemati R, Shooli H, et al. An aggressive functioning pituitary adenoma treated with peptide receptor radionuclide therapy. Eur J Nucl Med Mol Imaging 2020;47(4):1015–6.
22. Dutour A, Kumar U, Panetta R, et al. Expression of somatostatin receptor subtypes in human brain tumors. Int J Cancer 1998;76(5):620–7.

23. Kneifel S, Cordier D, Good S, et al. Local targeting of malignant gliomas by the diffusible peptidic vector 1, 4, 7, 10-tetraazacyclododecane-1-glutaric acid-4, 7, 10-triacetic acid-substance p. Clin Cancer Res 2006;12(12):3843–50.

24. Maggi CA. The mammalian tachykinin receptors. Gen Pharmacol 1995;26(5):911–44.

25. Królicki L, Kunikowska J, Bruchertseifer F, et al, editors. 225Ac-and 213Bi-Substance P analogues for glioma therapy. Seminars in nuclear medicine. Netherlands: Elsevier; 2020.

26. Lütje S, Heskamp S, Cornelissen AS, et al. PSMA ligands for radionuclide imaging and therapy of prostate cancer: clinical status. Theranostics 2015;5(12):1388–401.

27. Verma P, Malhotra G, Goel A, et al. Differential uptake of 68Ga-PSMA-HBED-CC (PSMA-11) in low-grade versus high-grade gliomas in treatment-naive patients. Clin Nucl Med 2019;44(5):e318–22.

28. Mitri Z, Constantine T, O'Regan R. The HER2 receptor in breast cancer: pathophysiology, clinical use, and new advances in therapy. Chemother Res Pract 2012;2012:743193.

29. Slamon DJ, Leyland-Jones B, Shak S, et al. Use of chemotherapy plus a monoclonal antibody against HER2 for metastatic breast cancer that overexpresses HER2. N Engl J Med 2001;344(11):783–92.

30. Brufsky AM, Mayer M, Rugo HS, et al. Central nervous system metastases in patients with HER2-positive metastatic breast cancer: incidence, treatment, and survival in patients from registHER. Clin Cancer Res 2011;17(14):4834–43.

31. Puttemans J, Dekempeneer Y, Eersels JL, et al. Preclinical targeted α-and β–-radionuclide therapy in HER2-positive brain metastasis using camelid single-domain antibodies. Cancers 2020;12(4):1017.

32. Linder MC, Hazegh-Azam M. Copper biochemistry and molecular biology. Am J Clin Nutr 1996;63(5):797S–811S.

33. Gupta A, Lutsenko S. Human copper transporters: mechanism, role in human diseases and therapeutic potential. Future Med Chem 2009;1(6):1125–42.

34. Gupte A, Mumper RJ. Elevated copper and oxidative stress in cancer cells as a target for cancer treatment. Cancer Treat Rev 2009;35(1):32–46.

35. Osborn S, Szaz K, Walshe J. Studies with radioactive copper (64Cu and 67Cu): abdominal scintiscans in patients with Wilson's disease. Q J Med 1969;38(4):467–74.

36. Peng F, Lu X, Janisse J, et al. PET of human prostate cancer xenografts in mice with increased uptake of 64CuCl2. J Nucl Med 2006;47(10):1649–52.

37. Zhang H, Cai H, Lu X, et al. Positron emission tomography of human hepatocellular carcinoma xenografts in mice using copper (II)-64 chloride as a tracer. Acad Radiol 2011;18(12):1561–8.

38. Jørgensen JT, Persson M, Madsen J, et al. High tumor uptake of 64Cu: implications for molecular imaging of tumor characteristics with copper-based PET tracers. Nucl Med Biol 2013;40(3):345–50.

39. Ferrari C, Niccoli Asabella A, Villano C, et al. Copper-64 dichloride as theranostic agent for glioblastoma multiforme: a preclinical study. Biomed Res Int 2015;2015:129764.

40. Sharma A, McConathy J. Overview of PET tracers for brain tumor imaging. PET Clin 2013;8(2):129–46.

41. Assadi M, Nemati R, Shooli H, et al. Peptide receptor radionuclide therapy for high-grade glioma brain tumors: variable clinical response in a pilot study. Barcelona, Spain: EANM'19; 2019.

42. Emrich JG, Brady LW, Quang TS, et al. Radioiodinated (I-125) monoclonal antibody 425 in the treatment of high grade glioma patients: ten-year synopsis of a novel treatment. Am J Clin Oncol 2002;25(6):541–6.

43. Zalutsky MR, Moseley RP, Coakham HB, et al. Pharmacokinetics and tumor localization of 131I-labeled anti-tenascin monoclonal antibody 81C6 in patients with gliomas and other intracranial malignancies. Cancer Res 1989;49(10):2807–13.

44. Merlo A, Hausmann O, Wasner M, et al. Locoregional regulatory peptide receptor targeting with the diffusible somatostatin analogue 90Y-labeled DOTA0-D-Phe1-Tyr3-octreotide (DOTATOC): a pilot study in human gliomas. Clin Cancer Res 1999;5(5):1025–33.

45. Nomura N, Pastorino S, Jiang P, et al. Prostate specific membrane antigen (PSMA) expression in primary gliomas and breast cancer brain metastases. Cancer Cell Int 2014;14(1):1–9.

46. Pruis IJ, van Dongen GA, Veldhuijzen van Zanten SE. The added value of diagnostic and theranostic PET imaging for the treatment of CNS tumors. Int J Mol Sci 2020;21(3):1029.

47. Seidlin S, Marinelli L, Oshry E. Radioactive iodine therapy: effect on functioning metastases of adenocarcinoma of the thyroid. J Am Med Assoc 1946;132(14):838–47.

48. Virgolini I, Britton K, Buscombe J, et al, editors. 111In-and 90Y-DOTA-lanreotide: results and implications of the Mauritius trial. Seminars in nuclear medicine. Netherlands: Elsevier; 2002.

49. Cordier D, Forrer F, Bruchertseifer F, et al. Targeted alpha-radionuclide therapy of functionally critically located gliomas with 213 Bi-DOTA-[Thi 8, Met (O 2) 11]-substance P: a pilot trial. Eur J Nucl Med Mol Imaging 2010;37(7):1335–44.

50. Królicki L, Bruchertseifer F, Kunikowska J, et al. Safety and efficacy of targeted alpha therapy with 213 Bi-DOTA-substance P in recurrent glioblastoma. Eur J Nucl Med Mol Imaging 2019;46(3):614–22.

51. Kratochwil C, Bruchertseifer F, Rathke H, et al. Targeted α-therapy of metastatic castration-resistant prostate cancer with 225Ac-PSMA-617: dosimetry

estimate and empiric dose finding. J Nucl Med 2017;58(10):1624–31.

52. Wei X, Schlenkhoff C, Schwarz B, et al. Combination of 177Lu-PSMA-617 and external radiotherapy for the treatment of cerebral metastases in patients with castration-resistant metastatic prostate cancer. Clin Nucl Med 2017;42(9):704–6.

53. Matsuda M, Ishikawa E, Yamamoto T, et al. Potential use of prostate specific membrane antigen (PSMA) for detecting the tumor neovasculature of brain tumors by PET imaging with 89 Zr-Df-IAB2M anti-PSMA minibody. J Neurooncol 2018;138(3):581–9.

54. Fragomeni RAS, Menke JR, Holdhoff M, et al. Prostate-specific membrane antigen–targeted imaging with [18F] DCFPyL in high-grade gliomas. Clin Nucl Med 2017;42(10):e433.

55. Bartolomei M, Bodei L, De Cicco C, et al. Peptide receptor radionuclide therapy with (90)Y-DOTATOC in recurrent meningioma. Eur J Nucl Med Mol Imaging 2009;36(9):1407–16.

56. Heute D, Kostron H, von Guggenberg E, et al. Response of recurrent high-grade glioma to treatment with (90)Y-DOTATOC. J Nucl Med 2010;51(3):397–400.

57. Cordier D, Forrer F, Kneifel S, et al. Neoadjuvant targeting of glioblastoma multiforme with radiolabeled DOTAGA-substance P--results from a phase I study. J Neurooncol 2010;100(1):129–36.

58. Seystahl K, Stoecklein V, Schüller U, et al. Somatostatin receptor-targeted radionuclide therapy for progressive meningioma: benefit linked to 68Ga-DOTATATE/-TOC uptake. Neuro Oncol 2016;18(11):1538–47.

59. Parghane RV, Talole S, Basu S. Prevalence of hitherto unknown brain meningioma detected on 68Ga-DOTATATE positron-emission tomography/computed tomography in patients with metastatic neuroendocrine tumor and exploring potential of 177Lu-DOTATATE peptide receptor radionuclide therapy as single-shot treatment approach targeting both tumors. World J Nucl Med 2019;18(2):160.

60. Poli GL, Bianchi C, Virotta G, et al. Radretumab radioimmunotherapy in patients with brain metastasis: a 124I-L19SIP dosimetric PET study. Cancer Immunol Res 2013;1(2):134–43.

61. Jansen MH, Veldhuijzen van Zanten SEM, van Vuurden DG, et al. Molecular drug imaging: (89)Zr-Bevacizumab PET in children with diffuse intrinsic pontine glioma. J Nucl Med 2017;58(5):711–6.

62. Rainer E, Wang H, Traub-Weidinger T, et al. The prognostic value of [123 I]-vascular endothelial growth factor ([123 I]-VEGF) in glioma. Eur J Nucl Med Mol Imaging 2018;45(13):2396–403.

63. Souweidane MM, Kramer K, Pandit-Taskar N, et al. Convection-enhanced delivery for diffuse intrinsic pontine glioma: a single-centre, dose-escalation, phase 1 trial. Lancet Oncol 2018;19(8):1040–50.

64. Tang X, Zhao S, Zhang Y, et al. B7-H3 as a novel CAR-T therapeutic target for glioblastoma. Mol Ther Oncolytics 2019;14:279–87.

65. Vallejo-Armenta P, Santos-Cuevas C, Soto-Andonaegui J, et al. 99mTc-CXCR4-L for imaging of the chemokine-4 receptor associated with brain tumor invasiveness: biokinetics, radiation dosimetry, and proof of concept in humans. Contrast Media Mol Imaging 2020;2020:2525037.

66. Unterrainer M, Fleischmann DF, Vettermann F, et al. TSPO PET, tumour grading and molecular genetics in histologically verified glioma: a correlative (18)F-GE-180 PET study. Eur J Nucl Med Mol Imaging 2020;47(6):1368–80.

67. Röhrich M, Loktev A, Wefers AK, et al. IDH-wildtype glioblastomas and grade III/IV IDH-mutant gliomas show elevated tracer uptake in fibroblast activation protein-specific PET/CT. Eur J Nucl Med Mol Imaging 2019;46(12):2569–80.

68. Corroyer-Dulmont A, Valable S, Falzone N, et al. VCAM-1 targeted alpha-particle therapy for early brain metastases. Neuro Oncol 2020;22(3):357–68.

69. Pappius HM, Savaki HE, Fieschi C, et al. Osmotic opening of the blood-brain barrier and local cerebral glucose utilization. Ann Neurol 1979;5(3):211–9.

70. Chakravarty R, Goel S, Dash A, et al. Radiolabeled inorganic nanoparticles for positron emission tomography imaging of cancer: an overview. Q J Nucl Med Mol Imaging 2017;61(2):181–204.

71. Webb S, Ott RJ, Cherry SR. Quantitation of blood-brain barrier permeability by positron emission tomography. Phys Med Biol 1989;34(12):1767–72.

72. Van Tellingen O, Yetkin-Arik B, De Gooijer M, et al. Overcoming the blood–brain tumor barrier for effective glioblastoma treatment. Drug Resist Updat 2015;19:1–12.

73. Lesniak WG, Chu C, Jablonska A, et al. A distinct advantage to intraarterial delivery of 89Zr-bevacizumab in PET imaging of mice with and without osmotic opening of the blood–brain barrier. J Nucl Med 2019;60(5):617–22.

74. Varrone A, Varnäs K, Jucaite A, et al. A PET study in healthy subjects of brain exposure of 11C-labelled osimertinib – a drug intended for treatment of brain metastases in non-small cell lung cancer. J Cereb Blood Flow Metab 2019;40(4):799–807.

Theranostics in Neuroblastoma

Margarida Simao Rafael, MD[a], Sarah Cohen-Gogo, MD, PhD[a], Meredith S. Irwin, MD[a], Reza Vali, MD, MSc[b],*, Amer Shammas, MD[b], Daniel A. Morgenstern, MB, BChir, PhD[a]

KEYWORDS

- Theranostics • Neuroblastoma • MIBG • MIBG therapy • PET-[18F]FDG

KEY POINTS

- Theranostics enables a precision medicine approach.
- The gold standard of theranostics in neuroblastoma is metaiodobenzylguanidine (MIBG).
- Non–MIBG-avid neuroblastomas are a challenge that fosters the improvement of techniques and utilization of new radiopharmaceuticals.
- Promising results have been obtained with emerging radiopharmaceuticals.

INTRODUCTION

Neuroblastoma

Neuroblastoma (NB) is the most common extra-cranial solid tumor in children. The median age at diagnosis is 19 months,[1] but it can be diagnosed from infancy to adolescence. NB arises from primordial neural crest cells that give rise to sympathetic neural ganglia and the adrenal medulla. Thus, it has a diverse pattern of clinical presentation, and primary tumors can occur anywhere along the sympathetic chain or as a retroperitoneal mass. Prognosis also is variable and ranges from spontaneous regression to aggressive metastatic tumors, with spread to bone marrow, bone, liver, and/or lymph nodes. The overall survival (OS) for patients with low-risk and intermediate-risk NB is excellent, greater than 90%, with relatively minimal surgical or medical interventions.[1] In contrast, despite multimodal therapy, long-term survival for patients with high-risk (HR) NB historically has been poor, with 5-year 40% to 50% event-free survival (EFS) rates for patients older than 12 months. The ability to identify early prognostic factors of response may significantly affect decisions about subsequent therapy and help identify the individuals who may benefit from augmented or alternative treatment.[2]

Neuroblastoma Risk Stratification

Over the past 2 decades, the incorporation of clinical, pathologic, biological, and, most recently, genetic factors has enabled the classification of patients based on the risk of recurrence and has enabled tailoring of therapy based on prognosis.[1]

NB patients are classified into low risk, intermediate risk, and HR, based on clinical and biological factors, such as age, stage, histopathology, DNA index (ploidy), MYCN amplification, and, increasingly, the presence of segmental chromosome aberrations.[3,4]

The International Neuroblastoma Risk Group (INRG) Staging System[3] was developed through international consensus to provide a presurgical staging system that uses clinical and imaging data to facilitate comparisons across international clinical trials (Table 1). Locoregional tumors are staged as L1 or L2 based on the absence or presence of Image-Defined Risk Factors, respectively, on cross-sectional imaging. In order to complete staging, bone marrow involvement is assessed

[a] Division of Haematology/Oncology, Department of Paediatrics, The Hospital for Sick Children, University of Toronto, 555 University Ave, Toronto, ON M5G 1X8, Canada; [b] Division of Nuclear Medicine, Department of Diagnostic Imaging, The Hospital for Sick Children, University of Toronto, 555 University Ave, Toronto, ON M5G 1X8, Canada
* Corresponding author.
E-mail address: reza.vali@sickkids.ca

PET Clin 16 (2021) 419–427
https://doi.org/10.1016/j.cpet.2021.03.006

Table 1
The International Neuroblastoma Risk Group Staging System

Stage	Description
L1	Localized tumor not involving vital structures as defined by the list of image-defined risk factors and confined to 1 body compartment
L2	Locoregional tumor with presence of 1 or more image-defined risk factors
M	Distant metastatic disease (except stage MS)
MS	Metastatic disease in children younger than 18 mo with metastases confined to skin, liver, and/or bone marrow

Note: Patients with multifocal primary tumors should be staged according to the greatest extent of disease.

by examination of aspirates and biopsies, and cross-sectional and iodine 123 (^{123}I) metaiodobenzylguanidine (MIBG) scans are used to determine metastatic spread.[5]

Metaiodobenzylguanidine Scans

MIBG is a sympathomimetic guanethidine derivative, a norepinephrine analog that can enter cells via the human norepinephrine transporter. It concentrates in adrenergic tissues and has demonstrated high sensitivity and specificity in NB detection.[6,7] In the past 3 decades, whole-body imaging using radiolabeled MIBG has become a standard of care method for staging and monitoring treatment response in NB.[8,9]

The physiologic biodistribution of MIBG includes uptake in salivary glands, thyroid, heart, liver, urinary bladder, bowel, normal adrenal glands, and, occasionally, brown fat[10,11] but is not expected in bone and bone marrow, which enables the identification of osseous metastatic disease in NB, resulting in increased rates of sensitivity for disease detection as well as confidence in interpretation compared with radionuclide technician bone scans.[12,13]

Iodine 131 (^{131}I) is a beta emitter with a physical half-life of 8 days.[14] [^{131}I]-MIBG, however, is not an ideal radiotracer for diagnostic imaging. The ^{131}I label is not compatible with conventional δ camera imaging. Moreover, the β emission decay does not contribute to image formation by δ cameras.[15] In the early 1980s, Wieland and colleagues[16] demonstrated that MIBG could be labeled with ^{123}I, which

has a principal δ photon energy,[15] no β emissions, and a shorter half-life.[17] As a result, images are less noisy and have a higher resolution, which consequently increase disease detection, mostly in soft tissue, bone, and bone marrow, compared with the radionuclide bone scan.[7]

Planar imaging is a standard part of ^{123}I-MIBG imaging. Acquisition of planar image routinely includes anterior and posterior whole-body images, acquired as either a whole-body acquisition or as overlapping spot images.[18,19] ^{123}I characteristics, however, allow for the performance of single-photon emission computed tomography (SPECT) or SPECT/computed tomography (CT) where a low-dose CT is added to SPECT images.[20–22] The addition of SPECT improves diagnostic accuracy, not only by distinguishing sites of physiologic uptake from those of disease but also by increasing sensitivity of detection, by identification of small lesions/metastatic disease.[23,24] Furthermore, the ability to reformat SPECT data in multiple planes facilitates correlation with and fusion to separately acquired CT and MR imaging.[23] SPECT/(CT or MR imaging) is now the gold standard approach for NB assessment at many centers.

Approximately 10% of NB tumors do not incorporate MIBG, likely because of lower expression of mature neural features and consequently lower or absent norepinephrine transporter expression.[25] Use of 18-fluorodeoxyglucose ([^{18}F]FDG)-PET imaging is recommended in such patients to assess for metastatic disease.

Metaiodobenzylguanidine Scoring Systems

In 1995, the first semiquantitative scoring system for evaluating MIBG scans was developed to assess the extent of disease and response to chemotherapy as a prognostic factor.[26]

After several studies,[27–31] the role of semiquantitative MIBG scoring as a prognostic indicator for HR NB has been reported in both institutional and cooperative group trials, including trials within the Children's Oncology Group (COG) and the International Society of Paediatric Oncology European Neuroblastoma (SIOPEN) Research Network.[8] The goal of these scoring systems is to use standard methodology that is reliable, reproducible, easy to use, and adaptable to multicenter use, to evaluate the prognostic significance of tumor burden at diagnosis as well as therapeutic response. Currently, there are 2 scoring systems used worldwide. The Curie score (CS), used in North America, divides the body into 10 segments, 9 bone and 1 soft tissue, each scored 0 to 3, depending on the extent of disease involvement, as assessed by MIBG uptake.[31] The maximum score is 30 (**Fig. 1**). The SIOPEN scoring method was validated in the early 2000s. In this method, the body is divided into 12 osseous segments (no soft tissue), each scored 0 to 6.[8] The maximum score is 72 (**Fig. 2**). Thus, the major difference between these 2 systems is that the CS includes the soft tissue tumor(s), such as primary tumor, whereas SIOPEN does not.

Metaiodobenzylguanidine Score Correlations with Outcome

In 2013, a study reported the prognostic impact of postinduction chemotherapy CS in HR NB,[31] and in 2018, further work reinforced the validation of this score as a prognostic marker of response and survival in a large, independent data set of patients with ^{123}I-MIBG avid, stage 4, newly diagnosed HR NB, within the European group.[32] Multiple studies,[6,30,33–35] demonstrated that a low MIBG score at diagnosis (less than or equal to 2 for CS, and less than or equal to 4 for SIOPEN score) correlates with significantly better EFS and OS. The investigators were able to demonstrate an optimum cutpoint after induction—a CS of 2. Patients with a CS of 2 or less after induction therapy had significantly better 5-year EFS and OS than patients with a CS of more than 2. These findings are important from an overall prognostic perspective, but they also potentially may identify patients who would benefit from alternative or intensification treatment to improve remission status following induction chemotherapy. No studies, however, have shown that additional treatments aimed at this group improve overall outcome. Furthermore, a majority of patients included in this study[35] did not receive immunotherapy with anti-GD2 monoclonal antibodies, now considered standard in the treatment of HR NB. Prognostic significance of CS at the time of initial diagnosis was not demonstrated in this study.[35]

Metaiodobenzylguanidine Therapy

The use of [131I]MIBG as a therapeutic agent began in the middle of the 1980s.[7] The potential to deliver high levels of absorbed radiation to tumor cells, the rapid clearance by kidneys and its metabolic stability, makes [131I]MIBG an ideal systemic tumor targeting therapeutic agent for NB.[36,37]

Until a few years ago, the focus had been on those patients with relapsed or refractory disease, as salvage or palliative treatment. Overall response rates of approximately 30% have been reported,[38] confirming [131I]MIBG therapy as one of the most active regimens in relapsed disease. Complexities of administration, such as the requirement for appropriate radio-isolation facilities and need for available peripheral blood stem cells to ensure marrow recovery post-treatment, have to an extent limited widespread availability. Beyond giving single-agent ^{131}I-MIBG, multiple studies also have explored options for enhancing efficacy through, for example, combining the radioisotope with radiosensitizing agents such as vincristine and irinotecan[39] or vorinostat.[40] Most recently, the NANT consortium undertook a randomized study comparing these approaches, with initial data indicating an improved response rate in patients treated with the combination of ^{131}I-MIBG and vorinostat compared with ^{131}I-MIBG alone or in combination with vincristine/irinotecan.[41] Further combinations currently are being explored in clinical trials, including in combination with the anti-GD2 antibody dinutuximab (NCT03332667) or in combination with anti-GD2

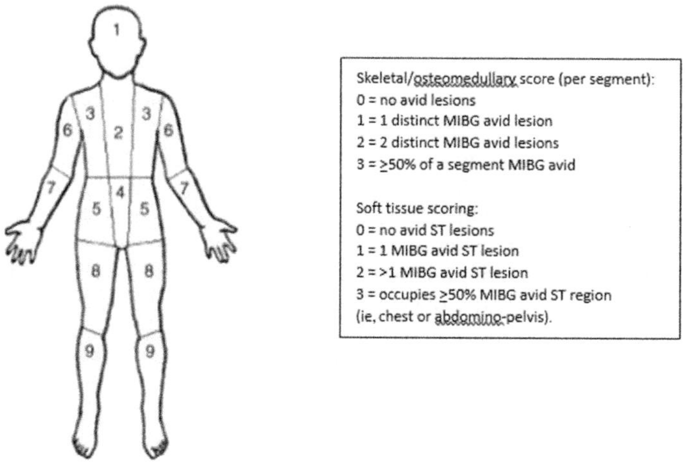

Fig. 1. Curie Score

Skeletal/osteomedullary score (per segment):
0 = no avid lesions
1 = 1 distinct MIBG avid lesion
2 = 2 distinct MIBG avid lesions
3 = ≥50% of a segment MIBG avid

Soft tissue scoring:
0 = no avid ST lesions
1 = 1 MIBG avid ST lesion
2 = >1 MIBG avid ST lesion
3 = occupies ≥50% MIBG avid ST region
(ie, chest or abdomino-pelvis).

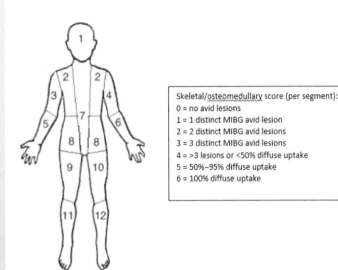

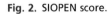

Fig. 2. SIOPEN score.

antibody dinutuximab-beta and immune check-point inhibitor nivolumab (NCT02914405).

[^{131}I]MIBG therapy also may have a role in the upfront treatment of MIBG-avid HR NB patients, an approach that was pioneered in the Netherlands.[42]

In North America, this concept was explored by COG in the ANBL09P1 trial, in which the last cycle of chemotherapy during the induction phase was replaced with [^{131}I]MIBG therapy (NCT01175356). This pilot study set the foundation for the current COG HR study, ANBL1531, which aims to determine in the context of a randomized trial whether the EFS of patients with newly diagnosed HR NB is improved with the addition of [^{131}I]MIBG during induction, before tandem autologous stem cell transplantation. In this study, patients with upfront MIBG-avid disease and no ALK aberrations are randomized between 3 therapeutic arms, 2 of them adding MIBG therapy to induction chemotherapy (NCT03126916).

In parallel, in Europe, the SIOPEN group is running the VERITAS study, an international multicenter phase II randomized trial for metastatic NB with a poor response to induction chemotherapy. It aims to evaluate and compare 2 intensification treatment strategies: ^{131}I-MIBG with topotecan, followed by busulfan and melphalan (BuMel) high-dose chemotherapy versus tandem high-dose chemotherapy using thiotepa followed by BuMel (NCT03165292).

DISCUSSION
Metaiodobenzylguanidine as Theranostics

Theranostics is the use of a successful combination in therapy and diagnostics to create a unique approach to each individual patient. The goal of the diagnostic phase is to identify certain biomarkers that can be predictive of therapy response and can be used for therapy monitoring. The approach usually is achieved using the same molecule, which is labeled either with different radionuclides or an identical one used at a different dosage.[7]

The most suitable radionuclides for the theranostic are the ones with both δ and β emissions. Although, in some cases, different radioisotopes can be used (**Fig. 3**), usually δ emitters are used for diagnosis and β-emitter or α-emitter for therapy.[43] Emerging positron emitters, such as iodine 124 (^{124}I), and emerging a emitters, such as astatine 211, or iodine 125, have shown better quality of imaging with PET and potentially more potent radiation in therapy, respectively, but more studies are needed for more concluding results.[43]

Since the introduction of SPECT/CT as a routine image modality, the introduction of other complementary PET tracers for correct identification of NB lesions in clinical practice has appeared particularly useful.[43] Moreover, the small proportion of non-MIBG avid tumors require other diagnostic strategies. Despite the high diagnostic accuracy of MIBG imaging, there are several disadvantages of MIBG imaging, such as limited spatial resolution and sensitivity in small lesions, need for 2 or even more acquisition sessions in the case of SPECT, and a delay between the start of the examination and results. Furthermore, in most cases, MIBG imaging is not sufficient for operative or biopsy planning.[43]

Most of these disadvantages potentially can be overcome with PET, due to its higher spatial resolution and the possibility of a whole-body

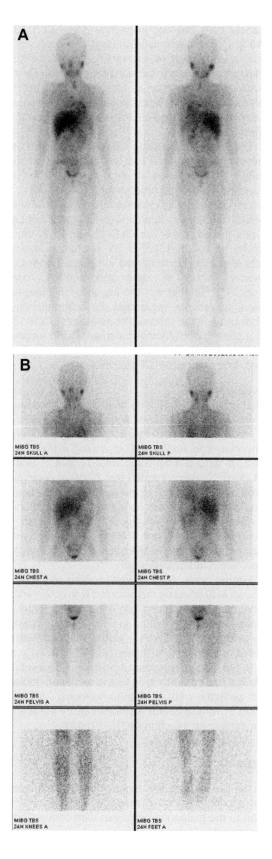

tomography versus SPECT with a limited field of view. PET or PET/CT is completed in 1 examination within 30 minutes to 60 minutes after injection versus [¹²³I]MIBG scintigraphy with SPECT or SPECT/CT requiring at least 18 hours to 24 hours to reach a desirable tumor-to-background ratio. The resulting shorter scanning time of PET has the potential for reducing the number or length of sedations.[44] Besides, MIBG needs an oral medication to be administered for thyroid protection, which makes it less patient-friendly. In recent years, different types of PET tracers have been used in NB and compared with [¹²³I]MIBG.[45]

18-Fluorodeoxyglucose PET–Computed Tomography

NB often is characterized by a high [¹⁸F]FDG uptake, as other malignancies.[44] Although data about the role of [¹⁸F]FDG in NB are limited and no prospective multicenter studies have been conducted, [¹⁸F]FDG PET-CT represents an important and widely available alternative to [¹²³I]MIBG scans, especially in cases of nonavid MIBG NB. However, 2011 INRG guidelines[46] for imaging and staging of NB did not recognize the diagnostic role of [¹⁸F]FDG PET-CT. The investigators underlined that the feasibility of PET-CT in young children, the associated radiation exposure, and the higher cost, in addition to those of MIBG scanning, may explain the limited use of this technique.[47] Recent studies[48,49] also are not conclusive as to which of the techniques is more sensitive or where the biggest differences fall on the detection of localized or metastatic disease. Established protocols for the management of patients with metastatic NC typically have been developed on the basis of response determination by MIBG evaluation, and thus the interpretation of [¹⁸F]FDG PET in evaluation of therapy response has considerably less evidence on which to base decision making.

Nevertheless, given that [¹⁸F]FDG PET-CT can identify disease in ¹²³I-MIBG negative lesions, it might serve as a complementary imaging modality in selected patients. Furthermore, [¹⁸F]FDG PET-CT imaging is helpful during follow-up, when ¹²³I-

Fig. 3. An 11-year old girl with multiple foci of [123I] MIBG activity in the skull, cervical, thoracic and lumbar spine, pelvis, and proximal left femur as well as an [123I]MIBG avid lesion in a left abdominal paraspinal soft tissue on [123I]MIBG scan (A). The patient was treated with 445-mCi [131I]MIBG. There was only a small focus of residual MIBG activity in the left abdominal paraspinal soft tissue on [123I]MIBG scan performed 2 months after therapy (B). TBS, total body scan.

MIBG scan/SPECT yield discrepant or inconclusive findings.[50] In contrast, if [18F]FDG PET-CT is negative but the 123I-MIBG scan is still positive, a biopsy might be placed to confirm a tumor's maturation or only its lack of metabolic activity.[46,49]

The principal limitation of [18F]FDG PET-CT remains the nonspecific bone marrow uptake during chemotherapy or administration of granulocyte-stimulating factor. This problem can be overcome by scheduling [18F]FDG PET-CT just before the course of chemotherapy.[46]

68-Gallium–DOTA-TOC([68Ga]Ga–DOTA-TOC)/ 68-Gallium–DOTATATE ([68Ga]Ga-DOTATATE) PET–Computed Tomography

The use of radiolabeled somatostatin analogs in NB involves a distinct and separate cell surface molecular target, different from the norepinephrine transporter molecule that takes up [131I]MIBG. Somatostatin receptor (SR) scintigraphy has been used for the assessment of NB in the past,[51,52] due to its overexpression of SR, mostly types 1 and 2. This rationale has been considered for the development of new PET tracers, such as [68Ga]Ga–DOTA-TOC.[52]

DOTATATE is the abbreviation used to describe a somatostatin analog, octreotide, linked with a chelator (DOTA), which binds radionuclides, such as gallium 68 (68Ga), useful for imaging, and lutetium 177 (177Lu) for therapy, both with high affinity for SR subtype 2. Kroiss and colleagues[52] found that the sensitivity of [68Ga]Ga–DOTA-TOC PET-CT was higher than that of 123I-MIBG imaging, and the primary NB lesion was better definable with the former than with the latter. These data are especially relevant for considering indication for therapy with radiolabeled somatostatin analogs. Another study[53] used [68Ga]Ga–DOTATATE PET-CT for diagnosing the presence of disease and 177Lu–DOTA-TATE ([177Lu]Lu–DOTA-TATE) for therapy in patients with relapsed or refractory NB and concluded that is a safe treatment. This study was the previous step for the phase IIa trial of molecular radiotherapy, with [177Lu]Lu–DOTA-TATE in children with primary refractory or relapsed HR NB carried out by the same group.[54] Despite the negative results of this study, peptide receptor radionuclide therapy leaves an open door to different theranostic imaging and treatment emerging radiopharmaceuticals targeting SR.

Emerging Therapies

CLR-131

Phospholipid ethers (PLEs) are naturally occurring molecules that accumulate in the membranes of cancer cells but not in healthy ones. CLR 131 (18-[p-(131I)-iodophenyl]octadecyl phosphocholine) is an investigational, radioiodinated therapy that use these tumor-targeting properties to selectively deliver radiation to tumor cells but not to normal tissues. The lipid raft regions of the cancer cell plasm membrane are involved in this selective mechanistic.[55]

The core PLE analog 18-(p-iodophenyl)octadecyl phosphocholine (CLR-1404) was radioiodinated with 131I due to its well-established in cancer therapy,[56,57] producing CLR 131.

The preclinical studies showed almost 100% of selective uptake in adult and pediatric cancer cell types tested, either for CLR-124 (used in diagnosis) and CLR-131.[56,57] Its antitumor activity has also been documented in several tumor cell models, either in adult and pediatric cancers,[55,58,59] confirming the capacity of target tumors universally, regardless its histopathology. That provide the rationale to investigate CLR 131 in a phase I pediatric clinical trial for solid tumors, which currently is open in the United States, Canada, and Australia (NCT02952508).

Omburtamab

Omburtamab is a murine immunoglobulin monoclonal antibody, 8H9, designed to target B7-H3, a surface immunomodulatory glycoprotein and important checkpoint that plays a role in the inhibition of natural killer cells and T cells.[60] Some studies[61–63] demonstrated that B7-H3 is preferentially expressed on a broad spectrum of pediatric and adult solid tumors compared with normal human tissues. Another group[64] demonstrated, in xenograft models, that 8H9 can suppress tumor cell growth by deliver therapeutic doses of radiation, when radiolabeled with 131I.

Furthermore, Grewal and colleagues[65] have shown 8H9 could be radiolabeled with other radiopharmaceuticals, such as 124I, and currently a phase I clinical trial is open with 124I 8H9, mostly for primary brain tumors or leptomeningeal metastases in adults and children (NCT01502917).

In NB, after a successful phase I, a phase II/III clinical trial currently is open and recruiting pediatric patients with CNS/leptomeningeal disease, with 131I-omburtamab administered by intracerebroventricular injection (NCT03275402).

SUMMARY

In the past 2 decades, most oncology treatments have followed a path of targeted therapies, mainly due to the plateau in outcomes with conventional treatments. These new therapies further highlight the importance of a multidisciplinary approach, linking the clinic with emerging techniques in nuclear medicine and molecular imaging, to offer the best treatment.

Theranostics is a personalized medicine concept, combining diagnosis and treatment in the same technique to achieve an individual treatment. MIBG is the gold standard in NB patients and one of the most well-established techniques, using the same molecule labeled with 2 different radionuclides, 1 for imaging—[123]I—and another for therapy—[131]I.

Not only have other imaging techniques, such as PET-CT or PET–MR imaging, emerged in the last decades, however, but also several new radiopharmaceuticals, with better radioactivity characteristics are emerging. Thus, building on the foundations of MIBG, both imaging and therapy options and ultimately outcomes for children with NB may be able to be improved.

DISCLOSURE

The authors have nothing to disclose.

Dr Daniel Morgenstern has received consultancy fees from ymAbs Therapeutics and Clarity Pharmaceuticals and travel expenses from EUSA Pharma.

REFERENCES

1. Irwin MS, Park JR. Neuroblastoma: paradigm for precision medicine. Pediatr Clin North Am 2015; 62(1):225–56.
2. Matthay KK, George RE, Yu AL. Promising therapeutic targets in neuroblastoma. Clin Cancer Res 2012; 18(10):2740–53.
3. Cohn SL, Pearson AD, London WB, et al. The international neuroblastoma risk group (INRG) classification system: an INRG task force report. J Clin Oncol 2009;27(2):289–97.
4. Pinto NR, Applebaum MA, Volchenboum SL, et al. Advances in risk classification and treatment strategies for neuroblastoma. J Clin Oncol 2015;33(27): 3008–17.
5. Monclair T, Brodeur GM, Ambros PF, et al. The international neuroblastoma risk group (INRG) staging system: an INRG task force report. J Clin Oncol 2009;27(2):298–303.
6. DuBois SG, Mody R, Naranjo A, et al. MIBG avidity correlates with clinical features, tumor biology, and outcomes in neuroblastoma: a report from the Children's Oncology Group. Pediatr Blood Cancer 2017;64(11).
7. Parisi MT, Eslamy H, Park JR, et al. ^{131}I-Metaiodobenzylguanidine theranostics in neuroblastoma: historical perspectives; practical applications. Semin Nucl Med 2016;46(3):184–202.
8. Lewington V, Lambert B, Poetschger U, et al. ^{123}I-mIBG scintigraphy in neuroblastoma: development of a SIOPEN semi-quantitative reporting, method by an international panel. Eur J Nucl Med Mol Imaging 2017;44(2):234–41.
9. Park JR, Bagatell R, Cohn SL, et al. Revisions to the international neuroblastoma response criteria: a consensus statement from the National cancer Institute clinical trials planning meeting. J Clin Oncol 2017;35(22):2580–7.
10. Shulkin BL, Shapiro B. Current concepts on the diagnostic use of MIBG in children. J Nucl Med 1998;39(4):679–88.
11. Boubaker A, Bischof Delaloye A. MIBG scintigraphy for the diagnosis and follow-up of children with neuroblastoma. Q J Nucl Med Mol Imaging 2008;52(4): 388–402.
12. Hadj-Djilani NL, Lebtahi NE, Delaloye AB, et al. Diagnosis and follow-up of neuroblastoma by means of iodine-123 metaiodobenzylguanidine scintigraphy and bone scan, and the influence of histology. Eur J Nucl Med 1995;22(4):322–9.
13. Parisi MT, Greene MK, Dykes TM, et al. Efficacy of metaiodobenzylguanidine as a scintigraphic agent for the detection of neuroblastoma. Invest Radiol 1992;27(10):768–73.
14. Wafelman AR, Nortier YL, Rosing H, et al. Renal excretion of meta-iodobenzylguanidine after therapeutic doses in cancer patients and its relation to dose and creatinine clearance. Nucl Med Commun 1995;16(9):767–72.
15. Liu B, Zhuang H, Servaes S. Comparison of ^{123}I-MIBG and ^{131}I-MIBG for imaging of neuroblastoma and other neural crest tumors. Q J Nucl Med Mol Imaging 2013;57(1):21–8.
16. Wieland DM, Brown LE, Tobes MC, et al. Imaging the primate adrenal medulla with [123I] and [131I] meta-iodobenzylguanidine: concise communication. J Nucl Med 1981;22(4):358–64.
17. Vallabhajosula S, Nikolopoulou A. Radioiodinated metaiodobenzylguanidine (MIBG): radiochemistry, biology, and pharmacology. Semin Nucl Med 2011; 41(5):324–33.
18. Matthay KK, Shulkin B, Ladenstein R, et al. Criteria for evaluation of disease extent by (123)I-metaiodobenzylguanidine scans in neuroblastoma: a report for the international neuroblastoma risk group (INRG) task force. Br J Cancer 2010;102(9): 1319–26.
19. Bombardieri E, Aktolun C, Baum RP, et al. 131I/123I-metaiodobenzylguanidine (MIBG) scintigraphy: procedure guidelines for tumour imaging. Eur J Nucl Med Mol Imaging 2003;30(12):BP132–9.
20. Rufini V, Giordano A, Di Giuda D, et al. [123I]MIBG scintigraphy in neuroblastoma: a comparison between planar and SPECT imaging. Q J Nucl Med 1995;39(4 Suppl 1):25–8.

21. Rufini V, Fisher GA, Shulkin BL, et al. Iodine-123-MIBG imaging of neuroblastoma: utility of SPECT and delayed imaging. J Nucl Med 1996;37(9):1464–8.

22. Rozovsky K, Koplewitz BZ, Krausz Y, et al. Added value of SPECT/CT for correlation of MIBG scintigraphy and diagnostic CT in neuroblastoma and pheochromocytoma. AJR Am J Roentgenol 2008; 190(4):1085–90.

23. Vik TA, Pfluger T, Kadota R, et al. (123)I-mIBG scintigraphy in patients with known or suspected neuroblastoma: results from a prospective multicenter trial. Pediatr Blood Cancer 2009;52(7):784–90.

24. Shusterman S, Grant FD, Lorenzen W, et al. Iodine-131-labeled meta-iodobenzylguanidine therapy of children with neuroblastoma: program planning and initial experience. Semin Nucl Med 2011;41(5): 354–63.

25. Streby KA, Shah N, Ranalli MA, et al. Nothing but NET: a review of norepinephrine transporter expression and efficacy of 131I-mIBG therapy. Pediatr Blood Cancer 2015;62(1):5–11.

26. Ady N, Zucker JM, Asselain B, et al. A new 123I-MIBG whole body scan scoring method–application to the prediction of the response of metastases to induction chemotherapy in stage IV neuroblastoma. Eur J Cancer 1995;31A(2):256–61.

27. Kushner BH, Yeh SD, Kramer K, et al. Impact of metaiodobenzylguanidine scintigraphy on assessing response of high-risk neuroblastoma to dose-intensive induction chemotherapy. J Clin Oncol 2003;21(6):1082–6.

28. Matthay KK, Edeline V, Lumbroso J, et al. Correlation of early metastatic response by 123I-metaiodobenzylguanidine scintigraphy with overall response and event-free survival in stage IV neuroblastoma. J Clin Oncol 2003;21(13):2486–91.

29. Messina JA, Cheng SC, Franc BL, et al. Evaluation of semi-quantitative scoring system for metaiodobenzylguanidine (mIBG) scans in patients with relapsed neuroblastoma. Pediatr Blood Cancer 2006;47(7):865–74.

30. Decarolis B, Schneider C, Hero B, et al. Iodine-123 metaiodobenzylguanidine scintigraphy scoring allows prediction of outcome in patients with stage 4 neuroblastoma: results of the Cologne interscore comparison study. J Clin Oncol 2013;31(7):944–51.

31. Yanik GA, Parisi MT, Shulkin BL, et al. Semiquantitative mIBG scoring as a prognostic indicator in patients with stage 4 neuroblastoma: a report from the Children's oncology group. J Nucl Med 2013;54(4):541–8.

32. Yanik GA, Parisi MT, Naranjo A, et al. Validation of postinduction Curie scores in high-risk neuroblastoma: a children's oncology group and SIOPEN group report on SIOPEN/HR-NBL1. J Nucl Med 2018;59(3):502–8.

33. Suc A, Lumbroso J, Rubie H, et al. Metastatic neuroblastoma in children older than one year: prognostic significance of the initial metaiodobenzylguanidine scan and proposal for a scoring system. Cancer 1996;77(4):805–11.

34. Perel Y, Conway J, Kletzel M, et al. Clinical impact and prognostic value of metaiodobenzylguanidine imaging in children with metastatic neuroblastoma. J Pediatr Hematol Oncol 1999;21(1):13–8.

35. Ladenstein R, Poetschger U, Boubaker A, et al. The prognostic value of semi-quantitative I-123 mIBG scintigraphy at diagnosis in high risk neuroblastoma: validation of the SIOPEN score method. Pediatr Blood Cancer 2011;57:732–3.

36. Sisson JC, Yanik GA. Theranostics: evolution of the radiopharmaceutical meta-iodobenzylguanidine in endocrine tumors. Semin Nucl Med 2012;42(3): 171–84.

37. de Kraker J, Hoefnagel KA, Verschuur AC, et al. Iodine-131-metaiodobenzylguanidine as initial induction therapy in stage 4 neuroblastoma patients over 1 year of age. Eur J Cancer 2008;44(4):551–6.

38. Wilson JS, Gains JE, Moroz V, et al. A systematic review of 131I-meta iodobenzylguanidine molecular radiotherapy for neuroblastoma. Eur J Cancer 2014;50(4):801–15.

39. DuBois SG, Allen S, Bent M, et al. Phase I/II study of (131)I-MIBG with vincristine and 5 days of irinotecan for advanced neuroblastoma. Br J Cancer 2015; 112(4):644–9.

40. DuBois SG, Groshen S, Park JR, et al. Phase I study of vorinostat as a radiation sensitizer with 131I-meta-iodobenzylguanidine (131I-MIBG) for patients with relapsed or refractory neuroblastoma. Clin Cancer Res 2015;21(12):2715–21.

41. DuBois SG, Granger M, Groshen SG, et al. Randomized phase II trial of MIBG versus MIBG/vincristine/irinotecan versus MIBG/vorinostat for relapsed/refractory neuroblastoma: a report from the New Approaches to Neuroblastoma Therapy Consortium. ASCO Abstract J Clin Oncol 2020;38 [suppl; abstr 10500].

42. Hoefnagel CA, De Kraker J, Valdés Olmos RA, et al. 131I-MIBG as a first-line treatment in high-risk neuroblastoma patients. Nucl Med Commun 1994; 15(9):712–7.

43. Filippi L, Chiaravalloti A, Schillaci O, et al. Theranostic approaches in nuclear medicine: current status and future prospects. Expert Rev Med Devices 2020;17(4):331–43.

44. Piccardo A, Lopci E, Conte M, et al. PET/CT imaging in neuroblastoma. Q J Nucl Med Mol Imaging 2013; 57(1):29–39.

45. Boyd M, Mairs RJ, Keith WN, et al. An efficient targeted radiotherapy/gene therapy strategy utilizing human telomerase promoters and radioastatine and harnessin gradiation-mediated by stander effects. J Gene Med 2004;6:937–47.

46. Brisse HJ, McCarville MB, Granata C, et al. Guidelines for imaging and staging of neuroblastic tumors:

consensus report from the International Neuroblastoma Risk Group Project. Radiology 2011;261(1): 243–57.

47. Bleeker G, Tytgat GA, Adam JA, et al. 123I-MIBG scintigraphy and 18F-FDG-PET imaging for diagnosing neuroblastoma. Cochrane Database Syst Rev 2015;2015(9):CD009263.

48. Sharp SE, Shulkin BL, Gelfand MJ, et al. 123I-MIBG scintigraphy and 18F-FDG PET in neuroblastoma. J Nucl Med 2009;50(8):1237–43.

49. Taggart DR, Han MM, Quach A, et al. Comparison of iodine-123 metaiodobenzylguanidine (MIBG) scan and [18F]fluorodeoxyglucose positron emission tomography to evaluate response after iodine-131 MIBG therapy for relapsed neuroblastoma. J Clin Oncol 2009;27(32):5343–9.

50. Melzer HI, Coppenrath E, Schmid I, et al. ^{123}I-MIBG scintigraphy/SPECT versus ^{18}F-FDG PET in paediatric neuroblastoma. Eur J Nucl Med Mol Imaging 2011;38(9):1648–58.

51. Albers AR, O'Dorisio MS, Balster DA, et al. Somatostatin receptor gene expression in neuroblastoma. Regul Pept 2000;88(1–3):61–73.

52. Kroiss A, Putzer D, Uprimny C, et al. Functional imaging in phaeochromocytoma and neuroblastoma with 68Ga-DOTA-Tyr 3-octreotide positron emission tomography and 123I-metaiodobenzylguanidine. Eur J Nucl Med Mol Imaging 2011;38(5):865–73.

53. Gains JE, Bomanji JB, Fersht NL, et al. 177Lu-DOTA-TATE molecular radiotherapy for childhood neuroblastoma. J Nucl Med 2011;52(7):1041–7.

54. Gains JE, Moroz V, Aldridge MD, et al. A phase IIa trial of molecular radiotherapy with 177-lutetium DOTATATE in children with primary refractory or relapsed high-risk neuroblastoma. Eur J Nucl Med Mol Imaging 2020;47(10):2348–57.

55. Weichert JP, Clark PA, Kandela IK, et al. Alkylphosphocholine analogs for broad-spectrum cancer imaging and therapy. Sci Transl Med 2014;6(240): 240ra75.

56. Mollinedo F, de la Iglesia-Vicente J, Gajate C, et al. Lipid raft-targeted therapy in multiple myeloma. Oncogene 2010;29(26):3748–57.

57. Macklis RM, Pohlman B. Radioimmunotherapy for non-Hodgkin's lymphoma: a review for radiation oncologists. Int J Radiat Oncol Biol Phys 2006;66(3): 833–41.

58. Baiu DC, Marsh IR, Boruch AE, et al. Targeted molecular radiotherapy of pediatric solid tumors using a Radioiodinated alkyl-phospholipid ether analog. J Nucl Med 2018;59(2):244–50.

59. Marsh IR, Grudzinski J, Baiu DC, et al. Preclinical pharmacokinetics and dosimetry studies of 124I/131I-CLR1404 for treatment of pediatric solid tumors in murine xenograft models. J Nucl Med 2019; 60(10):1414–20.

60. Modak S, Kramer K, Gultekin SH, et al. Monoclonal antibody 8H9 targets a novel cell surface antigen expressed by a wide spectrum of human solid tumors. Cancer Res 2001;61(10):4048–54.

61. Wang L, Zhang Q, Chen W, et al. B7-H3 is overexpressed in patients suffering osteosarcoma and associated with tumor aggressiveness and metastasis. PLoS One 2013;8(8):e70689.

62. Wang L, Kang FB, Zhang GC, et al. Clinical significance of serum soluble B7-H3 in patients with osteosarcoma. Cancer Cell Int 2018;18:115.

63. Zhang T, Wang F, Wu JY, et al. Clinical correlation of B7-H3 and B3GALT4 with the prognosis of colorectal cancer. World J Gastroenterol 2018;24(31): 3538–46.

64. Modak S, Guo HF, Humm JL, et al. Radioimmunotargeting of human rhabdomyosarcoma using monoclonal antibody 8H9. Cancer Biother Radiopharm 2005;20(5):534–46.

65. Grewal RK, Lubberink M, Pentlow KS, et al. The role of iodine-124-positron emission tomography imaging in the management of patients with thyroid cancer. PET Clin 2007;2(3):313–20.

Emerging Preclinical and Clinical Applications of Theranostics for Nononcological Disorders

Majid Assadi, MD, FASNC[a], Narges Jokar, MSc[a], Anna Yordanova, MD[b,c],
Ali Gholamrezanezhad, MD, FEBNM, DABR[d], Abdullatif Amini, MD[e],
Farhad Abbasi, MD[f], Hans-Jürgen Biersack, MD[b], Azam Amini, MD[g],
Iraj Nabipour, MD[h], Hojjat Ahmadzadehfar, MD, MSc[b,i],*

KEYWORDS

• Theranostics • Nononcological diseases • Infection • Inflammation • Sarcoidosis
• Rheumatoid diseases

KEY POINTS

• Along with the considerable results of theranostics in tumoral tissues, there has been a strong push to use this approach for nononcological diseases as well.
• Theranostics approaches may have efficient role in management of rheumatic and cardiovascular diseases, as well as the infections including viral, bacterial and fungal.
• There is an emerging need for randomized trials to specify the factors affecting validity and efficacy of theranostic approaches in nononcological diseases.

INTRODUCTION

Studies in nuclear medicine have shed light on molecular imaging and therapeutic approaches for oncological and nononcological conditions. Theranostic approaches using the same radiopharmaceuticals for the diagnoses and subsequent therapeutics of malignancies have continuously evolved for site-directed molecular imaging and therapy, especially in oncology. Theranostics, one of the remarkable consequences of the Human Genome Project, has added considerable value to personalized medicine as diagnostic and therapeutic methods are performed exclusively per personal genotypes and phenotypes. Molecular pathways and high-throughput omics platforms are used to recognize and extend small molecular probes for these conditions. Theranostic approach, however, has long been used in clinical practice, namely in

[a] Department of Molecular Imaging and Radionuclide Therapy (MIRT), The Persian Gulf Nuclear Medicine Research Center, Bushehr Medical University Hospital, School of Medicine, Bushehr University of Medical Sciences, Bushehr, Iran; [b] Department of Nuclear Medicine, University Hospital Bonn, Bonn, Germany; [c] Department of Radiology, Marienhospital Bonn, Bonn, Germany; [d] Department of Diagnostic Radiology, Keck School of Medicine, University of Southern California, 1520 San Pablo Street, Suite L1600, Los Angeles, CA 90033, USA; [e] Bushehr Heart Medical Center, School of Medicine, Bushehr University of Medical Sciences, Bushehr, Iran; [f] Department of Infectious Diseases, Bushehr Medical University Hospital, School of Medicine, Bushehr University of Medical Sciences, Bushehr, Iran; [g] Department of Internal Medicine, Division of Rheumatology, Bushehr Medical University Hospital, School of Medicine, Bushehr University of Medical Sciences, Bushehr, Iran; [h] The Persian Gulf Tropical Medicine Research Center, The Persian Gulf Biomedical Sciences Research Institute, Bushehr University of Medical Sciences, Bushehr, Iran; [i] Department of Nuclear Medicine, Klinikum Westfalen, Am Knappschaftskrankenhaus 1, Dortmund 44309, Germany
* Corresponding author. Department of Nuclear Medicine, Klinikum Westfalen, Am Knappschaftskrankenhaus 1, Dortmund 44309, Germany.
E-mail addresses: hojjat.ahmadzadehfar@ruhr-uni-bochum.de; nuclearmedicine@gmail.com

PET Clin 16 (2021) 429–440
https://doi.org/10.1016/j.cpet.2021.03.009
1556-8598/21/© 2021 Elsevier Inc. All rights reserved.

the use of radioactive iodine 131 (^{131}I) in thyroid patients.[1,2] The principle of this method involves the utilization of different imaging and/or therapeutic radionuclides labeled with the same or a very similar tracer as a specific vector for the diagnosis and individually tailored treatment of patients. An important value of the theranostic procedure is the identification of patients who likely will respond (or not) to a new specific or common nonspecific treatment approach and the monitoring of patients' responses to the treatment procedures.[3,4]

Noninvasive nuclear imaging techniques can quantify the concentration of intravenously injected radiopharmaceuticals using single-photon emission computed tomography (SPECT), positron emission tomography (PET), PET/computed tomography (CT) and, recently, PET/MR imaging. Nuclear molecular imaging contributes to the more precise localization and biodistribution of radiopharmaceutical compounds and thus individual dosimetry calculations. This enables prediction of the optimal therapeutic dosage through the diagnostic part of the theranostic twin and consequently selective delivery of the therapeutic agent. Among nononcological disorders, the most important infectious organisms, including fungal, bacterial, and viral, are pathogens that can multiply quickly, affect the whole body significantly, and decrease patients' survival. Inflammation is defined as a primary and sophisticated response through the cluster of immunologic and histopathologic events to tissue injuries and infections. Inflammation diseases mostly are relapsed, affecting quality of life and likely requiring long-lasting treatment techniques. Furthermore, there are increasing case report studies about the emerging nononcological applications of theranostic agents in sarcoidosis, including cardiac and another treatment-refractory sarcoidosis, as an inflammation disease. So it is time to implement a new emerging theranostic approach for the timely diagnosis and successful treatment of inflammations and infectious pathogens. Radioimmunotherapy (RIT) is a valuable approach that integrates the cytotoxic effect of radiation-emitting particles with a monoclonal antibody (mAb) to eradicate target cells; its development was initiated for malignancy treatment. Additionally, microbe-specific radiolabeled antibodies hold enormous potential for the diagnosis and treatment of inflammations and infections.[5]

Along with the considerable and useful results of theranostics in tumoral tissues, and given the encouraging results of theranostic reports in nontumoral tissues, there has been a strong push to use this approach for nononcological diseases as well. Researchers must perform different validation procedures and considerations for utilization of theranostic approaches in non-oncological diseases. In accordance with these reports, this article aims at enumerating important mechanisms, considerations, and studies about theranostic approaches in nononcological disorders, including inflammations and infections.

THERANOSTIC APPROACHES IN THE MANAGEMENT OF INFECTIONS
Mechanisms of Action

In addition to the development of RIT in the treatment of malignancies, intense research has been carried out for nonmalignant disorders. This process may be performed through different mechanisms, the most important of which are direct hit (binding to the microbial cell and emission cytotoxic radiation) or bystander effect/cross-fire effect (radiation emission from an adjacent or distant cell killing the infected cell [**Fig. 1**]).[6,7] The comparison of RIT processes in infectious and malignant cells demonstrated that due to the specified characteristics of infection, the delivery of cytotoxic dosage to the infected cell is facial, which is different from the oncology situations. Furthermore, one of the difficulties of RIT in the cancerous cell is the gradual penetration rate of antibodies into the target tissue, which results in decreased treatment efficiency. On the other hand, organism-specific antibodies absorb to the infectious site more rapidly due to better and greater capillary permeability at the location of the infection.[8] The antigen-antibody interaction in RIT is not affected by the complicacy of the multidrug-resistant mechanisms in the various microbial species. Moreover, there is no possibility of producing radiation-resistant strains in this approach; nevertheless, researchers are concerned about the probability risk of radiation in this method. Although this danger is minimal, the practical risk must be considered. The main purpose of the use of the antibodies in RIT is as delivery vehicles, so they do not protect in the same way as they do in the naked antibody treatment procedure. They are required only to be an appropriate reagent to attach to the targeted pathogen.[5] So, theoretically, RIT is useful for any kind of microbes reactive to radiation. RIT has been known to work favorably in the treatment of infectious diseases, including fungal, bacterial, and viral (human immunodeficiency virus [HIV]-1) infections.[9]

Some studies evaluated the feasibility of imaging or localizing the site of pathogens to detect infectious foci. Researchers injected radioiodinated intact mAb to *Candida albicans* and observed the

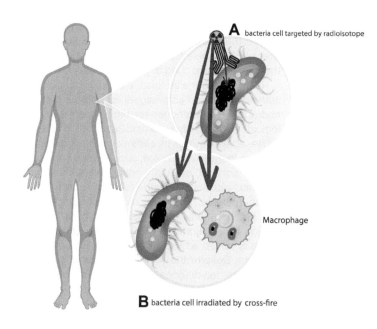

A bacteria cell targeted by radioisotope

Macrophage

B bacteria cell irradiated by cross-fire

Fig. 1. An illustration of the mechanisms by RIT. (*A*) A radiolabeled mAb binds to bacteria and delivers localized lethal dose. (*B*) Adjacent bacteria and infected macrophages also can be killed by a cross-fire effect.

adjustment of *Candida albicans*–specific mAb biodistribution to the anatomic extension of infection confirmed by the colony-forming unit per pathogen.[10] Several study groups managed to utilize specific immune imaging of the infectious agent with mAbs in both human and experimental animal studies; these findings indicate that this approach should be clinically applied.[11–15] The imaging can be achieved through low-energy radionuclides, such as technetium (^{99m}Tc) ($t_{1/2}$ = 6 h) or indium (^{111}In} ($t_{1/2}$ = 2.83 d) for localization of the infection by a planar gamma camera or SPECT, whereas the therapeutic aim can be achieved through rhenium ^{188}Re ($t_{1/2}$ = 16.98 h) or yttrium ^{90}Y ($t_{1/2}$ = 64.1 h).[16] Therapeutic radiations include alpha and beta radiations. Some advantages of β-emitters include relatively long-range emission, relatively low price, convenience, and extensive clinical experience of applications. ^{90}Y emits β⁻ radiation and ^{188}Re emits β⁻ and Y radiations that provides simultaneously visual information and therapeutic effect. Bismuth ^{213}Bi radionuclide ($t_{1/2}$ = 45.6 min) with the emission of alpha radiation results in potentially less radiation cross-fire to nontarget tissues via short range radiation and high linear energy transfer.

Fungal Infection

The standard antifungal treatments no longer are effective, especially in immunocompromised patients, so researchers are urgently attempting to find beneficial approaches. First of all, the feasible efficacy of RIT against fungal infectious diseases with *Cryptococcus neoformans* as a serious fungal

infection was evaluated.[17,18] Administration of ^{213}Bi and ^{188}Re-labeled mAbs to AJ/Cr mice infected with *C neoformans* delivered a lethal dose to the region of interest. So, the therapeutic applicability of this method against the infected lesions was confirmed, along with increasing survival and decreased organ fungal burden with minimum hematological toxicity. Also, Jiang and colleagues[19] reported that RIT is independent of the immune model of the host and can be used for any kind of host. Both findings are incentives to extend this procedure in the clinical treatment of medical conditions, including infections.[17,20–21] Dadachova and colleagues[22] identified ^{111}In and ^{188}Re as two of the best delivery carriers for RIT of *C neoformans* infections. Their study indicated that affinity for the target antigen is a crucial aspect to be considered for favored targeting of infected cells in vivo.

Another antimicrobial application of RIT was explored in a human infectious fungus called *Histoplasma capsulatum*, which causes fungal pneumonia in immunocompromised patients.[23] ^{188}Re-labeled mAb 9C7 (IgM) was used to treat *H capsulatum* in vitro. The results proved the application of ^{188}Re-RIT as a localized agent and therapeutic antifungal modality.[24,25] Also, ^{188}Re labeled to the immunoglobulin G mAbs was dramatically more effective than ^{90}Y and lutetium 177 ^{177}Lu for fungal RIT.[26] These encouraging results lay the foundation for future theranostic studies on fungal infections. An ongoing effort must be carried out to translate RIT of infection to common clinical applications. The cellular in vitro dosimetry calculations showed that RIT of

C neoformans and *H capsulatum* with alpha and beta-emitting radionuclides was more efficient than gamma emission (approximately 1000-fold and 100-fold more efficacious in the elimination of *C neoformans* and *H capsulatum* respectively), supporting the use of RIT as an antifungal approach.[27]

The antigen-antibody interaction yields high affinity and specificity to deliver the antibacterial composition to specific loci of infection. Radiolabeled antibodies deliver microbicidal radiation to pathogen agents. However, there is a considerable limitation in the usage of RIT for tumors that include a small number of antigenic differences between normal and malignant cells that result in non-targeted effects, but RIT of infectious diseases can easily detect antigenic differences between microbes and the host. This important property results in appropriate specificity for targeting microorganism with minimal or no toxicity to the host besides transient hematological toxicity.[16,28,29]

Bacterial Infection

Patients with immunodeficiency disorders, especially those subjected to immunosuppressive therapies, such as patients with AIDS, often are exposed to the increased outbreak of invasive pneumococcal disease.[28] There are different reasons for partial control of this disease, such as drug resistance type, which involves mostly older persons and patients with an impaired immune system. Accordingly, there is an emergent and inevitable need to develop new procedures for antipneumococcal treatment involving newly designed drugs, vaccines, and inactive antibody-based strategies. So, the successful results of RIT in fungal infection provided the impetus for adopting the probability of RIT for bacterial infection utilization of *Streptococcus pneumoniae* as the main cause of bacterial infections, such as meningitis, community-acquired pneumonia, and bacteremia. A study by Dadachova and colleagues[30] found that RIT can be applied to treat *S pneumoniae* infection in in vitro and in animal cases. Evaluation of ^{213}Bi-labeled pathogen-specific antibacterial mAbs (213Bi-D11) demonstrated that a large number of mice remained alive in the group treated with ^{213}Bi-D11 compared with the untreated group without weight loss and confirmed the probable use of RIT for bacterial pathogenesis. In contrast to chronic fungal infections, the replication rates of streptococcal pneumonia are more rapid than those of *C neoformans*. Thus, successful results for *Cryptococci* infections cannot be generalized to fungal studies. Alpha particle ^{213}Bi is selected as the most appropriate radionuclide due to having

a shorter half-life than ^{188}Re and delivering a high dose in the short time of bacterial replication. Moreover, ^{188}Re-labeled D11 should be considered a theranostic compound in future studies.[31,32]

RIT approach was also extended to *Bacillus anthracis* infection as an agent for anthrax disease and a powerful pathogen for bioterrorism and biological war. In vitro administration of ^{213}Bi- or ^{188}Re-labeled mAbs to anthrax toxins provided a suitable therapeutic choice; subsequently, the prolonged survival of A/JCr mice infected with *B anthracis* radiolabeled with 213Bi was confirmed.[33]

Tuberculosis (TB) is an old infectious disease that affects mainly the lungs. It occurs as a coinfection in a majority of HIV patients. Drug resistance is observed in approximately 10% of these patients. Despite the high prevalence of this disease, common diagnostics methods, such as conventional chest radiography and CT, are nonspecific and strictly insufficient to give an absolute diagnosis due to the highly heterogeneous manifestation of TB.[34] So, researchers have decided to design a specific probe for the diagnosis of TB. There are unique challenges and considerations regarding probe design in TB disease, including target selection, suitable pharmacokinetic and pharmacodynamic properties for the radioprobe, the short half-life and high specific activity of the radioisotope, the appropriate biochemical properties of the probe, developing a high-affinity probe for high signal-to-noise ratio, and optimal clearance rate.[35] The different diagnostic radiopharmaceuticals for conventional imaging of disease activity and the monitoring and evaluation of therapeutic response to TB infection include fluorodeoxyglucose F 18 ^{18}F-FDG, ^{125}I-DPA-713, ^{99m}Tc-DMSA (dimercapto succinic acid), ^{99m}Tc-MIBI (methoxyisobutylisonitrile), ^{64}Cu-ATSM, ^{99m}Tc-tetrofosmin, and sestamibi.[36] Other novel pathogen-specific probes and new interpreting techniques need to be developed for clinical management. There is a need to speed up the expansion of new therapeutic drugs or provide comprehensive preclinical details for the proper dosing of new TB drugs that can be applied in clinical studies or trials.

Some studies have detected specific somatostatin (SST) receptors (SSTRs) expressed in all patients with TB. The visualization of these receptors via somatostatin analog scintigraphy will prove advantageous in assessing the extent of immune-mediated diseases and treatment responses.[37] The collection of modified lymphocytes and macrophages, as well as fibroblasts and granulocytes, constitutes granulomas that occur in infectious diseases, such as mycobacterial disorders. Mycobacteria are a type of microorganism that has several strains. The most common species causes TB (*Mycobacterium tuberculosis*). The use of ^{111}In-octreotide for the visualization, localization, and more precise staging of granuloma lesions with SSTRs has been confirmed.[38] SSTRs are overexpressed in human immune cells and tissues, including lung (subtypes SSTR-1, SSTR-2, and SSTR-4) and bronchial gland (subtypes sst3), and, based on these encouraging results, the utilization of theranostic somatostatin analogs appears promising in preclinical and clinical imaging and therapeutic nuclear medicine studies.

Viral Infection

HIV is a major threat to an individual's health as the CD4 glycoprotein that attaches to human helper T cells in the early phases of acquired immunodeficiency syndrome (AIDS). The current complicated and toxic treatment, highly active antiretroviral therapy (HAART), cannot stop viral replication in vivo. Thus, an extra modality in combination with HAART is required to cause the death of HIV-1–infected cells. In addition, the treatment must have a significant effect on the steady reservoir of infected cells and drug-resistant HIV varieties. It has been suggested that RIT may show significant efficiency in targeting HIV-1–infected host cells.[39,40] Radiolabeling mAb 246-D with [213]Bi and [188]Re was evaluated; subsequently, reduction in the intensity of HIV-1–infected cells was observed. The results for 2 types of radionuclides were similar.[41,42] The confirmation of the usefulness of RIT against HIV supplied a fundamental principle for the treatment theory of viral infected cells. This approach potentially could be extended to other chronic viral condition, such as hepatitis.[27]

Moreover, it has been reported that the covering of HIV protein binds with CD4, a conserved protein region that includes chemokine receptors CCR5 (R5) or CXCR4 (X4), and interacts with it as another receptor. These second receptors are called coreceptors and are known to be a necessity for the HIV-1 infection process. CXCR4 is the most well-known chemokine receptor and plays a significant role in targeted treatments of numerous malignant diseases.[43–45] As of the time of this writing, multiple studies have demonstrated the remarkable opportunity for discovering drugs that exclusively target the binding and/or signaling paths of CXCR4, including its modulators (orthosteric, allosteric, cyclic, dimerized, or bivalent groups), which have an important role in the progression of malignancies, tumor metastases, and HIV-1 infections.[46] Moreover, the successful clinical results have reported CXCR4 as a molecular target in

cancerous cells via the imaging probe ^{68}Ga-pentixafor or ^{177}Lu-pentixather through peptide receptor radionuclide therapy (PRRT).[47,48] These results point out the clinical potential of the theranostic role of ^{68}Ga/^{177}Lu pentixather-based CXCR4 targeting in patients with AIDS. The utilization of RIT in infectious diseases will become optimized with specifications of the best effective dose to decrease the toxic and long-term effects of the disease.

THERANOSTIC APPROACHES FOR CARDIOVASCULAR DISEASES

Cardiovascular diseases continue to be the foremost cause of mortality and morbidity worldwide and present as numerous correlated cardiovascular symptoms. These disorders include vascular inflammation, cardiac sarcoidosis, thrombosis, plaque angiogenesis, and microclassification. The identification of molecular targets along with the development of noninvasive diagnostic and therapeutic approaches can assist in reducing rates of mortality and morbidity and improving quality of life. The emergence of safe and noninvasive imaging methods can allow early visualization of the important fundamental pathophysiologic processes of cardiovascular deficiencies and risk stratification as well as the identification of plaques vulnerable to rupture and individuals at higher risk of cardiovascular incidents.[49] It has been shown that atherosclerotic plaques express various promising targets for imaging biological actions. The most important radiopharmaceuticals used to specify the biological appearances of inflammations, such as cardiac sarcoidosis, are ^{18}F-FDG, ^{68}Ga-DOTATATE, and ^{68}Ga-pentixafor.[50–54] The intravenous injection of radiolabeled somatostatin analogs is most efficient for detecting malignant tissues, especially neuroendocrine tumors.[55,56] Nevertheless, there is increasing evidence about the potential value of somatostatin analogs in nononcological diseases. Sarcoidosis is a chronic non-caseating granulomatous disease with unknown etiology that can present in multiple organs and tissues, such as the heart, eyes, skin, neuroendocrine system, and lungs. According to the severity of the disease and the involved organ system, different modalities can be used to manage the symptoms, from no treatment to systemic therapy with cytotoxic and biological drugs.[57,58] The granulation tissues that characterize this disease are composed mostly of macrophages and T lymphocytes that make them a target for radionuclide molecular imaging and therapy. Many different studies have confirmed the potential value of cardiac 18F-FDG PET imaging for detecting metabolically active cardiac sarcoid lesions that occur as a consequence of granulomatous inflammatory cells. Despite common and extensive use of FDG, this method does not show an appropriate degree of specificity so it is not the best possible tracer for identifying myocardial inflammation. An ongoing attempt to recognize new potential molecular targets for the identification of sarcoidosis-specific radiotracers for diagnosis and assessing treatment response found overexpression of the SSTR subtype 2 in activated macrophages in sarcoidosis disease. ^{111}In-penteotride, ^{68}Ga-DOTATOC, ^{68}Ga-DOTATATE, and ^{68}Ga-DOTANOC are radiopharmaceuticals used for targeting and binding to SSR-2. They showed appropriate biodistribution for cardiac imaging, especially in the baseline condition of those who had not shown cardiac uptake.[54,59–62] Somatostatin analogs (such as those in octreotide scintigraphy) can detect the overexpression of SSTR-2, SSTR-3, and SSTR-5 (Fig. 2). Preferably, similar molecular targets for imaging and therapy are selected for precise detection and the most efficient treatment. Thus, it is possible to use a theranostic approach for inflammation as well. [99m]Tc-/^{111}In octreotide is used for oncological imaging purposes. Also, the usage of ^{68}Ga-DOTATATE imaging as an SSTR-2–labeled PET tracer led to the absorbance of this radiotracer in M1-primed proinflammatory macrophages of atherosclerosis patients.[63] In a retrospective analysis, the applicability of ^{68}Ga-DOTATATE PET/CT for specifying the biological activity of atherosclerotic plaque through the expression of SSTR-2 was speculated. The investigators found a decrease in atherosclerotic plaque inflammation using a DOTATATE-based radiopharmaceutical, including the theranostics twin ^{68}Ga/^{177}Lu DOTATATE as the SSTR-2–targeted. In this regard, each whole-body 68Ga-DOTATATE PET/CT scan was achieved after injection of 73 MBq $\pm$ 13 MBq of ^{68}Ga-DOTATATE intravenously along with the average therapeutic injected dose of 7.5 GBq $\pm$ 0.3 GBq of ^{177}Lu-DOTATATE.[64] This new exciting result should be validated and may serve as an incentive for subsequent studies on potential theranostic implications in anti-atherosclerotic and anti-inflammatory SSTR-directed endoradiotherapies in large homogenous groups of high-risk cardiovascular patients. Additional trials with currently known and other specific inflammation-targeted radiotracers are recommended. The results will provide comprehensive insights into the process of disease development, drug efficacy assessment, patient response, and implementation of personalized medicine.

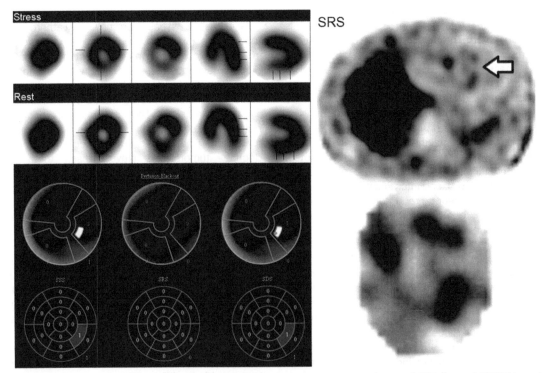

Fig. 2. Display of normal ^{99m}Tc-MIBI–SPECT in a 56-year-old patient versus abnormal SST-directed SPECT trough 99mTc-octreotide. Three lesions of atherosclerotic plaque using the expression of SSTR-2 is demonstrated. SSS; Summed Stress Score, SRS; Summed Rest Score, SDS; Summed Difference Score.

Fibroblast activation protein (FAP) is another promising tracer for clinical purposes. It is overexpressed in activated fibroblasts, allowing for the utilization of this agent as a target for radionuclide-based approaches in both diagnosis and treatment of malignant and nonmalignant diseases correlated with membrane-anchored enzymes.[65,66] Similar to the expression of activated fibroblasts in tumoral cells, this expression occurs in healing wounds and diseases associated with matrix remodelings, such as myocardial ischemia, lung and liver fibrosis, and chronic inflammation.[67] FAP imaging has been accompanied by labeling antibodies and an inhibitor particles with radionuclides. For diagnosis of atherosclerotic plaques, the boronic acid–based FAP inhibitor MIP-1232 has been applied in a preclinical study.[68] Also, noninvasive imaging using ^{68}Ga-FAPI-04 of activated fibroblasts in the injured myocardium in a rat model demonstrated that the FAP-positive myofibroblast is a promising radiotracer for in vivo imaging of post–myocardial infarction fibroblast activation. Thus, it may have considerable diagnostic and prognostic value in the management of patients who have suffered myocardial infarctions.[69] These emerging and novel targeted molecular imaging compounds may be exclusively labeled to drugs in a manner similar to therapeutic applications, wherein the physical half-life of the radioactive element must be modified to the retention time. Therefore, radionuclides with short half-lives, such as [188]Re ($T_{1/2}$ = 16.98 h), [153]Sm ($T_{1/2}$ = 46.3 h), [213]Bi ($T_{1/2}$ = 0.76 h), and [212]Pb ($T_{1/2}$ = 10.6 h), seem to be more suitable than those with longer half-lives.[68,70]

More recently, ^{68}Ga-pentixafor, with minimum risk of harm, was proved a valuable imaging probe for the detection of up-regulated CXCR4, which is detected in most malignancies. Also, ^{177}Lu-pentixather can be used as a theranostic twin for ^{68}Ga-pentaxifor in PRRT via CXCR4-targeting endoradiotherapy.[71] Primitive inflammatory cell collection and recruitment are organized by potential cytokine-directed and chemokine-directed therapeutic agents.[72] Clear overexpression of CXCR4 is indicated in the infarct region of patients in preliminary clinical studies. These sites demonstrated the highest uptake of gadolinium. The results of different studies, however, show discrepancies concerning the comparable up-regulation of CXCR4 in patient cohorts with inflammatory myocardial cells. Based on these results, a comprehensive throughput characterization of the target population is required; nevertheless, the findings indicate the possibility of the application of chemokine receptors as a therapeutic target.[73–76]

THERANOSTICS APPROACHES FOR RHEUMATIC DISEASE

Rheumatic disease (sometimes called musculoskeletal disease) is characterized by systemic inflammation and can involve bones, joints, tendons, ligaments, muscles, or even organs.[77] Also, sarcoidosis may present as a mimicker of different primary rheumatological diseases along with musculoskeletal complaints, and rarely it may be observed as a co-occurrence with them.[78,79] As far as using radiolabeled peptides is extended to malignancies, the increasing use of different somatostatin analogs that target SSTRs also has been considered in inflammatory diseases, especially rheumatoid arthritis. Various studies indicate the overexpression of SSTRs in immunologic and inflammatory cells as well as blood vessels for diagnostic and therapeutic purposes. Some studies have described the relationship of SSTR's expression in disorders, including the immune system.[38,80–82] Today, there are different synthetic compounds of pentetreotides (such as ^{68}Ga-DOTATATE, ^{64}Cu-DOTATATE, ^{68}Ga-DOTANOC, and ^{99m}Tc-hydrazinonicotinyl-Tyr3-octreotide (^{99m}Tc-EDDA/HYNIC-TOC)) that may be labeled with radionuclides for imaging purposes with a wider affinity for SSTR, in particular SSTR-2 and SSTR-5.[83] The in vivo and in vitro report by Vanhagen and colleagues[84] examined the expression of SSTRs for patients with rheumatoid arthritis for visualization of the synovial tissues. They confirmed the presence of these receptors in the synovial tissues of these patients due to activated lymphocytes and monocytes in synovial membranes.

As stated previously, the activated granuloma macrophages up-regulated SSTR-2 on the external cellular membrane, which could be targeted via, for example, receptor-directed PRRT for the detection and therapeutic advantages of patients with sarcoidosis centralized on the lung, mediastinum, hilar lymph nodes, and, newly, the heart.[85,86]

The first human case report study that showed well-tolerated therapeutic use of a single course of SST-directed PRRT in ongoing inflammatory disease is that of a 46-year-old woman with refractory sarcoidosis.[87] The pretherapeutic SSTR-PET/CT with ^{68}Ga-DOTATOC clearly showed a high accumulation of the tracer in the regions with numerous granuloma spots. Thus, clinicians decided to treat the patient with ^{177}Lu-DOTATOC. This method did not show any acute unfavorable effect on either the bone marrow or the kidneys. Moreover, another study described 2 patients with sarcoidosis, wherein 1 was treated with

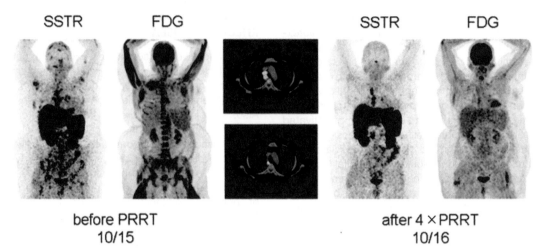

SSTR   FDG   SSTR   FDG

before PRRT   after 4 × PRRT
10/15   10/16

Fig. 3. Display of ^{18}F-FDG–PET/CT versus SSTR-directed PET/CT with ^{68}Ga-DOTATOC before and 1 year after initiation of PRRT with ^{177}Lu in the patient with treatment-refractory sarcoidosis. A total of 7.7 GBq in 4 treatment cycles have been administered. (*Adapted from* Lapa C, Kircher M, Hänscheid H, Schirbel A, Grigoleit GU, Klinker E, Böck M, Samnick S, Pelzer T, Buck AK. Peptide receptor radionuclide therapy as a new tool in treatment-refractory sarcoidosis - initial experience in two patients. Theranostics. 2018 Jan 1;8(3):644-649. https://doi.org/10.7150/thno.22161. PMID: 29344295; PMCID: PMC5771082.)

octreotide and showed good improvements in skin lesions and lymph node extent.[88]

Recently, a study observed the encouraging efficiency of a somatostatin analog in 2 patients with refractory multisystem involvement of sarcoidosis. The expression of SSTR in activated macrophages was proved by ^{18}F-FDG PET/CT and ^{68}Ga-DOTA-TOC–PET/CT. This approach was executed according to a guideline directing a total of 4 cycles of ^{177}Lu-DOTATATE. In the first patient, who suffered from skeletal involvement, SST-directed PET/CT and ^{18}F-FDG PET/CT showed high uptake of the tracer in the regions with active granulomas. Another case demonstrated high accumulation of ^{68}Ga-DOTATOC in lymphadenopathy spots, but minuscule pulmonary lesions and numerous osseous lesions showed no uptake at the SST expression sites; however, ^{18}F-FDG–PET/CT detected these lesions. None of the prescribed cycles of PRRT resulted in any acute harmful side effects or kidney malfunctions. The clinical and radiological responses were positive, and the continued well-being of the first patient, especially in the post-therapeutics evaluation via ^{18}F-FDG/^{68}Ga-DOTATATE PET/CT, was encouraging (**Fig. 3**). For the second patient, a reduction in serum activity factors was observed at the end of 4 sessions, but there was no considerable alleviation in pain. Additionally, the imaging methods demonstrated constant disease morphology with a slight decline in size.[89] This preliminary result verified that PRRT might be a valuable new approach for patients with treatment-resistant sarcoidosis. In this regard, according to the theranostic approach, pretherapeutic SSTRs targeting PET/CT can have potential value in the selection of patients for whom this method is appropriate. Lastly, there is an essential need for additional analysis of this new treatment choice in larger patient groups.

A preliminary study evaluated efficacy and safety of a long acting somatostatin analogue, octreotide, for refractory rheumatoid patients. The results showed significant clinical improvement for various symptoms, such as reducing pain and inflammation.[90,91] Thus, these studies showed the feasibility of using long acting somatostatin analogue in the treatment of patients with refractory rheumatoid arthritis. Additional large-scale research, however, is necessary.

FUTURE DIRECTIONS

To date, nuclear medicine has provided considerable clinical improvements in the diagnosis and treatment of malignancies. Additionally, major preclinical and clinical studies have shed light on emerging theranostics approaches for nononcological diseases. These recent accomplishments, however, require in-depth investigations, such as prospective, multicenter, randomized, and controlled studies to conduct specific dosimetric calculations and to monitor and assess side effects. Although some dosimetric data exist, it is crucial to ensure their reliability by quantifying the background activities in normal organs, absorbed target dose, chemical toxicity, in vivo stability of the probe, tracer biodistribution in patients, potential for pharmacologic action, physical toxicity, quality control, pharmacokinetics, and binding characteristics as well as the pharmacodynamics of new drugs through molecular imaging and the potential for the accumulation of radionuclides on repeated injection.[92] A commensurable and safe profile is a prerequisite for clinical utilization. Furthermore, serial imaging should be performed to indicate the progression of disease or treatment response and to assess whether the prescribed dose of the new treatment option should be modified or not. The protocols of the SPECT/PET imaging techniques should be defined exactly for newly developed radiotracers to identify and normalize the extent of the probe dose, absorbance period, and patient fasting time.[93] All of the studies should clarify the precise characterization of large-scale patient groups, dose range, number of treatment sessions, interval sessions, time clearances, and the effects of repeated administrations to assess which particular candidate theranostics twin is the most appropriate for nononcological applications. Resolving these challenges will require collaboration between physicians, technologists, medical physicists, and pharmacologic companies to overcome unprecedented problems and move forward toward clinical usage. Despite exciting progress in the preclinical phase, it is crucial to avoid any danger (eg, side effects) to patients, and the expenditure entailed by such modern systematic treatments should be curtailed, especially in patients with intractable infections or drug-resistant diseases.

SUMMARY

There is increasing evidence of the benefits of utilizing RIT and theranostics in nononcological disorders, including inflammation and infections. In accordance with the successful results of theranostics radiopharmaceuticals for oncological purposes and the positive results of RIT for infectious pathogens, more trials should be performed that include theranostics compounds in treating these diseases. The theranostic approach in nononcological disorders might augment the efficacy of treatments and personalize medicine as well. These findings should be replicated in large-scale multidisciplinary programs that focus on the validation and expansion of these techniques to exploit their treatment effectiveness while ensuring minimal side effects.

CLINICS CARE POINTS

The most important clinical care points are presented in the "future directions" section. These recent accomplishments, however, require in-depth investigations, such as prospective, multicenter, randomized, and controlled studies to conduct specific dosimetric calculations and to monitor and assess side effects. Although some dosimetric data exist, it is crucial to ensure their reliability by quantifying the background activities in normal organs, absorbed target dose, chemical toxicity, in vivo stability of the probe, tracer biodistribution in patients, potential for pharmacologic action, physical toxicity, quality control, pharmacokinetics, and binding characteristics as well as the pharmacodynamics of new drugs through molecular imaging and the potential for the accumulation of radionuclides on repeated injection.

DISCLOSURES

The authors have nothing to disclose.

REFERENCES

1. Seidlin S, Marinelli L, Oshry E. Radioactive iodine therapy: effect on functioning metastases of adenocarcinoma of the thyroid. J Am Med Assoc 1946; 132:838–47.
2. Stokkel MP, Junak DH, Lassmann M, et al. EANM procedure guidelines for therapy of benign thyroid disease. Eur J Nucl Med Mol Imaging 2010;37:2218–28.
3. Ballinger JR. Theranostic radiopharmaceuticals: established agents in current use. Br J Radiol. 2018 Nov;91(1091). 20170969. https://doi.org/10.1259/bjr.20170969. Epub 2018 Mar 12.
4. Yordanova A, Eppard E, Kurpig S, et al. Theranostics in nuclear medicine practice. Onco Targets Ther 2017;10:4821–8.
5. Dadachova E, Casadevall A. Antibodies as delivery vehicles for radioimmunotherapy of infectious diseases. Expert Opin Drug Deliv 2005;2:1075–84.
6. Maloney DG. Concepts in radiotherapy and immunotherapy: anti-CD20 mechanisms of action and targets. Semin Oncol 2005;32(1 Suppl 1):S19–26. Elsevier.
7. I Lin F, Iagaru A. Current concepts and future directions in radioimmunotherapy. Curr Drug Discov Technol 2010;7:253–62.
8. Becker W. The contribution of nuclear medicine to the patient with infection. Eur J Nucl Med 1995;22: 1195–211.
9. Dadachova E, Casadevall A. Treatment of infection with radiolabeled antibodies. Q J Nucl Med Mol Imaging 2006;50:193–204.

10. Poulain D, Deveaux M, Cailliez J-C, et al. Imaging of systemic Candida albicans infections with a radioiodinated monoclonal antibody: experimental study in the Guinea pig. Int J Rad Appl Instrum B 1991;18: 677–86.

11. Rubin RH, Young LS, Hansen WP, et al. Specific and nonspecific imaging of localized Fisher immunotype 1 Pseudomonas aeruginosa infection with radiolabeled monoclonal antibody. J Nucl Med 1988;29: 651–6.

12. Hazra D, Lahiri V, Saran S, et al. In vivo tuberculoma creation and its radioimmunoimaging. Nucl Med Commun 1987;8:139–42.

13. Malpani BL, Kadival GV, Samuel AM. Radioimmunoscintigraphic approach for the in vivo detection of tuberculomas—a preliminary study in a rabbit model. Int J Rad Appl Instrum B 1992;19:45–53.

14. Huang JT, Raiszadeh M, Sakimura I, et al. Detection of bacterial endocarditis with technetium-99m-labeled antistaphylococcal antibody. J Nucl Med 1980;21:783–6.

15. Goldenberg DM, Sharkey RM, Udem S, et al. Immunoscintigraphy of Pneumocystis carinii pneumonia in AIDS patients. J Nucl Med 1994;35:1028–34.

16. Dadachova E, Casadevall A. Radioimmunotherapy of infectious diseases. Semin Nucl Med 2009;39: 146–53. Elsevier.

17. Dadachova E, Nakouzi A, Bryan RA, et al. Ionizing radiation delivered by specific antibody is therapeutic against a fungal infection. Proc Natl Acad Sci U S A 2003;100:10942–7.

18. Larsen RA, Pappas PG, Perfect J, et al. Phase I evaluation of the safety and pharmacokinetics of murine-derived anticryptococcal antibody 18B7 in subjects with treated cryptococcal meningitis. Antimicrob Agents Chemother 2005;49:952–8.

19. Jiang Z, Bryan RA, Morgenstern A, et al. Treatment of early and established Cryptococcus neoformans infection with radiolabeled antibodies in immunocompetent mice. Antimicrob Agents Chemother 2012;56:552–4.

20. Bryan RA, Jiang Z, Howell RC, et al. Radioimmunotherapy is more effective than antifungal treatment in experimental cryptococcal infection. J Infect Dis 2010;202:633–7.

21. Bryan RA, Jiang Z, Morgenstern A, et al. Radioimmunotherapy of Cryptococcus neoformans spares bystander mammalian cells. Future Microbiol 2013; 8:1081–9.

22. Dadachova E, Bryan RA, Huang X, et al. Comparative evaluation of capsular polysaccharide-specific IgM and IgG antibodies and F (ab') 2 and Fab fragments as delivery vehicles for radioimmunotherapy of fungal infection. Clin Cancer Res 2007;13: 5629s–35s.

23. Dadachova E, Howell RW, Bryan RA, et al. Susceptibility of the human pathogenic fungi Cryptococcus neoformans and Histoplasma capsulatum to γ-radiation versus radioimmunotherapy with α-and β-emitting radioisotopes. J Nucl Med 2004;45:313–20.

24. Retallack DM, Woods JP. Molecular epidemiology, pathogenesis, and genetics of the dimorphic fungus Histoplasma capsulatum. Microbes Infect 1999;1:817–25.

25. Nosanchuk JD, Steenbergen JN, Shi L, et al. Antibodies to a cell surface histone-like protein protect against Histoplasma capsulatum. J Clin Invest 2003;112:1164–75.

26. Helal M, Dadachova E. Radioimmunotherapy as a novel approach in HIV, bacterial, and fungal infectious diseases. Cancer Biother Radiopharm 2018; 33:330–5.

27. Saylor C, Dadachova E, Casadevall A. Monoclonal antibody-based therapies for microbial diseases. Vaccine 2009;27:G38–46.

28. Pirofski L-A, Casadevall A. Use of licensed vaccines for active immunization of the immunocompromised host. Clin Microbiol Rev 1998;11:1–26.

29. Casadevall A, Scharff MD. Serum therapy revisited: animal models of infection and development of passive antibody therapy. Antimicrob Agents Chemother 1994;38:1695.

30. Dadachova E, Burns T, Bryan R, et al. Feasibility of radioimmunotherapy of experimental pneumococcal infection. Antimicrob Agents Chemother 2004;48:1624–9.

31. Argyrou M, Valassi A, Andreou M, et al. Rhenium-188 production in hospitals, by W-188/Re-188 generator, for easy use in radionuclide therapy. Int J Mol Imaging 2013;2013:290750.

32. Lepareur N, Lacœuille F, Bouvry C, et al. Rhenium-188 labeled radiopharmaceuticals: current clinical applications in oncology and promising perspectives. Front Med 2019;6:132.

33. Rivera J, Nakouzi AS, Morgenstern A, et al. Radiolabeled antibodies to Bacillus anthracis toxins are bactericidal and partially therapeutic in experimental murine anthrax. Antimicrob Agents Chemother 2009;53:4860–8.

34. Van Dyck P, Vanhoenacker F, Van den Brande P, et al. Imaging of pulmonary tuberculosis. Eur Radiol 2003;13:1771–85.

35. Johnson DH, Via LE, Kim P, et al. Nuclear imaging: a powerful novel approach for tuberculosis. Nucl Med Biol 2014;41:777–84.

36. Gupta V. The menace of tuberculosis and the role of nuclear medicine in tackling it. Now its time to tighten the loose strings. Hell J Nucl Med 2009;12:214–7.

37. Van Hagen P. Somatostatin receptor expression in clinical immunology. Metabolism 1996;45:86–7.

38. Vanhagen P, Krenning E, Reubi J, et al. Somatostatin analogue scintigraphy in granulomatous diseases. Eur J Nucl Med 1994;21:497–502.

39. Little SJ, Holte S, Routy J-P, et al. Antiretroviral-drug resistance among patients recently infected with HIV. N Engl J Med 2002;347:385–94.

40. Dadachova E. Radioimmunotherapy of infection with 213Bi-labeled antibodies. Curr Radiopharm 2008;1: 234–9.

41. Dadachova E, Patel MC, Toussi S, et al. Targeted killing of virally infected cells by radiolabeled antibodies to viral proteins. PLoS Med 2006;3:e427.

42. Ho DD, Moudgil T, Alam M. Quantitation of human immunodeficiency virus type 1 in the blood of infected persons. N Engl J Med 1989;321:1621–5.

43. De EC, Schols D. Inhibition of HIV infection by CXCR4 and CCR5 chemokine receptor antagonists. Antivir Chem Chemother 2001;12:19–31.

44. Deng H, Liu R, Ellmeier W, et al. Identification of a major co-receptor for primary isolates of HIV-1. Nature 1996;381:661.

45. Douek DC, Brenchley JM, Betts MR, et al. HIV preferentially infects HIV-specific CD4+ T cells. Nature 2002;417:95.

46. Choi W-T, Yang Y, Xu Y, et al. Targeting chemokine receptor CXCR4 for treatment of HIV-1 infection, tumor progression, and metastasis. Curr Top Med Chem 2014;14:1574–89.

47. Zaknun JJ, Bodei L, Mueller-Brand J, et al. The joint IAEA, EANM, and SNMMI practical guidance on peptide receptor radionuclide therapy (PRRNT) in neuroendocrine tumours. Eur J Nucl Med Mol Imaging 2013;40:800–16.

48. Brabander T, Nonnekens J, Hofland J. The next generation of peptide receptor radionuclide therapy. Endocr Relat Cancer 2019;26(8):C7–11.

49. Kastelein JJ, de Groot E. Ultrasound imaging techniques for the evaluation of cardiovascular therapies. Eur Heart J 2008;29:849–58.

50. Shimizu Y, Kuge Y. Recent advances in the development of PET/SPECT probes for atherosclerosis imaging. Nucl Med Mol Imaging 2016;50:284–91.

51. Langer HF, Haubner R, Pichler BJ, et al. Radionuclide imaging: a molecular key to the atherosclerotic plaque. J Am Coll Cardiol 2008;52:1–12.

52. Stacy MR. Radionuclide imaging of atherothrombotic diseases. Curr Cardiovasc Imaging Rep 2019;12:17.

53. Thackeray JT, Bengel FM. Translational molecular nuclear cardiology. Cardiol Clin 2016;34:187–98.

54. Gormsen LC, Haraldsen A, Kramer S, et al. A dual tracer 68 Ga-DOTANOC PET/CT and 18 F-FDG PET/CT pilot study for detection of cardiac sarcoidosis. EJNMMI Res 2016;6:52.

55. Hammad B, Evans NR, Rudd JH, et al. Molecular imaging of atherosclerosis with integrated PET imaging. J Nucl Cardiol 2017;24:938–43.

56. Dalm VA, Van Hagen PM, van Koetsveld PM, et al. Expression of somatostatin, cortistatin, and somatostatin receptors in human monocytes, macrophages, and dendritic cells. Am J Physiol Endocrinol Metab 2003;285:E344–53.

57. Piekarski E, Benali K, Rouzet F. Nuclear imaging in sarcoidosis. Semin Nucl Med 2018;48:246–60. Elsevier.

58. Baughman RP, Costabel U, du Bois RM. Treatment of sarcoidosis. Clin Chest Med 2008;29:533–48.

59. Bravo PE, Singh A, Di Carli MF, et al. Advanced cardiovascular imaging for the evaluation of cardiac sarcoidosis. J Nucl Cardiol 2019;26:188–99.

60. Lebtahi R, Crestani B, Belmatoug N, et al. Somatostatin receptor scintigraphy and gallium scintigraphy in patients with sarcoidosis. J Nucl Med 2001;42:21–6.

61. Nobashi T, Nakamoto Y, Kubo T, et al. The utility of PET/CT with 68 Ga-DOTATOC in sarcoidosis: comparison with 67 Ga-scintigraphy. Ann Nucl Med 2016;30:544–52.

62. Lapa C, Reiter T, Li X, et al. Imaging of myocardial inflammation with somatostatin receptor based PET/CT—a comparison to cardiac MRI. Int J Cardiol 2015;194:44–9.

63. Tarkin JM, Joshi FR, Evans NR, et al. Detection of atherosclerotic inflammation by 68Ga-DOTATATE PET compared to [18F] FDG PET imaging. J Am Coll Cardiol 2017;69:1774–91.

64. Schatka I, Wollenweber T, Haense C, et al. Peptide receptor–targeted radionuclide therapy alters inflammation in atherosclerotic plaques. J Am Coll Cardiol 2013;62:2344–5.

65. Garin-Chesa P, Old LJ, Rettig WJ. Cell surface glycoprotein of reactive stromal fibroblasts as a potential antibody target in human epithelial cancers. Proc Natl Acad Sci U S A 1990;87:7235–9.

66. de Haas HJ, van den Borne SW, Boersma HH, et al. Evolving role of molecular imaging for new understanding: targeting myofibroblasts to predict remodeling. Ann N Y Acad Sci 2012;1254:33–41.

67. Loktev A, Lindner T, Mier W, et al. A tumor-imaging method targeting cancer-associated fibroblasts. J Nucl Med 2018;59:1423–9.

68. Lindner T, Loktev A, Giesel F, et al. Targeting of activated fibroblasts for imaging and therapy. EJNMMI Radiopharm Chem 2019;4:16.

69. Varasteh Z, Mohanta S, Robu S, et al. Molecular imaging of fibroblast activity after myocardial infarction using a 68Ga-labeled fibroblast activation protein inhibitor, FAPI-04. J Nucl Med 2019;60:1743–9.

70. Lindner T, Loktev A, Altmann A, et al. Development of quinoline-based theranostic ligands for the targeting of fibroblast activation protein. J Nucl Med 2018; 59:1415–22.

71. Schottelius M, Osl T, Poschenrieder A, et al. [177Lu] pentixather: comprehensive preclinical characterization of a first CXCR4-directed endoradiotherapeutic agent. Theranostics 2017;7:2350.

72. Ridker PM. Anticytokine agents: targeting interleukin signaling pathways for the treatment of atherothrombosis. Circ Res 2019;124:437–50.

73. Thackeray JT. PET assessment of immune cell activity and therapeutic monitoring following myocardial infarction. Curr Cardiol Rep 2018;20:13.

74. Lapa C, Reiter T, Werner RA, et al. [68Ga] Pentixafor-PET/CT for imaging of chemokine receptor 4 expression after myocardial infarction. JACC Cardiovasc Imaging 2015;8:1466–8.

75. Thackeray JT, Derlin T, Haghikia A, et al. Molecular imaging of the chemokine receptor CXCR4 after acute myocardial infarction. JACC Cardiovasc Imaging 2015;8:1417–26.

76. Weiberg D, Thackeray JT, Daum G, et al. Clinical molecular imaging of chemokine receptor CXCR4 expression in atherosclerotic plaque using 68Ga-pentixafor PET: correlation with cardiovascular risk factors and calcified plaque burden. J Nucl Med 2018;59:266–72.

77. Firestein GS. Evolving concepts of rheumatoid arthritis. Nature 2003;423:356.

78. Kobak Ş, Sever F, Sivrikoz ON, et al. Sarcoidois: is it only a mimicker of primary rheumatic disease? A single center experience. Ther Adv Musculoskelet Dis 2014;6:3–7.

79. Kobak Ş, Karaarslan AA, Yilmaz H, et al. Co-occurrence of rheumatoid arthritis and sarcoidosis. Case Rep 2015;2015. bcr2014208803.

80. Sreedharan S, Kodama KT, Peterson KE, et al. Distinct subsets of somatostatin receptors on cultured human lymphocytes. J Biol Chem 1989;264:949–52.

81. Weinstock J. Production of neuropeptides by inflammatory cells within the granulomas of murine schistosomiasis mansoni. Eur J Clin Invest 1991;21:145–53.

82. Matucci-Cerinic M, Marabini S. Somatostatin treatment for pain in rheumatoid arthritis: a double blind versus placebo study in knee involvement. Med Sci Res 1998;16:233–4.

83. Anzola-Fuentes L, Chianelli M, Galli F, et al. Somatostatin receptor scintigraphy in patients with rheumatoid arthritis and secondary Sjögren's syndrome treated with Infliximab: a pilot study. EJNMMI Res 2016;6:1–9.

84. Vanhagen P, Markusse H, Lamberts S, et al. Somatostatin receptor imaging. The presence of somatostatin receptors in rheumatoid arthritis. Arthritis Rheum 1994;37:1521–7.

85. Armani C, Catalani E, Balbarini A, et al. Expression, pharmacology, and functional role of somatostatin receptor subtypes 1 and 2 in human macrophages. J Leukoc Biol 2007;81:845–55.

86. Kwekkeboom DJ, Krenning EP, Kho GS, et al. Somatostatin receptor imaging in patients with sarcoidosis. Eur J Nucl Med 1998;25:1284–92.

87. Lapa C, Grigoleit GU, Hänscheid H, et al. Peptide receptor radionuclide therapy for sarcoidosis. Am J Respir Crit Care Med 2016;194:1428–30.

88. Bokum T, Jong D, Lamberts J, et al. Immunohistochemical localization of somatostatin receptor sst2A in sarcoid granulomas. Eur J Clin Invest 1999;29:630–6.

89. Lapa C, Kircher M, Hänscheid H, et al. Peptide receptor radionuclide therapy as a new tool in treatment-refractory sarcoidosis-initial experience in two patients. Theranostics 2018;8:644.

90. Koseoglu F, Koseoglu T. Long acting somatostatin analogue for the treatment of refractory RA. Ann Rheum Dis 2002;61:573.

91. Paran D, Elkayam O, Mayo A, et al. A pilot study of a long acting somatostatin analogue for the treatment of refractory rheumatoid arthritis. Ann Rheum Dis 2001;60:888–91.

92. Choudhury RP, Fisher EA. Molecular imaging in atherosclerosis, thrombosis, and vascular inflammation. Arterioscler Thromb Vasc Biol 2009;29:983–91.

93. Ohno Y, Takenaka D, Kanda T, et al. Adaptive iterative dose reduction using 3D processing for reduced-and low-dose pulmonary CT: comparison with standard-dose CT for image noise reduction and radiological findings. Am J Roentgenol 2012;199:W477–85.

Theranostic Agents in Musculoskeletal Disorders

Sanaz Katal, MD, MPH[a], Antonio Maldonado, MD[b], Javier Carrascoso, MD[c],
Majid Assadi, MD, FASNC[d], Ali Gholamrezanezhad, MD, FEBNM, DABR[e,*]

KEYWORDS

- Theranostics ● Rheumatoid arthritis ● Osteoarthrosis ● Multiple myeloma ● Sarcoma
- Glucocorticoid-loaded liposomes ● Macrophage imaging ● Radiolabeled anti-CD38 antibodies

KEY POINTS

- Theranostic approaches combine a single agent's therapeutic and diagnostic characteristics to achieve a targeted molecular therapy, with little or no toxicity to normal tissues.
- Selective theranostic agents have shown potential for targeted imaging and therapy in a variety of musculoskeletal illnesses.
- Some of these strategies include macrophage-related tools in inflammatory arthritis, chemokine receptor agents in multiple myeloma, and endothelial antibodies (TEM-1) in sarcoma.

RHEUMATOID ARTHRITIS

Rheumatoid arthritis (RA) is a chronic autoimmune joint and soft tissue disease that affects approximately 0.5% to 1% of the world population.[1] It is a systemic inflammatory disease defined by polyarticular synovitis, causing irreversible joint damage and deformity, if not treated. Early diagnosis and treatment of RA remain a major clinical challenge. No definite curative treatments are available to date and the currently available drugs for RA only delay the disease progression. Symptomatic therapy and inflammation reduction with glucocorticoids (GCs), methotrexate (MTX), nonsteroidal anti-inflammatory drugs, azathioprine, tumor necrosis factor-α blockers, and minocycline is applied for symptomatic control of the disease.

The available medications used in the management of RA cause various short- and long-term side effects. Thus, there is a great need for biocompatible novel therapies with high targeted efficiency and minimal unwanted toxicity. Selective theranostic agents have shown potential for targeted imaging and therapy for inflamed joints, with the least collateral toxicity to the healthy tissues.[2,3]

Glucocorticoid-Loaded Liposomes in Rheumatoid Arthritis

As a well-documented anti-inflammatory drug, GCs are being used widely in the management of RA. However, they pose many side effects. To reduce the systemic toxicity of GCs and to enhance the RA treatment, encapsulation of GCs into long-circulating liposomes (LCLs) has been proposed. LCLs preferentially accumulate in the inflamed tissue, allowing selective targeting to diseased versus healthy tissue.

In-depth knowledge of the in vivo behavior of LCLs with molecular imaging may offer a great chance to monitor the drug biodistribution within the host body. Besides, it will also allow clinicians to select the best candidates for such therapies. This might be of great importance, because the kinetic properties of LCLs vary widely among different patients and also between different

[a] Department of Nuclear Medicine, Kowsar Hospital, Shiraz, Iran; [b] Department of Nuclear Medicine, Quironsalud Madrid University Hospital, 28223 Pozuelo de Alarcón, Madrid, Spain; [c] Department of Radiology, Quironsalud Madrid University Hospital, 28223 Pozuelo de Alarcón, Madrid, Spain; [d] Department of Molecular Imaging and Radionuclide Therapy (MIRT), The Persian Gulf Nuclear Medicine Research Center, Bushehr University of Medical Sciences, Bushehr, Iran; [e] Department of Diagnostic Radiology, Keck School of Medicine, University of Southern California (USC), Los Angeles, CA, USA
* Corresponding author.
E-mail addresses: A.gholamrezanezhad@yahoo.com; ali.gholamrezanezhad@med.usc.edu

PET Clin 16 (2021) 441–448
https://doi.org/10.1016/j.cpet.2021.03.008
1556-8598/21/© 2021 Elsevier Inc. All rights reserved.

lesions.[4,5] In this regard, molecular imaging with PET offers a great potential value to track and quantify the level of drug uptake over time and predicts the drug efficacy.

In a nonhuman study by Gawne and colleagues,[6] a preformed GC-loaded LCL nanomedicine (PEGylated liposomal methylprednisolone hemisuccinate [NSSL-MPS]) was radiolabeled using [^{89}Zr] Zr-oxinate$_4$ (^{89}Zr-oxine). PET imaging was obtained to image the labeled cells within the host body. ^{89}Zr-NSSL-MPS PET/computed tomography (CT) imaging demonstrated high tracer accumulation in the inflamed joints compared with the control joints. More importantly, the uptake level was clearly correlated with the degree of inflammation. Besides, mice receiving a therapeutic dose of the drug had a reduction in inflammation on follow-up PET/CT imaging. Indeed, a clear anti-inflammatory effect was observed from a single dose of NSSL-MPS. Consequently, they suggested that PET could track the GC-LCLs in the inflamed joints, thus providing insight into the mechanism of action and the potency of these agents. Furthermore, they suggested this liposome labeling technique followed by PET tracking could offer valuable chance in the preclinical development of anti-inflammatory liposomal theranostic agents in patients with various inflammatory diseases, including RA.

Macrophage Imaging in Rheumatoid Arthritis

The complex pathophysiology of RA involves the infiltration of various immune cells, along with the release of destructive immune cytokines and mediators into the synovium of the inflamed joints. As the primary promotors of RA, synovial macrophage infiltration is a characteristic hallmark of RA. This subset of inflammatory cells contributes to the disease activity in the acute and chronic stages of the disease. Besides, these biologic markers are a sensitive indicator to monitor the therapy response in RA.[7] Therefore, activated macrophages could serve as ideal targets for imaging and guiding therapy in this entity. To this end, folate-directed tracers have been examined, because folate receptors-typeβ (FRβ) are expressed selectively and abundantly on activated macrophages. Thus, radiotracer toward FRβs is able to map the macrophage activity in an ongoing active arthritic joint.

The first folate-based macrophage imaging was performed using [^{99m}Tc] Tc-folic acid (FolateScan with technetium-99m EC$_{20}$ [^{99m}Tc-EC20]) in rats with adjuvant-induced arthritis.[8,9] They found that ^{99m}Tc-EC20 was able to assess the disease activity in patients with RA and osteoarthrosis

(OA). They also demonstrated that FolateScan was a useful tool to predict clinical disease activity, more sensitive than physical examinations. Piscaer and colleagues[10] found similar results for folate-receptor imaging in osteoarthritis. They suggested that macrophage activation in OA could be monitored using dedicated folate-tracer single-photon emission CT (SPECT)/CT for targeting folate receptors, which are expressed on the activated but not resting macrophages.

Further studies found macrophage-targeted PET imaging to be a more useful tool compared with SPECT, as expected.[11] It would be able to detect active arthritis, quantify disease activity, and also monitor the therapy response with high accuracy. In this regard, various macrophage-specific folate-based PET tracers, such as [^{18}F]-fluorophenylfolate, [^{68}Ga]-DOTA-folate, [^{18}F]-fluoro-PEG-folate, and [^{18}F]-folate-PEG-NOTA-Al have been examined to detect folate receptor-expressing macrophages.[12]

Gent and colleagues[13] used [^{18}F]-fluoro-PEG-folate to target folate-receptors in a rat model with RA. [^{18}F]-fluoro-PEG-folate uptake was higher in arthritic knees compared with the control knees. Besides, the target to blood ratio was higher than those seen with the previous macrophage tracers, such as (R)-[^{11}C]PK11195.

In another study, [^{18}F]-fluoro-PEG-folate PET examination was used as a therapeutic monitoring tool of MTX therapy.[14] Subsequent PET studies were performed before and after MTX therapy. Significantly lower standard uptake values were seen in the inflamed knees after MTX therapy (approximating the levels in normal control subjects). Similar results were observed for the detection and monitoring of "systemic" inflammation in RA, reflected as reduced uptake in the liver and spleen after treatment.[15] PEG-folate has currently been tested in the clinical phase setting, to visualize arthritic joints in RA.[16] More recently, novel improved folate-PET agents have been introduced, such as ^{18}F-Folate-NOTA-Al with a faster labeling procedure. However, further evaluation is warranted regarding their usefulness.[17]

In addition to folate tracers, various other macrophage-specific PET tracers have also been proposed to visualize active arthritis, including [^{11}C]-PK11195. It is targeted against the translocator protein (TSPO) on activated macrophages, and was investigated in many preclinical models.[18,19] A clinical study has also displayed increased [^{11}C]-PK11195 uptake in the severely inflamed joints of RA.[20] However, [^{11}C]-PK11195 PET imaging suffers from limitations in detecting subclinical RA synovitis, specifically because of the high background uptake in the periarticular soft tissues.

Consequently, second-generation TSPO tracers were developed using $[^{11}C]$-DPA7$_{13}$ and $[^{18}F]$-DPA$_7$ with improved imaging characteristics. Clinical studies are still needed to confirm their application.

Apart from their efficacy for imaging purposes, folate receptors serve as excellent targets for drug delivery (folate antagonist and folate-conjugated drugs) to the pathologic macrophages. Folate receptors can bind and internalize antiarthritic therapeutics into the diseased cells.[21,22] Several therapeutic strategies for FRβ targeting have been suggested, including folate antagonists, folate-conjugated immunotoxins, folate-conjugated drugs, and folate-conjugated nanoparticles.[23] Therefore, the application of folate-target nanoparticles as drug delivery systems in RA is an interesting subject for future clinical research for antiarthritis therapy.

Overall, folate-linked imaging and therapeutic agents hold a promising role for early diagnosis, targeted therapies, and therapy response monitoring in RA, with little or no off-target toxicity to normal tissues.

OSTEOARTHROSIS

As a leading cause of disability, OA is a disabling, painful, multifactorial disease resulting from a combination of repetitive mechanical stress, aging, and trauma. OA lesions usually cause irreversible bone and cartilage damage. Currently, OA is not diagnosed until the intermediate to late stages, when it becomes symptomatic. Besides, no proven specific therapy exists for OA, and the current therapeutic (mainly symptomatic) strategies for chronic OA pain are also inadequate. Effective methods are needed for early diagnosing OA and monitoring its progression during early stages.[24] Theranostic nanoparticles have a great potential to noninvasively detect, track, and treat OA in its early stages.

Macrophage-linked imaging tools is one of these techniques. It may play a promising role in OA management. A small animal role model has studied the feasibility of macrophage imaging techniques (through FRβ) in experimental OA. They found that macrophage activation in OA is clearly imaged using folate receptors. They also suggested that this method allows monitoring of the disease progression over time, in which late-stage disease displayed less macrophage activation than early stages. Moreover, this tool might offer the potential to investigate the effect of specific folate antagonists, such as BCG-495 in OA, similar to RA.[25–28] However, it should be noted that the small number of activated macrophages present in OA joints makes the application of such methods more challenging (compared with RA, which is an inflammatory immune-related disease). Thus, further studies in this regard are still needed.

MULTIPLE MYELOMA
Chemokine Receptor Agents in Multiple Myeloma

Multiple myeloma (MM), a malignant plasma cell disorder, is the second most frequent hematologic malignancy, accounting for around 1% of all cancers. Despite recent therapy advances, such as immuno-modulatory drugs, proteasome inhibitors, and stem cell transplantation, MM essentially remains incurable with relapse rates greater than 90%.[29] Hence, novel therapeutic strategies enabling effective killing of myeloma cells are highly encouraged. Currently, developing targeted selective therapies using nanoparticle drug delivery systems is under investigation in various preclinical studies.

Recently, the role of chemokine receptor 4 (CXCR4) and its ligand (CXCL12) has been widely debated in several publications. CXCR4-activation plays a key role in numerous pathologic conditions. Overexpression of these receptors has been described in more than 30 different types of cancers,[30] including MM bone disease. Besides, the chemotactic CXCR4/CXCL12 interactions serve as a strong stimulator for tumor growth, angiogenesis, invasiveness, tumor progression, and distant metastasis to organs with high CXCL12-expressing stromal tissues.

Most recently, a radiolabeled CXCR4 ligand (^{68}Ga-pentixafor) has been developed for PET imaging.[31] [^{68}Ga]-pentixafor-PET represents a promising method for the in vivo assessment of the CXCR4 expression status in patients with cancer.

Studies have found that ^{68}Ga-CPCR4-2 (^{68}Ga-pentixafor) is a suitable PET tracer for targeting imaging of human CXCR4 receptor expression in vivo. ^{68}Ga-pentixafor PET imaging provides high-contrast sensitive tumor imaging, given its high uptake in tumors and rapid renal clearance.[32–34] These findings suggest promising clinical potential for ^{68}Ga-pentixafor/^{177}Lu or ^{90}Y-pentixather for CXCR4-directed theranostic approaches in MM and other diseases.

Currently, several potent CXCR4 antagonists are being investigated in several clinical trials for CXCR4-directed antitumor therapy.[35–37]

Other Agents in Multiple Myeloma

Radiolabeled anti-CD38 antibodies
Cluster of differentiation38 (CD38) is a cell surface proteoglycan involved in the MM cell signaling.

This antigen is currently considered as a standard biomarker of MM cell identification. Anti-CD38 immuno-PET serves as a potential tool for MM imaging, especially in lesions with low metabolic activity.

In this regard, preclinical studies[38,39] found that ^{64}Cu- and ^{89}Zr-labeled anti-CD38 antibodies (^{64}Cu-TE2A-9E7.4 and ^{89}Zr-DFO-9E7.4) could detect subcutaneous MM tumors and bone marrow lesions with high sensitivity, outperforming ^{18}F-fluorodeoxyglucose PET imaging.

In addition, anti-CD38 monoclonal antibodies have been clinically approved for the treatment of refractory/relapsing MM. Therefore, in a theranostic concept, radiolabeled anti-CD38 antibodies (eg, ^{89}Zr-DFO-daratumumab) could be applied for therapeutic planning targeting CD138. These emerging methods in PET may improve patient selection for further radioimmunotherapy.

^{89}Zr-TiO$_2$-Tf

Most recently, a novel theranostic nanoparticle (^{89}Zr-TiO$_2$-Tf) has been proposed for imaging and treating MM. This agent consists of reactive oxygen–generating titanium dioxide (TiO$_2$) nanoparticles, coated with a tumor-targeting agent, transferrin (Tf), and radiolabeled with a radionuclide (^{89}Zr).[40] PET/CT imaging revealed that a single dose of ^{89}Zr-TiO$_2$-Tf completely suppressed tumor growth in a mice model with disseminated MM, and doubled the survival. However, data in this field are still lacking.

SARCOMA
TEM-1-Targeted Agents in Sarcoma

The role of fluorodeoxyglucose PET/CT in sarcoma of musculoskeletal origin has already been widely debated.[41–43] Recently, the application of other imaging agents has been proposed, such as anti–tumor endothelial marker (TEM) antibodies.

TEM-1, also known as endosialin (or CD248), is a transmembrane glycoprotein, which is expressed on mesenchymal stromal fibroblasts and pericytes during tissue development, tumor neoangiogenesis, and progression. In most tumors, TEM-1 overexpression is observed in perivascular pericytes and stromal fibroblasts. Besides, it is associated with higher tumor aggressiveness and poorer prognosis.

TEM-1 is an attractive theranostic target, because of its high specificity, which provides a high target to background ratio and little toxicity to nontumoral tissues. Therefore, targeted TEM-1-therapy with antiendosialin immunotoxins is a promising theranostic approach for TEM-1-expressing tumors, especially soft tissue sarcoma (because of high antigen expression in both the tumor vasculature and tumor cells in sarcoma).[44,45] This is clinically important for patient management in sarcoma, because these aggressive tumors often present in the late unrespectable stages. Only a few patients might benefit from curative resection, and the current treatment of these patients is primarily based on palliative therapy approaches. Thus, novel theranostic strategies with nanoparticles will be greatly useful in this group.

Several anti-TEM-1 antibodies have been introduced for oncologic applications, such as the MORAb-004 antibody.[46] Radioiodinated MORAb-004 antibody (^{124}I-MORAb-004) has been found to display high contrast and sensitivity for the detection of the extracellular epitope of human TEM-1 (hTEM1) in preclinical studies.[47] This antibody is currently being tested in phase II clinical trial studies.

Other studies have investigated human TEM-1-antibody fragment (single-chain variable fragment [scFv]-Fc fusion protein [78Fc]) in human sarcoma cells.[48] They observed a specific in vivo targeting of labeled anti-TEM1 78FC to sarcoma xenografts. More importantly, anti-TEM1 78Fc with saporin (78Fc-Sap) was effective in killing in vitro TEM1-expressing sarcoma cells without apparent toxicity in vivo.

In a few other studies, the preclinical efficacy of a novel TEM-antibody drug conjugate (ENDOS/ADCs) has been tested.[49] ENDOS/ADC demonstrated a target-specific strong cytotoxic activity in a model of human osteosarcoma.

Recently, a fully human scFv-Fc-fusion (1C1m-Fc), conjugated to DOTA and labeled with ^{177}Lu, was also applied.[50] The study suggested that [^{177}Lu] Lu-1C1m-Fc is a potentially useful tool for diagnostic (SPECT) and therapeutic applications in sarcoma or other solid tumors.

In another study by Cicone and colleagues,[51] the scFv78-Fc was conjugated with the chelator p-SCN-Bn-CHX-A″-DTPA, followed by labeling with indium-111. They found specific binding of [^{111}In] CHX-DTPA-scFv78-Fc to endosialin/TEM1 antigen in vitro in sarcoma and neuroblastoma cells. Furthermore, the radiation dosimetry to humans was estimated to be in the range of other monoclonal antibodies radiolabeled with indium-111.

Taken together, TEM-1/endosialin is an emerging attractive theranostic target for the detection and therapy in patients with sarcoma.

Other Agents in Sarcoma

Osteosarcoma
Over the last few decades, radioimmunotherapy with rhenium-labeled small molecules (antibodies,

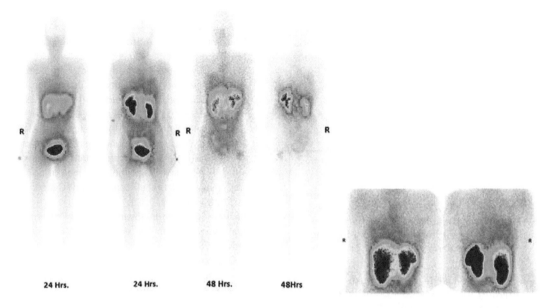

24 Hrs.   24 Hrs.   48 Hrs.   48Hrs

Fig. 1. A 20-year-old woman with refractory metastatic Ewing sarcoma presented with extreme severe pain. Some literature references suggest that somatostatin receptors (SSTRs) are present in about 80% of the soft tissue tumors, and reveal positive uptake in molecular imaging using PET and SPECT.[60–63] Accordingly, the patient underwent three cycles of therapy with Lutathera (lutetium-dotatate therapy), a radiolabeled somatostatin analogue that has been established to be an effective safe treatment of SSTR–positive neuroendocrine tumors.[60–63] Fig. 1 shows post-therapy ^{177}Lu-Dotatate whole-body studies (first row, 24 and 48 hours after the first course; second row, 24 and 48 hours after the third course). The study shows mild tracer uptake in the right hemithorax and left upper femur. Excellent tolerance was seen, as it has been previously reported. More importantly, the patient had a significant clinical improvement, better quality of life, and performance status.

peptides, particulates) has been investigated in a few studies.[52] Rhenium is a potent beta-emitter radioisotope that has been widely applied in therapeutic nuclear medicine, particularly for bone palliation in patients with widespread bone metastases (using either 188-rhenium [^{188}Re] or 186-rhenium [^{186}Re]).

In osteosarcoma, the overexpression of insulin-like growth factor-2 receptors (IGF2R) has been previously reported.[53] Thus, IGF$_2$ serves as a novel diagnostic/therapeutic target in this disorder. ^{188}Re-labeled IGF$_2$R-specific murine monoclonal antibody/MEM-238 (^{188}Re-MEM-238) has shown some promising results in this era.[54] ^{188}Re has also been used for labeling vascular endothelial growth inhibitor (VEGI) as a theranostic agent for radioimaging and radioimmunotherapy in fibrosarcoma xenografts (Re-NGR-VEGI), which has shown excellent tumor inhibition effect.[55]

As another potential theranostic target for metastatic osteosarcoma, integrin αvβ3-receptors have been investigated, which are labeled using ^{68}Ga/^{177}Lu pair radioisotopes (^{68}Ga-NODAGA-RGD$_2$ and ^{177}Lu-NODAGA-RGD$_2$).[56] The tripeptide Arg-Gly-Asp amino acid sequences (RGD) have been added to the radiotracer formulation, given their high affinity for αvβ3 integrins.

Synovial sarcoma

Frizzled homolog10 (FZD10) is a transmembrane receptor that is overexpressed in the synovial sarcoma cells. DTPA-^{90}Y-radiolabeled-OTSA101 (^{90}Y-OTSA101) associated with ^{111}In-OTSA101 SPECT/CT is a radiolabeled monoclonal antibody, targeting synovial sarcoma cells in a theranostic approach. In a study by Sarrut and colleagues,[57] patients with synovial sarcoma who had significant ^{111}In-OTSA101 tumor uptake and favorable biodistribution were treated with ^{90}Y-OTSA101. They found that a single intravenous injection of ^{90}Y-OTSA101 had remarkable antitumor activity, with minimal collateral toxicity.[57]

Moreover, a recent preclinical nonhuman model study revealed that radioimmunotherapy with an alfa-particle emitting anti-FZD$_{10}$-antibody agent (eg, astatine-211; ^{211}At-OTSA101) suppresses the tumoral growth more efficiently than those conjugated with the beta-emitter yttrium-90 tracers (^{90}Y-OTSA101), even though the absorbed doses were comparable.[58]

Pediatric sarcoma

18-(p-iodophenyl) octadecyl phosphocholine (CLR1404) is a novel antitumor compound that largely targets cancer cells. A preclinical study on xenograft models has shown that radioiodinated-CLR1404 (^{124}I-CLR1404 and ^{131}I-CLR1404) can be applied as a potential tumor-targeting theranostic agent for pediatric solid tumors, such as neuroblastoma, rhabdomyosarcoma, and Ewing sarcoma (**Fig. 1**).[59]

CLINICS CARE POINTS

- Liposome labeling techniques followed by PET tracking (using radiolabeled glucocorticoid-loaded liposomes, such as ^{89}Zr-NSSL-MPS) offer a valuable chance in the preclinical development of theranostic anti-inflammatory agents in various inflammatory diseases, including RA.

- Macrophage-specific tracers (such as those targeting folate receptors on activated macrophages) hold a promising role for early diagnosis, targeted therapies, and therapy response monitoring in inflammatory arthritis (RA and OA).

- Novel chemokine receptor antagonists (such as ^{68}Ga-pentixafor/^{177}Lu or ^{90}Y-pentixather as a CXCR4-directed agent) are being investigated in several clinical trials for theranostic approaches in multiple myeloma.

- Theranostic strategies using radiolabeled antibodies and nanoparticles have also been proposed for imaging and treating multiple myeloma.

- TEM-1/endosialin is an emerging attractive theranostic target for the detection and therapy in patients with sarcoma.

- Although the evolving field of theranostic medicine promises a novel approach to various disorders, further studies are warranted before drawing definite conclusions in this regard.

DISCLOSURES

The authors have nothing to disclose.

REFERENCES

1. Cross M, Smith E, Hoy D, et al. The global burden of rheumatoid arthritis: estimates from the global burden of disease 2010 study. Ann Rheum Dis 2014;73:1316–22.
2. Katal S, Gholamrezanezhad A, Nikpanah M, et al. Potential applications of PET/CT/MR imaging in inflammatory diseases. Part I: musculoskeletal and gastrointestinal systems. PET Clin 2020;15(4):547–58.
3. Gholamrezanezhad A, Basques K, Batouli A, et al. Non-oncologic Applications of PET/CT and PET/MR in Musculoskeletal, Orthopedic, and Rheumatologic Imaging: General Considerations, Techniques, and Radiopharmaceuticals. J Nucl Med Technol 2017. https://doi.org/10.2967/jnmt.117.198663.
4. Lee H, Shields AF, Siegel BA, et al. 64Cu-MM-302 Positron emission tomography quantifies variability of enhanced permeability and retention of nanoparticles in relation to treatment response in patients with metastatic breast cancer. Clin Cancer Res 2017;23:4190–202.
5. Lammers T, Rizzo LY, Storm G, et al. Personalised nanomedicine. Clin Cancer Res 2012;18:4889–94.
6. Gawne PJ, Clarke F, Turjeman K, et al. PET imaging of liposomal glucocorticoids using 89Zr-oxine: theranostic applications in inflammatory arthritis. Theranostics 2020;10(9):3867.
7. Haringman JJ, Gerlag DM, Zwinderman AH, et al. Synovial tissue macrophages: a sensitive biomarker for response to treatment in patients with rheumatoid arthritis. Ann Rheum Dis 2005;64:834–8.
8. Matteson EL, Lowe VJ, Prendergast FG, et al. Assessment of disease activity in rheumatoid arthritis using a novel folate targeted radiopharmaceutical Folatescan™. Clin Exp Rheumatol 2009;27(2):253.
9. Henne WA, Rothenbuhler R, Ayala-Lopez W, et al. Imaging sites of infection using a 99mTc-labeled folate conjugate targeted to folate receptor positive macrophages. Mol Pharm 2012;9:1435–40.
10. Piscaer TM, Müller C, Mindt TL, et al. Imaging of activated macrophages in experimental osteoarthritis using folate-targeted animal single-photon-emission computed tomography/computed tomography. Arthritis Rheum 2011;63:1898–907.
11. Gholamrezanejhad A, Mirpour S, Mariani G. Future of nuclear medicine: SPECT versus PET. J Nucl Med 2009;50(7):16N–8N.
12. Chandrupatla DM, Molthoff CF, Lammertsma AA, et al. The folate receptor β as a macrophage-mediated imaging and therapeutic target in rheumatoid arthritis. Drug Deliv Transl Res 2019;15(1):366–78.
13. Gent YY, Weijers K, Molthoff CF, et al. Evaluation of the novel folate receptor ligand [18 F] fluoro-PEG-folate for macrophage targeting in a rat model of arthritis. Arthritis Res Ther 2013;15(2):1.
14. Chandrupatla DM, Jansen G, Vos R, et al. In-vivo monitoring of anti-folate therapy in arthritic rats using [18 F] fluoro-PEG-folate and positron emission tomography. Arthritis Res Ther 2017;19(1):1–9.
15. Chandrupatla DM, Jansen G, Mantel E, et al. Imaging and methotrexate response monitoring of systemic inflammation in arthritic rats employing the macrophage PET tracer [18F] fluoro-PEG-folate. Contrast Media Mol Imaging 2018;2018:8092781.

16. Verweij N, Bruijnen S, Gent Y, et al. Rheumatoid arthritis imaging on PET-CT using a novel folate receptor ligand for macrophage targeting. Arthritis Rheumatol 2017;69.

17. Chen Q, Meng X, McQuade P, et al. Synthesis and preclinical evaluation of folate-NOTA-Al18F for PET imaging of folate-receptor-positive tumors. Mol Pharm 2016;13(5):1520–7.

18. Kropholler MA, Boellaard R, Elzinga EH, et al. Quantification of (R)- [11C]PK11195 binding in rheumatoid arthritis. Eur J Nucl Med Mol Imaging 2009;36: 624–31.

19. Narayan N, Owen DR, Taylor PC. Advances in positron emission tomography for the imaging of rheumatoid arthritis. Rheumatology 2017;56(11): 1837–46.

20. van der Laken CJ, Elzinga EH, Kropholler MA, et al. Noninvasive imaging of macrophages in rheumatoid synovitis using 11C-(R)-PK11195 and positron emission tomography. Arthritis Rheum 2008;58:3350–5.

21. Nogueira E, Gomes AC, Preto A, et al. Folate-targeted nanoparticles for rheumatoid arthritis therapy. Nanomedicine 2016;12(4):1113–26.

22. Lu Y, Stinnette TW, Westrick E, et al. Treatment of experimental adjuvant arthritis with a novel folate receptor-targeted folic acid-aminopterin conjugate. Arthritis Res Ther 2011;13(2):1–8.

23. Poh S, Chelvam V, Ayala-López W, et al. Selective liposome targeting of folate receptor positive immune cells in inflammatory diseases. Nanomedicine 2018;14:1033–43.

24. Gholamrezanezhad A, Basques K, Batouli A, et al. Clinical nononcologic applications of PET/CT and PET/MRI in musculoskeletal, orthopedic, and rheumatologic imaging. AJR Am J Roentgenol 2018; 210(6):W245–63.

25. Van der Heijden JW, Oerlemans R, Dijkmans BA, et al. Folate receptor β as a potential delivery route for novel folate antagonists to macrophages in the synovial tissue of rheumatoid arthritis patients. Arthritis Rheum 2009;60:12–21.

26. Xia W, Hilgenbrink AR, Matteson EL, et al. A functional folate receptor is induced during macrophage activation and can be used to target drugs to activated macrophages. Blood 2009;113:438–46.

27. Rajkumar SV. Multiple myeloma: 2016 update on diagnosis, risk-stratification, and management. Am J Hematol 2016;91(7):719–34.

28. Batouli A, Gholamrezanezhad A, Petrov D, et al. Management of primary osseous spinal tumors with PET. PET Clin 2019;14(1):91–101.

29. Behzadi AH, Raza SI, Carrino JA, et al. Applications of PET/CT and PET/MR imaging in primary bone malignancies. PET Clin 2018;13(4):623–34.

30. Lapa C, Lückerath K, Rudelius M, et al. [68Ga] Pentixafor-PET/CT for imaging of chemokine receptor 4 expression in small cell lung cancer: initial experience. Oncotarget 2016;7(8):9288–95.

31. Demmer O, Gourni E, Schumacher U, et al. PET imaging of CXCR4 receptors in cancer by a new optimized ligand. ChemMedChem 2011;6:1789–91.

32. Gourni E, Demmer O, Schottelius M, et al. PET of CXCR4 expression by a 68Ga labeled highly specific targeted contrast agent. J Nucl Med 2011;52: 1803–10.

33. Wester HJ, Keller U, Schottelius M, et al. Disclosing the CXCR4 expression in lymphoproliferative diseases by targeted molecular imaging. Theranostics 2015;5:618–30.

34. Philipp-Abbrederis K, Herrmann K, Knop S, et al. In vivo molecular imaging of chemokine receptor CXCR4 expression in patients with advanced multiple myeloma. EMBO Mol Med 2015;7:477–87.

35. Domanska UM, Kruizinga RC, Nagengast WB, et al. A review on CXCR4/CXCL12 axis in oncology: no place to hide. Eur J Cancer 2013;49:219–30.

36. Peled A, Wald O, Burger J. Development of novel CXCR4-based therapeutics. Expert Opin Investig Drugs 2012;21:341–53.

37. Mishan MA, Ahmadiankia N, Bahrami AR. CXCR4 and CCR7: two eligible targets in targeted cancer therapy. Cell Biol Int 2016;40(9):955–67.

38. Bailly C, Gouard S, Guérard F, et al. What is the best radionuclide for immuno-PET of multiple myeloma? A comparison study between 89Zr-and 64Cu-labeled anti-CD138 in a preclinical syngeneic model. Int J Mol Sci 2019;20(10):2564.

39. Ghai A, Maji D, Cho N, et al. Preclinical development of CD38-targeted [89Zr] Zr-DFO-Daratumumab for imaging multiple myeloma. J Nucl Med 2018;59(2): 216–22.

40. Tang R, Zheleznyak A, Mixdorf M, et al. Osteotropic radiolabeled nanophotosensitizer for imaging and treating multiple myeloma. ACS Nano 2020;14(4): 4255–64.

41. Katal S, Gholamrezanezhad A, Kessler M, et al. PET in the diagnostic management of soft tissue sarcomas of musculoskeletal origin. PET Clin 2018; 13(4):609–21.

42. Hancin EC, Borja AJ, Nikpanah M, et al. PET/MR imaging in musculoskeletal precision imaging: third wave after X-ray and MR. PET Clin 2020;15(4): 521–34.

43. wang HM, Khoradmehr A, Tamadon A, et al. Imaging of the muscle and bone from benchtop to bedside. Eur Rev Med Pharmacol Sci 2020;24(6): 3254–66.

44. Rouleau C, Curiel M, Weber W, et al. Endosialin protein expression and therapeutic target potential in human solid tumors: sarcoma versus carcinoma. Clin Cancer Res 2008;14(22):7223–36.

45. Thway K, Robertson D, Jones RL, et al. Endosialin expression in soft tissue sarcoma as a potential

marker of undifferentiated mesenchymal cells. Br J Cancer 2016;115(4):473–9.

46. Li C, Chacko AM, Hu J, et al. Antibody-based tumor vascular theranostics targeting endosialin/TEM1 in a new mouse tumor vascular model. Cancer Biol Ther 2014;15(4):443–51.

47. Chacko AM, Li C, Nayak M, et al. Development of 124I immuno-PET targeting tumor vascular TEM1/endosialin. J Nucl Med 2014;55(3):500–7.

48. Guo Y, Hu J, Wang Y, et al. Tumour endothelial marker 1/endosialin-mediated targeting of human sarcoma. Eur J Cancer 2018;90:111–21.

49. Capone E, Piccolo E, Fichera I, et al. Generation of a novel antibody-drug conjugate targeting endosialin: potent and durable antitumor response in sarcoma. Oncotarget 2017;8(36):60368–77.

50. Delage JA, Faivre-Chauvet A, Fierle JK, et al. 177Lu radiolabeling and preclinical theranostic study of 1C1m-Fc: an anti-TEM-1 scFv-Fc fusion protein in soft tissue sarcoma. EJNMMI Res 2020;10(1):98.

51. Cicone F, Denoël T, Gnesin S, et al. Preclinical evaluation and dosimetry of [111In] CHX-DTPA-scFv78-Fc targeting endosialin/tumor endothelial marker 1 (TEM1) [published correction appears in Mol Imaging Biol]. Mol Imaging Biol 2020;22(4):979–91.

52. Lepareur N, Lacœuille F, Bouvry C, et al. Rhenium-188 labeled radiopharmaceuticals: current clinical applications in oncology and promising perspectives. Front Med (Lausanne) 2019;6:132.

53. Hassan SE, Bekarev M, Kim MY, et al. Cell surface receptor expression patterns in osteosarcoma. Cancer 2012;118(3):740–9.

54. Geller DS, Morris J, Revskaya E, et al. Targeted therapy of osteosarcoma with radiolabeled monoclonal antibody to an insulin-like growth factor-2 receptor (IGF2R). Nucl Med Biol 2016;43(12):812–7.

55. Ma W, Shao Y, Yang W, et al. Evaluation of (188) Re-labeled NGR-VEGI protein for radioimaging and radiotherapy in mice bearing human fibrosarcoma HT-1080 xenografts. Tumour Biol 2016;37(7): 9121–9.

56. Sui J, Shao G, Zhang L, et al. Theranostics of osteosarcoma and lung metastasis with new integrin α v β 3 receptor targeted radiotracers 2019;33(2):170–6 [In Chinese].

57. Sarrut D, Badel JN, Halty A, et al. 3D absorbed dose distribution estimated by Monte Carlo simulation in radionuclide therapy with a monoclonal antibody targeting synovial sarcoma. EJNMMI Phys 2017;4(1):6.

58. Li HK, Sugyo A, Tsuji AB, et al. α-Particle therapy for synovial sarcoma in the mouse using an astatine-211-labeled antibody against frizzled homolog 10. Cancer Sci 2018;109(7):2302–9.

59. Marsh IR, Grudzinski J, Baiu DC, et al. Preclinical pharmacokinetics and dosimetry studies of 124I/131I-CLR1404 for treatment of pediatric solid tumors in murine xenograft models. J Nucl Med 2019; 60(10):1414–20.

60. Frühwald MC, O'Dorisio MS, Pietsch T, et al. High expression of somatostatin receptor subtype 2 (sst2) in medulloblastoma: implications for diagnosis and therapy. Pediatr Res 1999;45(5 Pt 1):697–708.

61. Giannakenas C, Kalofonos HP, Apostolopoulos D, et al. Scintigraphic imaging of sarcomatous tumors with [111In-DTPA-Phe-1]-octreotide. Oncology 2000;58(1):18–24.

62. Crespo-Jara A, Manzano RG, Sierra ML, et al. A patient with metastatic sarcoma was successfully treated with radiolabeled somatostatin analogs. Clin Nucl Med 2016;41(9):705.

63. Friedberg JW, Van den Abbeele AD, Kehoe K, et al. Uptake of radiolabeled somatostatin analog is detectable in patients with metastatic foci of sarcoma. Cancer 1999;86(8):1621–7.

Printed and bound by CPI Group (UK) Ltd, Croydon, CR0 4YY

03/10/2024

01040307-0014